T0357242

THE INTERMEDIARIES

THE
INTERMEDIARIES

A Weimar Story

BRANDY SCHILLACE

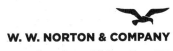

W. W. NORTON & COMPANY

Independent Publishers Since 1923

For information about permission to reproduce selections from this book,
write to Permissions, W. W. Norton & Company, Inc., 500 Fifth Avenue,
New York, NY 10110

For information about special discounts for bulk purchases, please contact
W. W. Norton Special Sales at specialsales@wwnorton.com or
800-233-4830

Manufacturing by Lakeside Book Company
Book design by Lovedog Studio
Production manager: Lauren Abbate

Library of Congress Cataloging-in-Publication Data is available.

ISBN: 978-1-32403-631-9

W. W. Norton & Company, Inc., 500 Fifth Avenue, New York, NY 10110
www.wwnorton.com

W. W. Norton & Company Ltd., 15 Carlisle Street, London W1D 3BS

10 9 8 7 6 5 4 3 2 1

It is absurd to say that the age of miracles is past. It has not yet begun.

—OSCAR WILDE

CONTENTS

THE INTERMEDIARIES

INTRODUCTION

MAY 6, 1933. THE NAZIS WERE COMING.

At half past nine in the morning, trucks began to arrive at In den Zelten 10 on Tiergarten Square, home of the Institut für Sexualwissenschaft, or Institute for Sexual Science. The gardens in front, awash with dew, would be crushed under the marching feet of Nazi students—and a full brass band. They had come to purge Germany of its enemies, they said.

In brown shirts emblazoned with the swastika, students emptied ink-wells on the Institute's carpets and tore down paintings. They threw a life-sized anatomical model out of the window, smashing it to pieces on the ground below. They overturned shelves, ransacked drawers, broke glass. They destroyed equipment in the consulting rooms. And the band played on, and on, and on. The students themselves did not confiscate property—they left that to the SA, Hitler's Storm Troops, who entered the premises at three in the morning and seized truckloads of books and manuscripts, whole volumes of journals, and the materials of the first ever World League for Sexual Reform. Valuable manuscripts, unpublished work, rare and unique editions—all gone. Up to 20,000 books in total, 35,000 photographs, and 40,000 case studies disappeared.[1] Some would be sold at auction. The rest would be committed to the flames.[2]

Four days later, the Institute's library lay piled on the Opernplatz, the square in front of the Berlin opera house. Wooden pallets rose like Jenga bricks, each filled with books and papers—a framework for destruction. Film crews were on hand to record the event, with Nazi chief propagandist Joseph Goebbels encouraging the crowd to embrace the "strong, great and symbolic undertaking" of "entrust[ing] to the flames the intellectual garbage of the past."[3] The carnage flickered over German newsreels and then those across Europe: here were officers, students, civilian men and women, throwing stacks of books at the twisting, heaving flames.

The Institute for Sexual Science had offered safe haven to homosexuals and those we today consider transgender for nearly two decades. It had been built on scientific and humanitarian principles established at the end of the nineteenth century, which blossomed into the sexology of the early twentieth century. Founded by Magnus Hirschfeld, a Jewish homosexual, the Institute supported tolerance, feminism, diversity, and science. As a result, it became a chief target of the Nazis: "It is our pride," they declared, to strike a blow against the Institute; "we oppose love being sold off in scientific clubs."[4] As for Magnus Hirschfeld, Hitler would label him the "most dangerous Jew in Germany."[5] It was his face that Hitler put on his anti-Semitic propaganda; his likeness that became a target; his bust that was committed to the flames on the Opernplatz.

You may have seen the images. You may have watched the towering inferno that roared into the night. The burning of Hirschfeld's library has been immortalized on film reels and in photographs, representative of the Nazi imperative, symbolic of all they would destroy. Yet few remember what they were burning—or why. Magnus Hirschfeld had built his Institute on powerful ideas, still in their infancy: that sex and gender characteristics existed on a vast spectrum, that people could be born this way, and that, as with any other diversity of nature, these identities should be accepted. He would call these people intermediaries.

TODAY, WE WOULD UNDERSTAND the term "intermediaries" to include those who are transgender. Gay, lesbian, intersex, and transgender people existed then as now, though different words were used even by members of those communities. I will note the historical antecedents, but I will prefer current terminology that respects the hard-won fight for proper representation. Words make the world; how we use them matters. The term "sexuality" itself, meaning "possession of sexual powers, or capability of sexual feelings," first entered the English language in 1879.[6] It became increasingly central to individual identity, while its related terms exploded: "sex" might mean sex acts, biological sex, gender identity, or sexual orientation.[7] The very first use of the words "homosexual" and "heterosexual" occurs in an 1868 letter—and they don't mean what you'd expect. (In 1892, Dr. James G. Kiernan used "hetero-sexual" to mean those with "abnormal manifestations of the sexual appetite.")[8] When Jonathan Ned Katz revisited his groundbreaking book *The Invention of Heterosexuality* a decade after its publication, he wrote, "I now think that human beings use words as tools to create particular sexualities as specific kinds of phenomena, and that the reality of a particular sexuality is dependent on and inseparable from the different words we use socially to describe it."[9]

Magnus Hirschfeld used a variety of words to try to convey the complexity of sexuality, from the unusual and now-forgotten "urning" to terms such as "homosexual," "transvestite," "psychical hermaphrodite" (transgender as opposed to intersex), and even "transsexual." Yet he would return frequently to "intermediary," in part because of its resonance with biological sciences. Nature creates intermediary forms, he would claim, as part of natural diversity. Included beneath the "intermediary" umbrella were those he considered "situational" and "constitutional" homosexuals—a recognition that there is often a spectrum and bisexual practice—as well as what he termed "transvestites." This group included those who wished to wear the clothes of the opposite sex, but also those who "from the point of view of their character" should be considered as the opposite sex. Perhaps even more surprising was Hirschfeld's inclusion of those with no fixed gender at all, akin to today's concept of gender-fluid or nonbinary identity (he counted the French novelist George Sand among them). Most importantly for Hirschfeld, these men and women were acting "in accordance with their nature," not against it. Intermediaries carried no stigma and no shame; these sexual and gender nonconformists had a right to live, a right to thrive. They also had a right to joy.

Science would lead the way, but this history unfolds as an interwar thriller—patients and physicians risking their lives to be seen and heard even as Hitler began his rise to power. Many weren't famous; their lives have not been celebrated in fiction or film. Born into a late-nineteenth-century world steeped in the "deep anxieties of men about the shifting work, social roles, and power of men over women,"[10] they came into their own just as sexual science entered the crosshairs of prejudice and hate. The Institute's community faced abuse, blackmail, and political machinations; they responded with secret publishing campaigns, leaflet drops, pro-homosexual propaganda, and alignments with rebel factions of Berlin's literati. They also developed groundbreaking gender affirmation surgeries and the first hormone cocktail for supportive gender therapy. Nothing like the Institute for Sexual Science had ever existed before it opened its doors—and despite a hundred years of progress, there has been nothing like it since.

Retrieving this tale has been an exercise in pursuing history at its edges and fringes, in ephemera and letters, in medical texts, in translations. Understanding why the Institute became such a target for hatred tells us everything about our present moment, about a world that has not made peace with difference, that still refuses the light of scientific evidence most especially as it concerns sexual and reproductive rights.

This book contains a nexus, perhaps a collision, of three different stories. It offers a comprehensive scientific history of sex hormones and genes and their impact on medicine—for better and for worse. It chronicles the rise of homosexual rights from 1890 to 1933, which culminated in the founding of Magnus Hirschfeld's Institute for Sexual Science and its fall at the hands of Nazi forces. And—perhaps most importantly—it tells the astounding story of the first patient to undergo gender affirmation surgery, way back in 1931. She wasn't glamorous like Lili Elbe (the subject of the book and film *The Danish Girl*); she wasn't well off, or well supported, or well known. In fact, her name has largely vanished from history, her personal narrative hidden away in the typed onionskin pages of an interwar German dissertation buried deep in the archives of Humboldt University in Berlin. She called herself Dora Richter; Hirschfeld would call her Dorchen, his little Dora. Unassuming and mild-mannered, she nevertheless helped to change the shape of Hirschfeld's research.

Taken together, these narratives race through the tumultuous political climate from the precipice of the twentieth century to the coming storm of fascism and genocide to answer questions that seem as important today as ever they did. What are the seeds of prejudice and fear that turn a populace against their brothers and sisters? Who watered them and made them grow? Put more succinctly and more urgently: How do we first begin to hate? And what can we do, as citizens, as scientists, as human beings, to counter hate with acceptance?

Scientific progress can be slow and ponderous, but science—so said Magnus Hirschfeld—would lead at last to justice. The Institute, like the Weimar Republic itself, existed from 1919 to 1933, but its story begins much earlier. Without breakthroughs in sexology and endocrinology— that is, the study of sex and of hormones—the Institute would never have existed, nor would Hirschfeld's battle against anti-homosexual laws have had any backing. Only the burgeoning understanding of homosexuality and gender nonconformity as congenital—as natural variation present from birth—could support his claims for equality. This science doesn't begin with sterile labs, test tubes, and Petri dishes, however. The first hint at a future where those who don't fit into the boxes of conformity could live free lives came not with the advent of psychology or surgery, but with physiology, six roosters, and the burgeoning science of very small things.

1

THE SCIENCE OF SMALL THINGS

HIS NAME WAS ARNOLD ADOLPH BERTHOLD, AND HE HAD AN ABIDING interest in testicles. A professor, physiologist, and director of zoology at the University of Göttingen, his studies in 1849 increasingly centered upon glands. Today we know there are nine types of glands in the endocrine system: hypothalamus, pineal, and pituitary, located in the brain; thyroid and parathyroids; the islets of Langerhans, located in the pancreas; adrenals; ovaries and testes.[1] This last pair captured Berthold's attention; clearly, they had something to do with sex—but what? Berthold wasn't thinking of sexuality or of gender. For the scientist, "sex" meant the distinction *between* and the operation *of* the genitals. He wanted to know how an organism changed from its nubile to its fertile state. How much work were those testicles doing?* Where did the messages for pubescent change come from, and how were they received?

Nineteenth-century scientific understanding of the human body resembled, to a degree, political hierarchy. It also owed a lot to René Descartes and the seventeenth-century concept of mind–body dualism. There were three substances, in this view: God (uncreated), soul or mind (created but immaterial), and body (material).[2] In healthy people, the mind and by association the brain and nervous system directed the body; therefore, all important functions were connected in some way to the nervous system. Berthold wasn't setting out to overturn this idea, at least not at first. He wanted to establish how the brain and glands

---

* The word "testes" (singular "testis") refers only to the gland. The word "testicles" refers to testes along with epididymis, a coiled tube just outside the testes, responsible for temporary storage and nourishment of sperm.

communicated with each other. And so, in 1848, he took home six young roosters and began a series of very peculiar experiments.

Roosters might not be the most usual lab animal, but they're easy to get hold of. In early summer, farmers typically butcher superfluous male chickens before they become a boisterous, rowdy problem. Berthold needed them before they began this one-way march through puberty—and he had his pick. From the first two roosters, he removed both testes entirely and left the birds to grow into adults without them. From the next two, he removed only one testis and reimplanted it in the same bird, to see whether it would survive implant. With the last two, he removed the testes from both roosters and swapped them, to see if they would work in another animal. Stranger yet, in both these pairs, he didn't implant the testes where they belonged, but instead sliced open a pouch in the belly.[3] Exactly why he did so would have confused his colleagues: what was the point, after all? For Berthold, the belly transplant would allow him to answer a curious question about *how* gland secretions traveled through the body.

The birds without any testes did not go through puberty. They didn't produce bright combs and wattles or long tail feathers. They lost their muscle tone, too, and put on significant amounts of weight; in a short time, both were round, soft, and henlike. They behaved like hens, as well. These castrated roosters (or capons) did not crow, did not mate with females, and lacked all aggression.[4] By itself, the experiment strengthened the idea that glands must in some way communicate with the nervous system, since the birds failed to develop secondary sex characteristics. (The scientific understanding of the time maintained that all bodily functions and changes were carried out via nerves.) This much had been observed in human *castrati*, men who were castrated before puberty to preserve their high singing voices.[5] So far, so good. Berthold went on to his two further experiments, transplanting the testes. He was in for a surprise.

When Berthold removed the testes, he made sure to cut vascular and nerve fibers as well. Even so, once reimplanted into the coils of the intestines, the testes enabled each rooster to develop normally. That made no sense to Berthold, because the glands were now unhooked from what was thought to be the all-powerful nervous system. Yet, according to Berthold, the roosters "crowed lustily, often engaged in battle with each other and other roosters," and showed the "usual" amorous attentions to hens in the chicken yard. After several months, Berthold killed and dissected the birds with belly testicles to find that the testes had attached to the intestinal wall, developed a substantial blood supply, and nearly doubled in size.[6] Under the microscope, slices of the gland revealed active spermatozoa. What his careful search did *not* find was any trace of nerve fibers. Somehow, the testicle had transferred its potency through the blood as a secretion, a chemical. The sexual maturation of these roosters hadn't required the action of the nervous system at all.[7]

Berthold's experiments uncovered a strange and secret property, an unnamed something in the body's juices. It may seem a small alteration in theory, but it had enormous consequences.

Sex, more than any other human behavior, fell into classifications both scientific and moral in the nineteenth century. The European morality of the time favored conceptual hierarchies of "good/natural" and "evil/unnatural," and influenced early sexual scientists and proto-endocrinologists alike.[8] Under this system, what we call heterosexuality was "natural" and therefore good; homosexuality was "unnatural" and therefore evil. Because the mind was supposed to govern the will (and everything else), sexual deviations were diagnosed as "moral insanity," a term coined by English physician James Cowles Prichard in 1835. Bad behavior, wrote Prichard, or any "erroneous notion," might be impressed on the mind like a seal into wax.[9] By decreeing heterosexual, procreative sex the natural state (and privileging male desire), anything else became a perversion, a disease—which meant it was also a contagion that could spread simply by proximity, influence, or familiarity.

Berthold's findings, published in a paper titled "Transplantation der Hoden" (testes), went entirely against the natural/unnatural argument. His fellow scientists didn't pay much attention at the time, but his claims—1) that testes and their secretions were transplantable, 2) that they continued to produce secretions once transplanted, and 3) that the secretions were not part of the nervous system but rather blood-borne messengers—opened the door to a brand-new understanding of sexuality. Sex characteristics and behaviors were influenced by the biological action of the body. And if they were biological, they were natural.

BORN AND NOT MADE

Karl Heinrich Ulrichs stood transfixed. It was the late 1830s, and he'd gone to a ball at Münden, Germany, as was his habit, to sit with a mix of young ladies and gentlemen between dances. No one there had turned his eye; no one had so much as attracted his notice. Now, however, he could scarcely move or even breathe. Twelve young men, "well developed and beautifully uniformed forestry students," took their turn on the ballroom floor. He could not look away and found himself mute with restraint the whole evening. "I should have liked to fling my arms around their necks," he wrote in a letter; "I suffered torments in my bedchamber . . . lonely and unseen by anyone, only moved by the memory of those beautiful young men."[10] His own sister would rebuke him, complaining that he had somehow been corrupted. But how could that be, Ulrichs wondered; his inclinations had arisen at the onset of puberty, when he resided in a quiet provincial town. No tragedy had befallen him; he'd been subject to no ill influence. Those inclinations must, he concluded, have been within him from birth.

Ulrichs had always disliked boys' games, avoided competition and fights, and had what others regarded as "girlish" preoccupations. "How often did I hear my mother complain, 'You are not like other boys!'"[11] He had the good fortune to grow up in relative affluence in the kingdom of Hanover, more permissive than other German polities (at this point, the German states were not yet united), where homosexual acts—then referred to as sodomy—were discouraged but not outlawed. But his family was Lutheran, his grandfather and brother-in-law clergymen; he'd grown up with a moral code that denounced homosexuality long before he arrived at the University of Göttingen (where Berthold would later do his experiments). "It cost me much inner struggle," he wrote to his family members, but he had come to believe that his sexual feelings were "innate" and not the product of "sinful inclinations."[12]

Ulrichs referred to himself as an *urning*, a word he coined after the myth of Aphrodite's birth by Uranus—a male god, but the player of both male and female parts in her creation.[13] He would go on to study Greek and Roman examples of "uranism" not just as acts, but as identities; he referred to "lasting covenants of love" among the ancients, and also scientific and medical studies of *zwitter*, the German word for hermaphroditism (what we today call intersex, or having reproductive anatomy that doesn't strictly fit into the categories of male or female).[14] We would not, today, consider homosexual, transgender, or intersex persons the same, but much of Ulrichs's thinking was influenced by strictly enforced gender roles. Because in nineteenth-century Germany it was thought that only women loved men, Ulrichs assumed that his desire for other men must be due to an internal "womanly" quality. Though not physically intersex, he believed he was psychically feminine, with a female soul, and that uranism was a new kind of *zwitter*. As a result, Ulrichs called himself and others like him a "third sex," a man-woman, with a nature "present in the mother's womb."[15] How could this be a sin?

His ideas did not impress his family. And yet, they did not cast him out; Ulrichs lived with his sister after 1854, when he lost a good position in the Ministry of Justice because of his homosexuality. Though it was not a crime (not yet, not in Hanover), it was still a punishable offense. Ulrichs was very much alone, surrounded by people who refused to see his desires as natural and isolated from others like himself. If he wanted community, he'd have to build it himself, so he took to print.

We think of our modern world as far removed from that of these early pioneers, but plenty of homosexual young people today find their first communities at a distance. Where today people gather online, Ulrichs drew a community together through the written word. He published his findings in twelve volumes over the next decades. All centered on the novel idea that the body, not the mind, had the greatest influence over sexual character. God, he asserted, had created intermediate forms: men-women and women-men. And why should we be surprised? Men retain nipples, as do all manner of male mammals, and there are people born with both male and female genitals. Ulrichs anchored the urn-ing to nature; as with Berthold's assertions about the power of chemical secretions, Ulrichs claimed that something innate in the biological body led to a natural variation of the form. As "natural" was equated with "good" in moral philosophy, it was, he wrote, an "unpardonable injus-tice" to abuse those with uranian natures or to build a society purely on normative terms.[16]

It was Ulrichs's friend Karl Maria Kertbeny who, in a letter to Ulrichs, coined the terms "homosexual" and "heterosexual," using the Greek *homos*, meaning "same," and *heteros*, meaning "other." But Ulrichs wanted to reach beyond denotations to the mythopoetic origins of fused beings; having homosexual sex was "doing," while for Ulrichs, uranism was "being." Thus, he formed the practice of "same" sexual orientation into an identity—something truly new.

The small led the great, a notion which, at a critical moment in Ger-man history, had the connotation of an organized populace making making democratic decisions for itself. The piecemeal structure of Ger-many, with its different kingdoms, principalities, and city-states, had begun to give way to united, nationalist sentiments. Ulrichs supported nationalism, but he also feared that the anti-sodomy law of Prussia (the dominant actor in the confederacy) might ultimately become wide-spread. He had already been writing, as a jurist, to the various depart-ments of justice on behalf of urnings, but no one had taken up the cause. Ulrichs collected correspondence from other homosexuals, making their accounts his evidence. Many agonized, anonymous letters spoke about how hard the writers had tried to conform; some had married, only to trap themselves and their spouses in loveless partnerships. Others wrote about the horrors of blackmail. "You have boldly broken open the clos-ets," wrote an Austrian soldier in a letter that ends, "please help me."[17] Urnings had no rights, no voice.

In August 1867, Ulrichs went to the Odeon in Munich to speak before law professionals of the German Confederation. He knew he would be the first to speak publicly about his sexual identity; he knew that it would threaten his future. Yet he could think of no way to argue for the naturalness of homosexuality without reference to himself. As a result, this would be the first coming-out in modern history.

Ulrichs approached the platform with dreadful apprehension. There was still time, he knew, to change his mind. But so many had entrusted their stories to him, expecting that he would speak for their rights; he could not "answer their trust with cowardice."[18] When he took the stand, he expressed his firm belief that uranism was a natural state that should not be penalized under the law. He spoke of the rights of homosexuals, their citizenship, and of how many had been shamed into suicide. The room erupted in shouts and hisses. "Crucify him!" the audience cried, pounding upon the benches. Ulrichs was forced to flee without finishing his speech.

Even so, his argument that the criminal code of a single province should not be applied unilaterally had support. A Swiss physician wrote to him the following month that "the initial blow has been made," in that the subject had come up for debate, even if the jurists had refused to hear it. This was but the beginning.[19] The Justice Ministry ultimately received over a hundred petitions against the anti-sodomy statute, and in March 1868 it hinted that anti-sodomy laws might be excluded from the new penal code. But it wasn't to be.

When Germany unified in 1871, the law Ulrichs feared most was imposed. Paragraph 175 of the German penal code outlawed love between those of the same sex and a host of other behaviors considered aberrant: "Unnatural fornication, which is committed between male persons or between people with animals, is to be punished with prison; loss of civil rights can also be recognized." Sodomy would be considered a "willful perversion," the product of bad upbringing, excessive mas-turbation, or other sexual excess. "I raised my voice in free and open protest," Ulrichs declared; unfortunately, "Hatred alone has enjoyed freedom of speech."[20] His words would echo into the future. They are still echoing.

Ulrichs's battle provided the bass line, the notes on which a move-ment would be built. It underscores, too, just how close—how astonish-ingly close—Germany came to leading the world in a progressive view of sexual nonconformity. It would have that chance again, spearheaded by unlikely allies in the science of small things.

BUILDING A HUMAN

In 1883, German embryologist August Weismann proposed a radical theory of heredity. Darwin's theory of evolution had taken hold, but it was not without inherent problems. It was all well and good to say a finch changed its beak to suit the available seeds, but no one really understood how. Darwin's own solution was pangenesis: the idea that the body produced particles of information called gemmules, which could be influenced by the environment, modified, and then collected in sperm and egg.[21] A famous example suggested that giraffes stretch their necks to reach things all their lives, and somehow the body reads this and translates the "need to stretch" into instructions for offspring. This somewhat vague theory was a departure from the religious framework, but it didn't travel very far; instead of a creative and sentient God directing the course of growth and change, semi-sentient "messages" were reading the world outside the body and passing the information along.

Weismann (and others) had grown increasingly dissatisfied with this mystical notion. If it were true, he theorized, then if you cut off a mouse's tail and the body communicated that information to the gonads, then it would surely give birth to tailless mice. He set out to prove or disprove this, with the aid of 901 unfortunate mice. Despite repeated efforts and careful study controls, the babies of the surgically altered mice were (not surprisingly to us) born with tails just as before.[22] Traits did pass from generation to generation, but the hereditary information must, therefore, be contained only and exclusively in the sperm and the egg, what Weismann called germ-plasm. Again, however, the problem had just been moved a bit further down the line. What were the "germs" of germ-plasm? How did they create the information from which to grow a human?

The answer came from nature. Peas, to start with. Unknown to most of the world, in a quiet Austrian monastery, Gregor Johann Mendel had been trying to understand hybrids decades earlier. That work would be taken up by Dutch botanist Hugo de Vries. From 50,000 primrose seeds, de Vries noted 800 new variants and occasional rare "freaks."[23] Within the flower, sperm cells are produced in the stamen via pollen; egg cells develop in ovules at the base of each pistil. Here at last was proof of spontaneous variation in nature, inheritable variant qualities carried in egg and sperm. Some variants provided an advantage and produced more offspring; others died away. None of them were "unnatural," and certainly not "sinful" (morals were rarely ascribed at all in natural science). De Vries had determined that each trait of a species was governed by a single particle of information—what he called a pangene.[24] English biologist William Bateson, who like de Vries had been deeply influenced by a rediscovery of Mendel, would call the field "genetics" in a private letter in 1905, effectively (if not officially) coining the word "gene"—though that would not appear publicly until 1909, when Danish botanist Wilhelm Johannsen adapted Bateson's "genetics" to refer to the information particles as genes.

Genes carry inheritable messages through sperm and egg. Hormones communicate messages as chemicals released into the body by glands to influence traits. In both cases, it was becoming evident that something very small, only visible under a powerful microscope, was pulling the strings of human development—and it's not by coincidence that the terms "genetics" and "hormones" were coined in the same year, 1905. With his rooster experiments, Berthold had proven that hormones need not be produced by the originating animal, or administered in the original location, to be effective. As a result, by the end of the nineteenth century, human patients were being given experimental treatments using extracts from animal thyroids, adrenal glands, and even the pancreas.[25] Illness might be cured by the manipulation of these small chemical messengers. The same train of thought had been steadily gathering steam among another group of thinkers led by British psychologist Francis Galton.

A Victorian conservative, Galton did not believe that human beings were created equal. He liked the idea of hereditary qualities, and, already a classist thinker, determined that some humans must therefore be inherently better than others. If traits could be passed down, it was best to start from good breeding stock, and for Galton that carried racial, sexual, and cultural meanings. The best people, in his mind, would be those whose race, sex, and class were just like his own. Whereas Ulrichs had argued that urnings, or uranians, were merely different—variants, but without a judgment about value—Galton and his cohort saw that difference as something to be rooted out.

Richard von Krafft-Ebing, the leading sexologist of the nineteenth century, agreed that homosexuals (and other sex and gender noncon-formists) were indeed "born that way," but even so he considered them pathological. His name will come up again and again in this history, and his works would remain bestsellers into the 1920s. But the theory he put forth was deeply flawed; homosexuals, he said, were sick, an instance of morbid nature. For the record, he borrowed heavily from Ulrichs's writing, even taking the terms "homosexual" and "heterosexual" from him (and Kertbeny). In Kertbeny's writing, it was the heterosexuals who had "unfettered" desires. Krafft-Ebing's definitive work *Psychopathia Sexualis* reverses this idea, lionizing "heterosexual" as healthy, norma-tive, natural—and, above all, preferred for the betterment of the nation. Far from recognizing the right of homosexuals to live and be treated humanely, the growing consensus was that all people who were not het-erosexual ought somehow to be removed from the gene pool altogether, along with any others considered substandard by those with the power to enforce it. If that sounds familiar, it should. This idea returns in the 1930s, with the force of Nazi-supported genocide.

Ulrichs wanted a world created for all, but Galton's ideas about heredity aligned very neatly with a concept that would become popular in interwar Germany: *Rassenhygiene*, or race hygiene (a term coined by German biologist Alfred Ploetz). Hormone science would go on to become sexology and endocrinology; control of heredity would become known—infamously—as eugenics.

The sciences of small things began as intimately intertwined: gene and cell, sexual hormones and chemical messengers. Unfortunately, Galton's eugenics, an unsupported social theory he himself compared to a religion, would be given the gravitas of a science along with the burgeoning field of genetics. The two were frequently conflated, muddying the early years of research into gene expression. Eugenics would go on to bend genetic science to make it fit politically expedient conclusions—ones that would eventually be embraced by Adolf Hitler and lead to the mass extermination of millions. The new science of sexual hormones, by contrast, would be taken up by researchers and physicians in support of a brand-new and progressive idea: if glandular secretions—as invisible chemical messengers—controlled sex behavior, characteristics, and secondary sexual traits, then nonconformity was congenital. How could nonconformity be considered immoral if it came not from the mind but from the body?

A contest between two sciences (endocrinology and genetics) and two very different social movements (homosexual rights and eugenics) had begun, and it's important to look at origins. The hatred that would engulf Germany in 1933 and lead to the Second World War developed from small seeds planted in the nineteenth century. But so, too, did the seeds of rebellion against it.

THE ASTONISHING RETURN OF SECRETIONS

Genetics got its start in Mendel's monastery garden with pea hybrids, but before de Vries and Bateson stumbled upon his papers, Mendel had been largely forgotten and researchers plodded their way to his conclusions in their own weary course. The same would happen with Berthold's breakthrough concerning the blood-borne chemical messengers secreted by sex glands. Not even Karl Ulrichs, who went to the same university and would probably have met Berthold on more than one occasion in the small campus community, knew about his roosters. Instead, the work would have to be done again by someone else—someone with greater impact on the scientific community, as well as a good showman's crowd appeal. He stepped onto a Paris stage in 1889 under the provocative billing "Elixir of Life."

Aged seventy-two, with a prodigious forehead and properly grizzled beard, Charles-Édouard Brown-Séquard proclaimed the "miraculous" results of his own self-experimentation. Stump speeches by quack doctors proffering cures were nothing new, but Brown-Séquard was not a quack. His scientific career included the discovery of localized function in the brain, advances in the understanding of epilepsy, and the naming of Brown-Séquard syndrome, a neurological condition characterized by a lesion in the spinal cord.[26] He would also be granted the appellation "father of endocrinology" (a single-parent birth almost as mythic as Athena's leap from the forehead of Zeus). When he took the stage that spring day in Paris, it was to proclaim that "dynamical influences" contained in the "active principles [of] testicular fluid" could be introduced to, and travel through, the blood.[27] He had duplicated Berthold's findings in experiments with dogs, cats, and guinea pigs. By injecting the "internal secretion of glands" into old animals, he renewed their vigor: the aged dog grew sportive and lusty, the aging cat's coat gleamed once more. It was Brown-Séquard's assumption that the substance, whatever it was, must travel through the blood to give strength and vitality to the nervous system. The audience listened with interest—and well they might; after all, the good doctor claimed to be his own test case.

He had begun with a mixture of three parts: the vascular blood of dog testicles, semen, and "juice extracted from a [dog] testicle" (freshly crushed).[28] Importantly for the strength of the preparation, all animals used were young, healthy, and vigorous. He injected one cubic centimeter, or around 1 ml or 1,000 mg; this was not pure testosterone, which in HRT may be used at 50 to 200 mg per week, but it would have been a considerable dose all the same. He gave himself a total of ten injections and, begging to be excused for the personal nature of the comments, proceeded to give an account of the results. After his injections, he reported, strength and vitality returned. He had an appetite once more, he could stand for hours in his lab, he ran rather than walking up and down stairs. He also praised his ability to spurt a "jet of urine" when relieving himself, as well as improvements in the "expulsion" of feces during bowel movements.[29] But for Brown-Séquard, the most important and impressive qualities had to do with the impact of "spermatic fluid" on the mind—and his speech and subsequent publication attest strongly to his renewed acuity, memory, and mental capacity. He'd just turned the accepted mind–body communication on its head.

Brown-Séquard's conclusions were met with applause by the public, and copied by a few patent-medicine quackery specialists. His research galvanized scientists to action as well, not so much in an effort to build upon his work as to overturn it. His "elixir of life" did not enjoy its fame for long; no one could replicate the results, and Brown-Séquard died five years later, his injections notwithstanding. But new discoveries followed in one important respect: the chemical messengers, whether adrenal, pancreatic, or emitted by the sex glands, clearly affected the brain rather than being ruled by it.[30] In 1896, Ernest Starling would begin his own research into the endocrine system and would later (with William Bayliss) discover and name the chemical messengers "hormones," from a Greek word meaning to arouse or set into motion. Starling first uses the word in print in 1905, the same year that Bateson named his field of study genetics.

Ulrichs was right; the small could lead the great. It was his fondest hope to inspire scientific conversation and to find a means of bringing that science—the work of men like Berthold, Brown-Séquard, and Starling—together with social reform. He died in 1895, in exile in Italy. At the time, the child who would come to be known as Dora Richter was four years old and was already distraught at having to wear boy's clothes. By the time she was an adult, the world would know all about hormones and urnings; they would know about Ulrichs, too. His work didn't have to wait decades to be appreciated, like that of Mendel or Berthold; it would be cherished and resurrected, edited and reprinted, by a young doctor named Magnus Hirschfeld.

THE MAKING OF A SEXOLOGIST

Youthful, engaging, and endlessly curious, Hirschfeld had only just set himself up as a doctor in the Berlin district of Charlottenburg. He had received his degree in 1892 from Friedrich-Wilhelms-Universität (today, Humboldt University) in Berlin, and his medical license a year later in Würzburg. He was also a man attracted to men, a writer, and the friend of poets. "The natural sciences have always left aside the most important aspect of life, which is love; that has been left to the artist," he wrote; "my true inclination had always been . . . to spend my life in the society of journalists, writers, poets, and artists."[31] He had made good on his inclinations, working as a journalist to cover the World's Columbian Exhibition of 1893 in Chicago with his friend and fellow reporter Johannes Gaulke. He had returned to Germany with some reluctance, settling first in Magdeburg-Neustadt and then in Charlottenburg. By 1896, he would be an ardent medical pioneer of sexology and leader of a movement that championed homosexual rights. A letter, a desperate plea—and a single gunshot—would change everything.

In the summer of 1895, the postman delivered a parcel just as Hirschfeld sat down to coffee and his morning paper. He was distracted; a grim headline shocked him terribly. A young man had killed himself the night before, and Hirschfeld recognized the name. It was one of his patients, a young man with a bright future.* The account rendered the details painfully stark: in the apparent grip of "mental disorder," the young lieutenant had shot himself dead on the eve of his wedding.[32]

The news was grave enough, but the newly delivered package provided no distraction. It bore the lieutenant's name, and the covering letter was addressed to Hirschfeld. "I did not have the strength to tell my parents," the letter read. They had "been urging me, their only child, for years to marry a childhood friend. I could not object to the marriage and confess the truth. They would never have understood me anyway."[33] Hirschfeld unwrapped the parcel to find the papers and letters of a man who loved other men. Unable to change his nature, he considered himself—and

---

* We know relatively little about Hirschfeld's early practice. He was interested in hydrotherapy, and some sources suggest (though without much evidence) that he was also interested in gynecology. He had earned a medical degree, which covered a relatively wide area of expertise at the time. It's difficult to know for what, exactly, he had been treating the patient.

his life—a curse. Suicide, he felt, was his only choice, so that his parents might never know "that which nearly strangled my heart." The letter, and its final plea for a future "when the German fatherland will think of us in more just terms," didn't just move Hirschfeld as a doctor; it shook him as a fellow homosexual man, subject to the same fears and pressures. How could this young officer, "highly honored, scientifically and socially profoundly educated," with "impeccable character," be brought to such a state of torment and nervous exhaustion that death was his only recourse—and Hirschfeld his only confidant?

The German term for suicide, *Selbstmord*, has no exact English equivalent. It resembles and nearly means "self-murder," but the word has greater criminal connotations in German. It casts the victim as a violent perpetrator punishable by law, not a victim. It misses entirely the source of the problem—society's castigation and pressure to conform—and the fact that many who committed suicide thought they were sacrificing self for others, usually a family they didn't want to shame. Hirschfeld made good on the soldier's request to publish his story; Hirschfeld calls him a "victim of human ignorance."[34] He was "murdered," yes, but not by his own choice. The man, and many others like him, had been forced into suicide by a society that refused his desires, his identity, his authenticity. These men did not suffer because they felt same-sex desire; they suffered because society would not accept them—would not recognize the authenticity of their lives. If Hirschfeld intended to save the "young men," as he referred to them, he would have to change society first.

2

TROUBLED ALLIANCES

THE COLD LONDON WINTER OF 1895 CLUNG ON AS THOUGH UNEND-
ing. The river Thames ceased to flow, bringing a halt to shipping, mass
unemployment, and a number of skating parties.[1] The poet, playwright,
and playboy Oscar Wilde spent the bitter February nights in the warmth
of his London club, the Albemarle. Known for his wit, fashion sense, and
scandalously luxuriant dark hair, Wilde had already been embroiled in
his share of controversy. Only a few years earlier, Max Nordau, a Hun-
garian physician, had condemned Wilde as a "degenerate" and "morally
insane" for his excesses and also for his sexuality.[2] Wilde had married
and fathered children, but he also kept company with men. He didn't
identify as an urning or a homosexual, but his tempestuous love affair
with Lord Alfred Douglas was something of an open secret, providing
plenty of grist for the rumor mill.

Pale and delicate of features, Lord Alfred had all the charm of a "golden
boy" and all the petulance of a spoiled child. As described by his biog-
rapher Douglas Murray, the young poet's relationship with Wilde was a
stormy one, with frequent fights and breakups, sometimes "savagely bitter."[3] The older Wilde, who had actively courted Douglas, always forgave,
and soon the two were paired again. However, both Wilde and Douglas
entertained careless relations with "rent boys," young male prostitutes.
One of Douglas's night guests stole a bundle of letters, among them love
notes from Wilde. The playwright would be plagued by blackmailers,
and eventually the story became semi-public. The charge of homosexuality alone could be ruinous to reputation, but worse was coming. The scandal reached the ears of Douglas's father, the violent and mercurial John

Douglas, 9th Marquess of Queensberry.* Known for thuggish behavior, violence, and anti-Semitism—he once referred to the prime minister, Benjamin Disraeli, as an "underbred disgusting Jew pimp"—the marquess made for a dangerous enemy.[4] He especially hated what he called sodomites—a common derogatory term for homosexuals that focused on the act. The law referred to it as gross indecency, with different punishments meted out for those considered the active and the passive parties.

In Britain, same-sex desire was considered a sinful and degrading choice, not an identity; regardless, it carried a gender-specific stigma. A century earlier, effeminate homosexual men had been maligned as "Mollies," their meeting places known as Molly houses. To a man like the Marquess of Queensberry, the link to effeminacy couldn't be borne. His loathing was rooted in a prevalent British misogyny and neurasthenic fears of emasculation, lack of virility, and "semen loss." He even called presumably heterosexual men "snob queers" if they appeared at all feminine in appearance or manner. How dare his own son be among them? The marquess first demanded that Alfred give up Wilde or be disinherited. He would later burst in on Wilde at his home and called him "every foul word he could think of," but refrained from actually slandering or directly accusing him.[5] The relationship continued, as did the marquess's descent into more manic behavior. He stalked the pair, declared that Alfred should have the "shit kicked out of him," and wrote in a letter that Wilde should be shot in the street.[6] He attempted to intercept Wilde at the theater (where he planned to hand him a bouquet of phallic vegetables), but was denied entry; thus stymied, he set out for the Albemarle Club to settle matters in writing.[7] He left a furiously scrawled letter with the porter, which read: "For Oscar Wilde, posing sodomite."[8] Wilde retaliated by bringing a case of libel against the marquess—but he'd picked the wrong adversary and a losing fight. In the end, it would cost Wilde everything.

* The Queensberry Rules of boxing were named after him.

Oscar Wilde suffered through three humiliating trials. The pur-
loined letters between Wilde and Lord Alfred Douglas were submitted as evidence, but other blackmailers happily testified against him,
too. To make matters worse, Douglas did not come to Wilde's defense.
The Crown prosecutors painted him as Wilde's victim—and astonish-
ingly, they considered the blackmailers to be his victims too. It was, they
claimed, far worse for Wilde to have committed sodomy on sex workers than it was for them to extort money in return.[9] The jury agreed,
and the public that had so recently celebrated Wilde's work now castigated him as a pederast, or child sex predator—a favorite slur thrown
at homosexuals then as now.[10] The court sentenced Wilde to two years'
hard labor, his books were pulled from shelves, and his estate largely
liquidated. Alone, abandoned by his lover, and in failing health, Wilde
penned "The Ballad of Reading Gaol," a stanza of which would be
inscribed on his tomb:

> And alien tears will fill for him
>> Pity's long-broken urn,
> For his mourners will be outcast men,
>> And outcasts always mourn.

Far away in Germany, those lines affected Magnus Hirschfeld vis-
cerally. Still emotionally raw from the suicide of his patient, he felt the
impact of Wilde's words as *markerschütternd*: as translated by historian
Heike Bauer, the splinter-shatter of bone marrow.[11] He wasn't alone;
writers and even scientists wrote petitions on Wilde's behalf, demanding his release. Perhaps more surprising, Wilde's works, banned in Britain, were performed, translated, and published en masse in Germany.
Booksellers couldn't keep them on the shelves, and the renewed (and
lucrative) interest in Wilde as a sexual minority also led to the publication of nonfiction works about homosexuality by others.

Homosexuality was illegal in both Britain and Germany, so why were
responses so different? Publishers in Germany had access to something
their counterparts in Britain did not: a press largely free of censorship.

The fact that Germany's press had such freedoms is surprising, and nearly didn't come to pass. Both Kaiser Wilhelm II and the Catholic Center Party, who were then in power, privileged traditional, conservative ideas. Some things were countenanced as long as they stayed out of the public eye, such that certain types of publications existed in a gray area between legality and illegality. That had changed in 1891, when a Berlin pimp named Heinze murdered a nightwatchman. His trial became both scandal and spectacle; seemingly the entire Berlin underworld turned out in "ostentatious" attendance. Even members of the press found themselves shocked by details of what went on in Berlin's darker corners, and by October the Kaiser demanded that immediate steps be taken to curb the spread of "moral corruption."[12] At his behest, the Heinze Law would drastically expand censorship, threatening everything from theatrical performances to contraception advertisements.[13] It would also have limited any scientific publications about sexuality, and homosexuality in particular. Rash and reactionary, the law sparked the longest (and possibly most passionate) debate about literature and the arts Germany had ever witnessed. Artists, writers, lawyers, members of the Social Democratic Party, and many thousands of middle-class Germans staged a protest, and the government's attempts to enact the law were blocked by "a campaign of obstruction unprecedented in [Germany's] history."[14] The law would be gutted before going into effect—a triumph for intellectual freedom.

In the end, so long as a text depicting homosexuality could be considered to have scientific or educational merit, the government could not stop it being published.[15] Emboldened, publishers such as Max Spohr, with his business acumen (and imperial mustache), decided to take every advantage. He published German translations of Oscar Wilde's collected works, along with Otto de Joux's *Die Enterbten des Liebesglückes oder das dritte Geschlecht* (Those Dispossessed of Love, or the Third Sex).[16] In doing so, he became the first publisher to specialize in "sexual minorities"—and Wengler & Spohr one of the first presses to produce such works in large quantities.

Even more than Ulrichs's revolutionary pamphlets, Wilde's traumatic fall from grace created a climate of acceptance for treatises on homosexuality.[17] More important, it provided "a collective sense of belonging" among homosexual men that helped to solidify the identity—even, or perhaps especially, for closeted ones like Hirschfeld.[18] When the term "homosexual" replaced "urning" in the late nineteenth and early twentieth century, it carried with it Ulrichs's original sense of inborn identity, and it would do so in print. Publication had become the weapon of the marginalized in Germany, and especially of gender and sexual minorities. All that was needed was a figure like Wilde around which to coalesce—and a cause, like the overturning of anti-sodomy laws, to champion. Against this emotive backdrop, Magnus Hirschfeld wrote his first book, more of an extended pamphlet, though bound for sale: *Sappho and Socrates: How Does One Explain the Love of Men and Women to Persons of Their Own Sex?*

SAPPHO AND SOCRATES

"At all times, among all peoples and everywhere," Hirschfeld wrote, there have always been those attracted to their own sex "in true love."[19] Same-sex desire was neither fad nor modern turn; its roots run so deep that the ancient Greek figures of Sappho, the lesbian poet, and Socrates, the homosexual philosopher, lent it classical validity. And yet, this love was illegal under German law. In Hirschfeld's first foray into print, he leaned heavily upon Karl Ulrichs. He even used Ulrichs's term "urning," though he would alter his terminology in later publications.

Why is it, he asked, that urnings are arrested and blackmailed for consensual acts, while the married heterosexual man who "destroys" a governess through seduction or rape goes unpunished? He quoted Oscar Wilde's statement to the judge at his trial: "The love that in this century dare not speak its name is such a great affection of an elder for a younger man, as there was between David and Jonathan, such as Plato made the basis of his philosophy, and such as you find in the sonnets of Michelangelo and Shakespeare." A powerful argument, but to no avail; love between those of the same sex would be punished, while blackmailers and violent offenders went free. "Where is the consequence," Hirschfeld demanded; "where is justice at the end of our much-celebrated century?" *Sappho and Socrates* supported the resurrection of Wilde's reputation, and with it the honor and dignity of same-sex love.[20]

Max Spohr suggested that Hirschfeld choose a pseudonym and present himself as an unbiased, presumably heterosexual doctor. So, the book presented its case as "the scientific exploration of a question" rather than a personal essay. If among all people, and at all times, there have been same-sex lovers, from where does the impulse come? It cannot be a product of culture; it cannot be the result of a modernizing world. Instead, wrote Hirschfeld, homosexuality comes as part of biological human development: sexual nature begins in the womb.

At the time of Hirschfeld's writing, sex chromosomes had yet to be discovered. The first to make the leap would be Nettie Maria Stevens, an American research scientist, in 1905.[21] (The lofty subjects were mealworms; she found that males made reproductive cells with both X and Y chromosomes whereas females made cells with only X.) We know now that human beings receive their chromosomes at the moment of fertilization, but genital or reproductive differences don't develop until week fourteen, or about 100 days of gestation.[22] Since early embryologists couldn't see into the chromosomal world, they assumed that no sex difference existed in earlier stages. "The human fruit," Hirschfeld writes, "is wholly asexual (or better, dual sexual)" in the first three months, because it is "impossible to distinguish whether the individual in question should become a boy or a girl." On the face of it, we know the assumption isn't accurate, at least not in most cases. Chromosomes do not always work as expected; in the case of Swyer syndrome, for instance, the Y of an XY pair doesn't initiate the development of male genitals—it doesn't turn on, so to speak. As a result, the fetus develops female genitals, even a uterus (though without fertile ovaries); the raw material for a female reproductive system is there.

Hirschfeld's argument doesn't hinge entirely upon external sex characteristics, however. He writes that the "mental center of the sexual sensations" does not develop immediately in the fetus. In other words, there is no sex orientation in utero. Most of us would probably agree; we don't think of a fetus, or a baby, as a particularly sexual being (though Freud would muddy those waters). For Hirschfeld, the infant self exists as a sexual possibility; it might love and desire in any direction—or in all of them. All humans, he explained, are thereby "physically and emotionally mixed (hermaphroditic)."[23]

Hirschfeld's use of the term "hermaphrodite," with its history of abusive connotations, requires addressing. The word originates in classical Greek myth. A nymph named Salmacis pursues Hermaphroditus, the son of Hermes and Aphrodite. He rejects her love but she begs the gods to "unite" them, which they do by causing them to inhabit a single body. The word frequently referred to intersex characteristics, but would also become a disparaging epithet—and "hermaphroditism" would be pathologized by most sexologists, including Krafft-Ebing. Ulrichs and Hirschfeld used the same word, but they deployed it in a new way. Neither was referring to physical genitalia or chromosomal difference. Ulrichs suggested that a homosexual man had a male body and a female soul.[24] Hirschfeld used the word to mean those with the psychic—or mental and emotional—capacity to love, and to be, both men and women. Both were moving toward the understanding that biological sex and gender are not one and the same. "Hermaphrodite" became a much-used and overloaded term precisely because the binary categories of male and female didn't provide room for variations.

Limited as much by lack of language as by the limits of science, Hirschfeld largely followed the convention of hetero-, homo-, and bisexuality in this, his earliest work. But he found a way around their narrow limits. "From the point of view of developmental history," he stated, "we can now consider six possibilities of the regulation of desire"—and by enumerating six, he asserted diversity.[25] Complete with illustrative tables, Hirschfeld made a case for states of being that, instead of being static, are aligned along a spectrum. In the first category, Hirschfeld included the "male" with "normally developed" sex organs—and the word "normal," with all its problems, continues to appear in this earliest publication.

Hirschfeld repeatedly argued that sexuality is not pathological but natural. In his desire to show sexual variations as natural, he compared them to equally natural but atypical physical formations, which, unfortunately, are not entirely free of accidental pejorative. At one point, he compared homosexuality to a cleft lip, which, in addition to being an egregious example of ableism, reinforces the notion of normative/non-normative. Hirschfeld provided a way out of that binary, however, in his assertion that the "normal man"—that is, the heterosexual man—is bisexual in utero. Before birth, he claimed, the forming human might love either men or women; after birth, the "instinct toward men" is "stunted" among heterosexuals.[26] Similarly, heterosexual women are those in whom attraction to other women has atrophied during development. The terminology has been swapped such that Hirschfeld can describe the "normal" in aberrant terms (stunted, atrophied).

At the other end of the spectrum from "normal," Hirschfeld placed men who love men and women who love women (categories 5 and 6). In between were those whose desires might be for neither or both. In providing for degrees of strength or weakness of desire (which he tied biologically to the production of the as-yet-unnamed "secretions"), Hirschfeld posited a continuum. It was the first step toward later and far more robust theories.

Copies of *Sappho and Socrates* were eagerly snapped up. The book would go into a second and a third printing, with a new foreword and Hirschfeld's real name as author. He had committed himself to this path and was ready to shed whatever protection anonymity afforded. It was time to make alliances, and to form a new association that would fight for homosexual rights.

ON MAY 15, 1897, three men gathered in a small apartment in Charlottenburg, trading commentary by lamplight. Perhaps they had dined together; perhaps they now shared a drink or smoked cigarettes in Hirschfeld's sitting room. Eduard Oberg, with his oversized mustache, several centimeters wider than his thin face, had met Hirschfeld the year before. He wasn't an academic or a doctor—he worked as a railway official—but he had been deeply affected by *Sappho and Socrates*. His encouragement had brought them together that night, and Max Spohr would provide the platform. That's why Hirschfeld chose them as co-founders of a new organization which would campaign for homosexual rights. They called themselves the Wissenschaftlich-humanitäres Komitee, the Scientific Humanitarian Committee (SHC).

The task that night was to draft the SHC's Articles of Association. The Committee would have six statutes in total. It would research homosexuality "and allied variations" in their "biological, medical, and ethnological significance" as well as "legal, ethical, and humanitarian situation." It would seek to change public opinion through the publication (thanks to Spohr) of the first sexual science journal, *Jarbüch für sexuelle Zwischenstufen* (Yearbook for Sexual Intermediaries). It would build a library and archive available to both students and laypersons. It would admit anyone as a member, regardless of sex, politics, or religion, and members would eventually include women as well as men. Oversight would come from a board of members, elected on five-year terms, drawn from all sectors of the public. The staff presiding over business were required to live in Berlin, and a general assembly would meet at least once a year and whenever emergency required.

The SHC existed for the furtherance of sexual science, the emancipation of the homosexual, and above all the overturning of Paragraph 175, the anti-sodomy law—and it soon had enthusiastic members. Prussian army officer Franz Josef von Bülow and Richard Meienreis, a philologist at the University of Königsberg, were early members; so too was attorney Hermann Freiherr von Teschenberg. Teschenberg, like Hirschfeld, was homosexual; unlike him, he openly acknowledged this and even wore women's clothing. He had been forced to leave the country once for kissing a soldier in public, but had returned to Berlin and often gave public talks. Even police commissioner Leopold von Meerscheidt-Hüllessem agreed to join them.[27] It may seem bold to have invited the police, since the society opposed a significant legal statute—it existed, in fact, to demand the statute's abolition. But if an officer of the law could see the value of repealing Paragraph 175, Hirschfeld reasoned, then surely so could the Reichstag.[28] One of the SHC's members, at least, agreed. August Bebel, leader of the Social Democratic Party, offered to submit a petition against Paragraph 175 to the Reichstag as an opening volley in the fight for rights. The SHC set to work on its first petition. Soon it would become the center of an entire movement.

The SHC held together through written communications, with the *Yearbook* acting as a vital outlet for promotion and organization. The core message was: 1) Hirschfeld's utter conviction that biology determined sexual orientation, and 2) that the congenital argument was the most effective means of changing the law. The argument from biology eventually made allies (if not friends) of Dr. Richard von Krafft-Ebing and even Dr. Albert Moll, whose theory of homosexuality was at odds with Hirschfeld's own, as he considered it deviant. But not everyone— not even among homosexuals—agreed.

LOOKING FOR SUPERMAN

Adolf Brand, with his dark sweep of thick hair and smoky eyes, had spent his youth near the artists' commune in Friedrichshagen. A quiet, bucolic landscape that unfurled along the Müggelspree river and hugged the lakeside, it was a meeting place for poets, avant-garde artist anarchists, and bohemians. The Poets' Circle of Berlin–Friedrichshagen and the Neue Gemeinschaft (New Community) combined Nietzschean philosophy with its own independent strand of socialism.[29] The Circle introduced the young Brand to the works of philosopher Max Stirner and to Friedrich Nietzsche's concept of the *Übermensch*.

Nietzsche's "superman," as the word roughly translates, isn't the sort to go rescuing Lois Lane from burning buildings. The *Übermensch* rises above the masses by thinking of himself only. He resists the social order and strives above all for self-expression. Similarly, the super-individual characterized by Stirner's egoist* likewise refuses ideologies. He must resist the laws of God, morality, and state to achieve self-realization.[30] Supermen succeed by their selfishness. They take and do not give; they follow only the rules that serve them; they have carte blanche to do exactly what they want, whenever, wherever, to whomever. (It isn't surprising that the free-living community at Friedrichshagen embraced the idea wholeheartedly.) *Übermensch* philosophy enjoyed publication and circulation under the same freedom from censorship as Wilde and Hirschfeld did. Even as Hirschfeld was writing *Sappho and Socrates*, Adolf Brand launched his own publishing endeavor: a journal he called *Der Eigene*, meaning "self-owner"[31] or "Ego." "Egoists unite," Brand wrote, and "we will make our own empire, our own earth."

This new earth would be made in man's image—literally by and for and about men. Brand and his followers rejected everything feminine and were notable for their misogyny. As masculinists, they believed that men who loved other men were more virile than most, and counted among their number Alexander the Great and other military and political figures. Women, by contrast, were seen as mere vessels of reproduction.[32] To love a woman, they believed, was to love something less than yourself. Homosexual practice, in this context, was an act of radical choice, not of biology. Brand read *Sappho and Socrates* with something like horror; Hirschfeld's theory—that in homosexual men, a bit of the woman remained—deeply offended his masculinist ideals. He wasn't alone.

Brand had supporters among anarchists, most especially the monied zoologist and philosopher Benedict Friedländer and a physician named Edwin Bab. Friedländer asserted that women had colluded with priests in forcing men to suppress their homoerotic natures—and that scientific medicine was little more than the modern iteration of a repressive church.[33] "No one doubted that the male sex on average was the more intelligent, wise, and just," he wrote; no one even thought to write

---

* From *Der Einzige und sein Eigentum* (translated variously as *The Ego and his Own*, *The Ego and Its Own*, and *The Unique and Its Property*).

about it among the ancients, because it was never in dispute. Now, he feared, Germany was threatened by "gynecocracy," and the male, he deemed, must be saved from women's tyranny.[34] (This, despite the fact that women in Germany could not vote, much less participate in other aspects of culture.) The hatred of women and the hatred of effeminacy in men—and certainly disdain and disgust for those born male who considered themselves partly female—set the masculinist homosexuals against all other sex and gender nonconformists. Like them, they opposed Paragraph 175 and rejected the idea that homosexuality was pathological; unlike them, they championed homosexuality as the highest expression of masculinity.

The inaugural issue of *Der Eigene* appeared in 1896, and the title, not wholly translatable in English, provides layers of meaning, vacillating among "own," "self," and "same." It was Brand's way of expressing homosexuality in a non-pathologizing, non-medical manner.[35] Gay sex, erotic writing, and even nude photos of adolescent boys (as well as personal advertisements for lovers) all appeared in the artistically rendered publication. Brand aspired to the Greek concept of mentor and ephebe: an older man would form a sexual relationship with an adolescent boy, sharing his knowledge and culture and helping the youth enter into the elite society of men.[36] Only after reaching adulthood (and, frequently, marrying) would ephebes take on their own young men. The Greeks did not have a word for homosexuality as an identity. They did, however, think of men as far superior to women—such that love for another man, whether physical or not, was superior to love for a woman (even if the "penetrated" continued to be denigrated as feminized).[37] That was a concept that Brand and his self-owners, with their fear of empowered women, could get behind.

Hirschfeld had his *Yearbook*, Brand his *Der Eigene*; together they represented opposing sides of an ongoing debate about what it meant to be homosexual. For Brand, Bab, and Friedländer, homosexuality represented the "right of personal freedom" and the "sovereignty of the individual to the farthest consequence."[38] Paragraph 175 should be opposed not because it unjustly criminalized people for an inborn predilection, but because no law should be allowed to penalize individual, voluntary behavior—a more radical idea by far. But despite these bold beliefs, Brand and his associates did not support equal rights for homosexuals. They championed, instead, the rights of men such as themselves, of the same economic, ethnic, and social class. The "movement for a male culture," wrote Bab, should not be confused with Hirschfeld's attempt to assign "uranian petticoats to profound minds and heroes."[39] In some respects, the masculinist attempt to determine "proper" homosexual culture had affinities with Galton's eugenics: the point was to bring about a reigning minority of the elite.

To the masculinists in Brand's circle, Hirschfeld had done all homosexuals a grave disservice: he had made them seem like patients, a return to pathologizing. In their view, homosexuality was a choice, not a condition. Brand used *Der Eigene* to poke holes in Hirschfeld's arguments from roughly 1899 onward, but the SHC was bigger and more influential. And at least as far as Paragraph 175 was concerned, their aims aligned. Despite their misgivings, Brand and Friedländer joined the SHC shortly after it was formed in 1897—and Hirschfeld welcomed them. In the fight to decriminalize homosexuality, they decided upon a truce.

It wasn't to last.

A PATH OVER CORPSES

By 1900, three sexologists had taken the limelight from Richard von Krafft-Ebing. His work would remain in print, popular, and widely read, but the man himself became associated with the nineteenth century rather than with the promising future. Hirschfeld, with his growing Scientific Humanitarian Committee, had established himself as a pragmatic, capable pioneer in the field, and Sigmund Freud had begun to formulate his theories of sexuality. But the man regarded as Europe's foremost expert on sex and its disorders was Albert Moll.

Moll, a fellow Jewish physician (though a Lutheran convert), was one of the earliest signatories to the petition against Paragraph 175. His monograph on homosexuality, *Conträre Sexualempfindung* (later translated as *Sexual Inversion*), had been published in 1897, the same year as *Sappho and Socrates*. He had also published an extensive work on heterosexuality that preceded Freud's 1905 *Three Essays on the Theory of Sexuality*, and from which Freud likely borrowed. Finally, Moll had edited—to the point of completely "overhauling"—Krafft-Ebing's *Psychopathia Sexualis*. He agreed with some of the SHC's principles: that the sexual drive should be considered natural even beyond the need for procreation, and that heterosexuals have latent homosexual tendencies (and vice versa). He likewise agreed with Hirschfeld that penalizing homosexuality made no sense. But, on almost everything else, the two men entirely diverged.[40]

Moll held the title of Privy Councillor of Health, and he considered himself an "objective truth-finder." Volkmar Sigusch, director of the modern-day Institute for Sexual Science at Goethe University, describes Moll's approach as theoretical and Hirschfeld's as hands-on: "Moll wanted to be a scholar and representative of pure science," while Hirschfeld was "a reformer and representative of the . . . homosexual movement." As a result, though Moll agreed to sign the petition against Paragraph 175, he felt that Hirschfeld's homosexuality (still unacknowledged but an increasingly open secret) disqualified him as a sexologist. His nature made him biased, Moll complained; it led him away from science and into "political agitation." Moll wasn't wrong about Hirschfeld's motivation; he did seek to agitate the political status quo, and his identity as a homosexual gave him both insight and passion. But because Moll considered science to be apolitical (something the coming decades would violently disprove), he felt that Hirschfeld had crossed a line. As Sigusch writes: "How should [Hirschfeld], unmanly, soft, effeminate, and an object of science himself, become the protagonist of sincere and objective research?" (Moll may also have been deeply offended, as he was by Freud, by the fact that neither man accepted Moll's leadership.)

In his writing, Moll encouraged homosexuals to look for sympathy instead of rights. Otherwise, the only option was violence and "to reach their goals over a mountain of corpses"—not of their enemies, but of members of their own community. Push too hard, or out too many people in a climate of prejudice, and there will be extortion, suicide, and worse. Moll meant his warning, written in 1902, to bring an end to the normalization of homosexuality. But the "path over corpses" acted as a veritable clarion call for Adolf Brand.

August Bebel made good on his promise; he took the SHC petition against Paragraph 175 before the Reichstag, where it sparked a full debate and flared tempers. The Social Democrats moved to overturn the law, but they didn't have the votes. In response, the SHC used Spohr's publishing house to print and mail a pamphlet called "Eros before the Imperial Court," along with the original petition and list of signatories, to every official, attorney, and legal scholar for whom they could find an address. They then went after 7,500 Catholic priests and 28,000 doctors. They collected more and more signatures, and more members, too.[41]

Correspondingly, the meetings of the SHC had far outgrown Hirschfeld's apartment, so the biannual meeting in July 1903 took place at a prominent hotel. The month began hot, with a rocketing high of 33.1° Celsius (91° F), but abated to more comfortable and breezy temperatures—and a good thing, too. Members pressed into one of the larger meeting rooms, cigarette smoke wafting with each successive speech. They had important business: following recent elections, the Reichstag had commissioned eight law professors to perform a comprehensive review of the criminal code. If the SHC could move them, perhaps Paragraph 175 could be scratched from legal record.

Hirschfeld had targeted all eight with SHC materials ahead of the meeting—but unfortunately, only two had responded favorably. There wasn't much point in trying to turn the other six; they were far too conservative. Besides, putting pressure on politicians might damage the SHC's scientific credibility. They'd tried to maintain political neutrality, partly to appease Albert Moll, but they'd hit an impasse: even though they presented scientific evidence and offered the supportive arguments of leading scientists and sexologists, the conservative members of the Reichstag flatly refused to listen. The SHC had tried using the influence of important public figures, equally to no avail. Even

Moll's strategy of leaning upon pathology for sympathy—the same idea that disgusted Brand—had been ineffectual. What could be done that hadn't been tried?

Brand fumed in irritation. This, he reasoned, is what comes of letting medical professionals lead the way. What good was a scientific organization if the government wasn't swayed by science? They needed an aggressive political strategy. Brand didn't respect Moll's authority any more than Hirschfeld's, but he did believe Moll was right about one thing: a path over corpses would definitely get people's attention. He knew (or believed he knew) that many officials were themselves closeted homosexuals. Why not reveal the truth?

At the meeting, Brand argued for staging a mass self-outing. If enough closeted homosexuals in positions of power (and there were plenty) made their sexuality public, it would cause a crisis. The authorities couldn't arrest everyone, especially when some might be in positions of legal power themselves. The strategy appealed to Brand precisely because it struck at the heart of his endeavor: the free sexual expression of all men. He also felt that, with great numbers of men from all walks of life expressing their freedom, they could shed the pathologization of same-sex love on which Moll's work, and Hirschfeld's early attempts, were based. And if these officials refused to identify themselves as homosexuals? Well, then Brand would out them anyway.

His words had a chilling effect on the room—not because the SHC members couldn't imagine such a scenario, but because they did not have to. The public outing of a prestigious homosexual had already taken place. It had ended in scandal, prejudice, and tragedy.

SCANDAL IN HIGH SOCIETY

Friedrich Alfred Krupp had grown up sickly but affluent, the only son of German steel magnate Alfred Krupp. Friedrich joined the Krupp family firm in 1875, and duly took on the role of mediator between his father, who lived an increasingly isolated life, and the board of directors.[42] He enlarged the company, added chemical engineering labs, and expanded the range of products to include armor plate, ships, submarines, and diesel engines. In 1897, Bernhard von Bülow, future Reich chancellor, delivered an address on Germany's "place in the sun," envisioning Germany as a colonial power with a strong navy. Krupp obliged by turning out vessels for Kaiser Wilhelm II's High Seas Fleet. By then, he had also married a member of the aristocracy, Margarethe von Ende, daughter of the Prussian baron August Freiherr von Ende. Known as the "Cannon King," Krupp became close friends with Kaiser Wilhelm II.[43] He could scarcely have been a more influential member of German society, but he would be brought down by a single, well-placed newspaper article.

Though married with two daughters, Krupp spent much of his time in the company of adolescent boys. Illegal on two counts—because of its homosexuality and because his sex partners were minors—Krupp's behavior had been cataloged for years by police commissioner Leopold von Meerscheidt-Hüllessem; cataloged, but not acted upon. Hüllessem kept a series of index cards with the names of prominent homosexuals, many of whom he safeguarded for fear that increased exposure to blackmail would destabilize the state. Shortly before his death, he sent the index cards to Wilhelm II. The Kaiser refused to open the package. It was better not to know, better that no one knew. As a result, the Krupp scandal would erupt not in Berlin but on the island of Capri.[44]

Unlike Germany, Italy did not have anti-homosexual legislation. It did, however, criminalize sex with minors. In 1902, the Italian authorities ejected Krupp from Capri for his offenses, and what had been largely kept quiet in Germany became an international sensation. Attempts at a cover-up failed, and a blackmail letter threatening to expose more details arrived addressed to Krupp's wife, Margarethe.[45] Worried and dismayed, she sought the help of the Kaiser. It was an ill-conceived decision. Apprised of his friend's behavior and alerted to his plight, Wilhelm did not suddenly agitate for homosexual freedom. Instead, he destroyed the blackmail letter and arranged for four psychiatrists to have Margarethe committed briefly to an asylum for the insane* in the hope of burying the story. That didn't work either.

The socialist newspaper *Vorwärts* (Forward) named Krupp as a homosexual and pederast, and the quiet story became an uproar. Krupp sought to sue for libel but was advised against it by the new police commissioner, Henning von Tresckow, because he might be forced to perjure himself in court—a delicately phrased warning that Krupp's accusers had reasonable evidence against him. A day later, Krupp was dead. The official cause of death was a stroke, and at the funeral the Kaiser rebuked newspapers and the Social Democrats for causing stress to Krupp's delicate health, but it was universally assumed that he had taken his own life. *Vorwärts* defended their intentions, saying that they (much like Brand) had merely meant to demonstrate the hypocrisy of Paragraph 175. That only stirred hostilities further. Far from bringing about equity, the Krupp case served as ample evidence that money and power were no protection against the consequences of being outed unwillingly.

For his part, Brand considered the Krupp affair a bungled opportunity; the solution, as he saw it, was to scale up. Instead of hiding in shame, they should out everyone. They just needed to out the right people, and enough of them, to sway public opinion, he claimed, but Hirschfeld (and most others at the SHC meeting) summarily dismissed the idea. To threaten the lives, careers, families, and security of innocent citizens was anathema to Hirschfeld: look at what it had done to Oscar Wilde; look at what it had done to Krupp. And then there were the suicides of patients he knew personally, the letters he had received attesting to more, and the slow compilation of a grief-ridden register in which he entered every name.

Observation and record-keeping—not brute force—were the tools of science. Hirschfeld rejected aggressive tactics and insisted that they

---

* Happily, Margarethe continued to run the company in trust as manager, reserving the stock for her eldest daughter. She would start several successful charities and die at the age of seventy-six.

needed data, concrete facts about the sex preferences and practices of everyday Germans. He had drafted an anonymous public survey to be distributed to young and old, student and wage worker, to find out what percentage of the population was in fact homosexual. Now it was Brand and Friedländer's turn to be incensed. What did Hirschfeld mean by "homosexuality"? More of his "emasculating" and pathologizing? The rift had always been there; now it broke into the open.

What counted as homosexuality? The term "homosexual" had replaced "urning," and the term "gay," though in use, was not widespread. That doesn't mean it went undisputed. The masculinists who espoused the *Übermensch* idea of friend-love among virile men refused to be grouped with "female-souled" men or "psychic hermaphrodites." They took further issue with Hirschfeld's broad application of the term. What about sex acts between men who did not think of themselves as homosexual at all? Did a sex act count as homosexual only if you felt desire? What about bisexuality? What if you were effeminate but not attracted to men? (And yes, there is a notable absence of women in these early discussions.) Hirschfeld had expected there would be questions, but he didn't address the controversy aroused by his term. Instead, he gave the floor to a Dutch psychiatrist named Lucien von Römer, who had surveyed 600 university students and come to the conclusion that 2 percent of the male population had intercourse only with members of their own sex.[46] There was precedent; the SHC could use the same survey technique.

If Brand's proposal for widespread outing came with the grim specter of collateral damage, Hirschfeld's suggested endless headaches. An attending attorney cited "difficult legal situations" that would make it impossible for people to reply openly; a Berlin merchant suggested that young people would give misleading responses and skew the study.[47] But Friedländer and Bab gave the most pointed criticism: inclination, not merely activity, should be measured. Hirschfeld, however, maintained that they had to start somewhere. If the percentage of those who had sexual acts only with their own sex could be determined—and this time, he meant to survey women as well as men—then one could extrapolate from that data. The members of the SHC were not wholly convinced, but Hirschfeld's study would go ahead.

Brand would not attend another SHC meeting for two decades. If the committee didn't support a mass outing, he would take matters into his own hands—and he would start with members of the ruling political party. Rumors had been circulating around the leading member of the Catholic Center Party, a priest by the name of Georg Friedrich (Kaplan) Dasbach. *Vorwärts*, not satisfied with the damage wrought on Krupp, had carried the story of an unsuccessful blackmail against Dasbach; an adolescent male prostitute in Cologne had demanded 100 marks from the priest, who refused to pay and reported him to the authorities. The boy went to prison, and Dasbach, who claimed his only contact with prostitutes was in efforts to convert them, escaped with his reputation intact—at least, for the time being.[48]

Brand began sending copies of *Der Eigene* to Dasbach and, when he received no reply, demanded a meeting. Dasbach reluctantly agreed. Brand, emboldened, dispensed with niceties. He claimed to have proof that Dasbach had purchased nude photographs of young boys. Own yourself, Brand demanded. Come into the open and claim your sexuality—or, so went the veiled threat, someone else will. Dasbach, enraged, ended the meeting. Brand responded by publishing a pamphlet about Dasbach's homosexuality; Dasbach responded by suing for libel. Brand ultimately withdrew the publication, but it had already sold in large numbers. Dasbach would be chased by scandal and lose his position in 1905 after another press story accused him of frequenting a hotel known for its homosexual prostitutes. He would, like Krupp, die under mysterious circumstances in 1907, another in the path of corpses.

Following Brand, Friedländer pulled his support from the SHC and formed a splinter organization, the Sezession des WHK (Secession SHC). It kept the name but not the theoretical grounding, aligning instead with Bab, Brand, and the masculinists, a community of "hyper-virile, homophilic supermen."[49] The first rupture in Hirschfeld's movement had fully materialized—a separate organization, with a separate publication. Neither would eclipse the work of Hirschfeld's SHC, but the split demoralized the movement and made it difficult for members to choose sides.

Brand had been right about one thing, however: Hirschfeld's attempts to win rights for homosexuals also had a tendency to pathologize them. His focus on homosexuality as a condition used medical terminology, and sexology, as a science of sex, tended to treat the homosexual person as an object of study rather than as a human being. His intention had been to build upon natural diversity, but in practice, this had not helped their cause. It may even—as suggested by a Munich chapter subcommittee—have damaged it.

There would be much more work to do if science were to bring about justice, but, ever the pragmatist, Hirschfeld responded by joining forces with the one group Brand and his ilk would never dream of approaching: women. The SHC had welcomed women since at least 1901, and outspoken feminist Anna Rühling delivered an address at the 1904 annual meeting, gazing out over a packed house and demanding that women (and especially lesbians) join in the fight for homosexual emancipation. At the time, female homosexuals were not actively punished under the law. Rühling's impassioned message was a warning: do not trust that this will last. If the state comes for male homosexuals, they will come for lesbians, too; they will not stop. And she wasn't wrong. By 1909, amendments were already being brought before the Reichstag to criminalize sexual relations between women. Hirschfeld joined Rühling and other powerful feminists like Helene Stöcker, Rosa Mayreder, and Hedwig Dohm, leaders of the German women's suffrage movement, in the fight against anti-lesbian legislation.[50] Stöcker had helped to found the progressive League for the Protection of Mothers (and sexual reform), and she now joined the SHC board of directors. She and Hirschfeld would begin a joint campaign for homosexual rights and for the right to birth control and abortion.[51] Hirschfeld would need to be fully persuaded that women and men were equals (Rühling, Stöcker, and Dohm would see to that), but he immediately saw women as critical allies in the fight for homosexual emancipation and the rights of sex and gender nonconforming people as human beings in need of a refuge.

Hirschfeld's newest allies would ultimately be some of his strongest and most long-lasting, but Brand and Moll would continue to be tenacious, and ultimately dangerous, adversaries. And worse, the trouble left brewing after the Krupp and Dasbach scandals had just come to a rolling boil. Another of the Kaiser's closest friends—and the chief advisor to his court—was about to fall foul of the gossip mill. Brand, and soon Hirschfeld himself, would end up right in the thick of it.

3

THE THIRD SEX ON TRIAL

IN THE FAR SOUTH OF SAXONY, ALONG THE CZECH-GERMAN BORDER, rises a Hercynian block, the tilted after-effects of a tectonic plate collision. Like a mountain heaved onto its side, the geography presents a stunningly steep escarpment to Bohemia, and a gentle rolling landscape to the German interior. Known as the *Krušné hory* in Czech and the *Erz* in German for the ore located within, this sideways spine held secret riches. Cobalt and copper, silver and zinc—but also the uranium used in thermal spas and colored glass, the mineral behind "mountain sickness" which would one day be responsible for scorched earth and atom bombs. This was an isolated, rural, fable-shrouded region, and Dora Richter was born on the steep side of the mountain.[1]

The village of Seifen stood at an elevation of around 3,000 feet. Despite its location on the Czech side of the border, most of the residents were German, and Catholic. On April 17, 1892, a Rudolf Richter was entered in the baptismal records of the parish, second child of Josef and Antonia, a musician and a lacemaker.[2] Antonia had wanted—prayed and wished for—a girl. Reproductive superstitions clung on in the late nineteenth century, and for a time these wishes were thought to have transferred to the child, who was a cherubic creature, small and delicate, taking after her mother in looks and personality.

Dora* was born two years into the marriage, which had already soured. Josef drank. He raged. There were more children on the way, and money would always be a problem. Antonia taught Dora and her

---

* Dora was christened Rudolf and known by that name as a child, but I have chosen to use the name she gave herself.

sisters lace-making. Boys were expected to take work and help the family, but Josef prohibited Dora from practicing this trade openly, as it was considered women's work. He insisted that Dora wear trousers, like a boy, instead of dresses; she didn't understand why. She took to sneaking her sisters' dresses, even after scoldings and beatings by her father. Why couldn't she do as her sisters did? Then, when she was around nine years old, she happened to see the genitals of a girl playmate her own age and realized in horror that they weren't anything like her own. Over the next few years, the first signs of puberty began to appear, and Dora's body differed more and more from the other girls she knew. She determined to do something about it.

Dora's mother had once treated a wart by tying a string around it so tightly that it atrophied and fell off. Perhaps, Dora thought, a string might do the same for the dangling bit of flesh between her legs. She snuck a piece of yarn from one of her sisters' lace-making workboxes (she had been denied her own, despite her skill at the craft) and tied it around her penis, but her parents discovered it in time to prevent complications or necrosis. She next considered her father's smooth, flat, straight razor. That would do it. But she'd seen how the smallest cut made the blood flow and was too afraid to try. Inconsolable, she feigned illness and stayed at home while the family went to church. Then she took a large piece of bread, stuck it with nails, and swallowed it. Dora was lucky; the bread sufficiently coated the nails and she passed them without puncturing her stomach or intestines.

It was the first of her suicide attempts. She was thirteen years old. She would spend the next two decades trying to conform, struggling and alone in a small town far from Berlin. That great city possessed a thriving—though underground—community of sexual intermediaries, but even surrounded by the throng, comfort, security, and support were in short supply.

THOUGH TWO AND A half million strong, early twentieth-century Berlin squeezed itself into oddly narrow communities with boundaries that were seldom crossed. Those living in the north and east of the city might never visit the south; those in the west lived and died without ever visiting the east. The unbroken urban skyline rose like a gray tide, enclosing its denizens and keeping them isolated all at once. It made disappearing easy; it made finding the lost impossible. Parents in search of estranged children could apply to Room 361 at police headquarters, with its 10 million alphabetical scraps of paper keeping track of the living and dead—or not, as was frequently the case. For every anxious mother seeking a distant son, there were plenty of sons (and daughters) for whom no one bothered to look.

On Christmas Eve, 1903, one such wanderer huddled alone in the cold dark.[3] A student in west Berlin, with fine features and dark hair, he wasn't yet twenty. Crouching in a dirty alley, he spied upon a distant window. From within its warm glow, he heard the laughter of his younger siblings. They were no doubt gathered around a tree, peeking at wrapped gifts and tinsel paper, but the youth was no longer welcome. His father, a respected member of Berlin society, had disowned him as a homosexual. This was as close as he dared get, waiting and watching until he saw the face of his mother as she pressed her forehead to the glass and peered out at the gloom.

This was too much to bear. The young man left his hiding place, sought out the nearest bar to drink away his pain, and returned to his rooms alone. Once inside, he tore them apart, thrashed himself against the furniture, and hurled a burning oil lamp to the floor. The flames went out; having failed at self-immolation, he severed two arteries on the jagged glass and lay down to die. By the time Hirschfeld arrived on Christmas morning, the boy was pale and mute, weak from loss of blood, the room "filled with scraps and pieces of furniture, torn clothes, books and papers, all doused in blood, ink, and petroleum [lamp oil]." A fit of apoplexy, said the housemaster. Hirschfeld looked into the boy's desperate eyes and saw suffering instead. He bandaged the wounds and hoped this would be a life saved among many losses—because there was hope, and support too.

The young man's Christmas Eve and Hirschfeld's couldn't have been more dissimilar, but the comparison shows just how much there was to live for, just how large and supportive the still-underground community could be. Twelve hours earlier, Hirschfeld had dusted the snow from his coat and enjoyed the warm welcome of a fellow townsman. The man, whom Hirschfeld never names, owned a large house and opened it every Christmas Eve to disowned homosexuals with nowhere else to go. He decorated a large fir tree with silver garlands and white candles, snow-flakes, glass globes, and "angels' hair," a tinsel that linked branch to branch like spiderwebs. He always decorated it himself, even negotiating a long ladder to attach the topmost star with its trumpeting angel calling for "peace on Earth to all." Provided with a warming drink and encouraged to make himself comfortable by the fire, Hirschfeld watched his friend wrap tiny presents so that everyone might have something: a chain ring, a hand mirror, even a mustache trainer to achieve the perfect curled corners. The servants helped by dressing the table and laying out silver and crystal, with a name card and a single flower for every guest; the servants had a table, too, and would enjoy the same luxurious banquet. Most surprising of all, in the home of an established bachelor, were the children. Hirschfeld watched them playing, the washing lady's children and the concierge's grandchildren among others. That was most important, his friend explained. The children would open presents under the bright tree, bringing something like the real joy of the holi-day to everyone present. It was beautiful, Hirschfeld agreed. Beautiful and heart-wrenchingly painful.

"Far, far back wander the thoughts of the uranians," he wrote (still using the term interchangeably with "homosexual"), "to the time when this day was a family celebration, when there was nothing yet to indi-cate a fate so different from [their] siblings." Parents went to their graves without accepting their homosexual child—or worse, parents lived on but considered their child dead to them. A dressmaker with the nick-name Lanky Emily wept openly in front of Hirschfeld, tears falling to the sound of small voices singing "Holy Night." Hirschfeld knew most of those present were longing for family, dwelling on hopes shattered by prejudice. Here, they grieved together. Here, they were safer from the agonizing solitude that had led an Austrian chemistry student to take cyanide the year before, after requesting that the pianist play Koschat's "Forsaken." His death had been listed as "suicide, reasons unknown."

Hirschfeld partook of dinner and recorded the sentiments of those who asked why homosexuals should be outcast from the Savior who had supposedly come to save all. Then he went home, only to be summoned a few hours later to the wounded student's rooms. The extraordinary feeling of joy and despair wrapped together in the bestowed light of Christmas finery comes to us directly from his writing, even down to the carols sung by the children. It's from Hirschfeld we learn of the youth crouching in the shadows and longing for his mother and from him, too, that we hear of Room 361 at police headquarters in Alexanderplatz. The description of a city that swallows humanity like a tide, and of its divided geography—as well as the tears that fall from Lanky Emily— all appear within a slim volume published on December 1, 1904.

Berlin's Third Sex: Gays and Lesbians Around 1900 was the first comprehensive sociological work on homosexual life in the new century. The foreword explains that Hans Ostwald, publisher of the Metropolis Documents—fifty-one volumes intent on capturing the sudden rapid expansion of Berlin—had asked Hirschfeld personally to write it. Berlin was now almost twenty times larger than it had been at the dawn of the previous century, staggering under the mind-bending pace of change in an industrial age. What were people's real lives like? And how did these urban vicissitudes affect the most marginalized amid the glitz that was upper-crust Wilhelmine society? With a broad (and largely educated) audience, the series offered Hirschfeld a chance to reach the public with his enduring, if still forming, message: "The great vanquisher of all prejudice is not humanity [that is, compassion, charity], but science."[4]

Wissenschaft, the German word for "science," is more inclusive than the Anglo-American idea of science. At the time of its emergence, *Sexualwissenschaft*, sexual science, was interlinked with other classifiable forms of knowledge, such as human psychology, psychoanalysis, ethnography, anthropology, criminology, physiology, social activism, and the still nascent field of endocrinology.[5] Hormones would ultimately be deeply important to Hirschfeld's work, particularly in arguments about the natural, biological, and congenital origins of sexuality. Oddly, they would not be critical in the work of the period's other rising sexologist, Sigmund Freud.

In 1905, Freud published *Three Essays on the Theory of Sexuality*. Anchored in the explosion of scientific studies at the end of the previous century, the collection offered an original take on what Freud termed "aberrant" or deviant sexuality.[6] The first essay, "Aberrant Sexuality," delineates a distinction between sexual object (the object of affection) and sexual aim (the intentions toward that object), and notes that there may be deviations from the norm in either. More important, these deviations exist in so-called normal people: the "constitution" contains the "seeds of all perversions" even in childhood.[7] The latter two essays, "Infant Sexuality" and "The Changes of Puberty," introduce the concepts of penis envy and the Oedipus complex. The essays would have enormous impact, and they align with Hirschfeld's emphasis on how widespread sexual "deviance" truly is. Freud proposed the first psychological view of sexuality but remained far more interested in the unconscious than in the body or its secretions. This would become a principal difference between the work of Freud and of Hirschfeld—though not the only one.

Hirschfeld's interest in the body preceded most of the technologies for exploring the science of small things. He didn't have Petri dishes or slides under microscopes. Instead, he worked from the laboratory of clinical and personal experience—and a more or less open invitation to all the homosexual establishments in town. Would they fill out his questionnaire?

Based upon the extensive questionnaires completed in 1903–04, Hirschfeld estimated the homosexual population of Berlin to be something over 50,000. For those stunned by the number, Hirschfeld reminded readers of the city's urban anonymity; people in the front of an apartment building didn't know who lived in the rear, "let alone what those inhabitants get up to."[8] Utterly unlike Dora Richter's experience of small-town life, the sprawling metropolis hosted thriving subcultures unseen by the uninitiated. In fact, most could not even be visited without a guide. Hirschfeld had already served in this role for sexologist Dr. Iwan Bloch and professor of neurology Dr. Albert Eulenburg, and had won both of them over to the SHC fight against Paragraph 175.[9] With the publication of *Berlin's Third Sex*, he intended to do the same for a much larger audience, offering himself up as Dante's Virgil to casual readers, guiding them on a journey through the underworld. Meet the elegant woman of the "Parisian demi-monde" revealed later to be "a man, and not even homosexual," or the Berlin lady at the Philharmonic who, at home, wore the appearance of a young and engaging gentleman, or even the youth with "no sexual impulses toward either women or men."[10] In fact, "when this study mentions homosexuals, one should not think of any type of sexual act," he writes; "what matters here is the essence of the uranian," a nature, unchangeable, from birth.

Berlin's Third Sex offers less a scientific theory than a grand invitation to see with fresh eyes. Hirschfeld had already understood that "homosexual" as a term didn't cover all the diversity he encountered. As a group, these people were not easily identifiable, did not fit into boxes, spent much of their time concealing their true selves. Let us, Hirschfeld wrote, speak of them as a third sex.

The word "sex" could mean the sex act or the sexual organs—mainly referring to type of genitalia. Slowly, it also came to mean something closer to gender, that is, the "womanness" of those with female genitalia. Many a treatise on propriety in the eighteenth and nineteenth century had been addressed to the Female Sex, by which the authors simultaneously meant "women" and "those whose genitalia include ovaries and a uterus." As a result, sex as act, sex as genitals, and sex as an identifier for gender were often conflated. Karl Ulrichs had begun the necessary work of dividing doing from being, and Hirschfeld built upon that work, claiming that "sex" was an identity unrelated to reproductive activity or physical traits—effectively separating gender, sex characteristics, and sexuality. This flew in the face of Adolf Brand's insistence upon personal choice rather than innate sexuality and popularized the idea of sexual identity. "Do you know for sure that among those closest to you, whom you love most tenderly, those you adore above all, whether among your best friends, your sisters and brothers—that not one is a uranian?"[11] We are everywhere. We always have been.

The homosexual bars and hotels frequented by male prostitutes were generally the establishments most raided by the police (and thus most often in the papers). Berlin's police commissioner, Leopold von Meerscheidt-Hüllessem, had been raiding gay bars such as the famous Seeger's Restaurant for a decade by then—and new ones promptly opened in their place and carried on as before. Yes, this was the same man who had agreed to sign Hirschfeld's petition against Paragraph 175, but it's not the hypocrisy it at first seems. Robert Beachy argues in *Gay Berlin* that Hüllessem's Department of Homosexuality served as much to soften, countenance, and tolerate homosexual activity as to police it. Hüllessem may even have helped indirectly to create the homosexual community by knitting together various activities under his department's purview.[12]

In Berlin, most homosexual activity was permitted so long as it remained quiet and out of sight. That doesn't make an environment of acceptance, nor even one of tolerance, but implicit was an understanding that such persons existed. Treated as an underclass, like sex workers (with whom they occasionally overlapped), the rule of law meant only to keep homosexuals in their "proper place." As a result, the city supported numerous gay bars as well as coffeehouses and patisseries where lesbians gathered to read, drink coffee, play chess, and speak about current events, unmolested by either police or intervening men. Hirschfeld listed the establishments in order to normalize them, demonstrating their tenure and their sheer number as if to say that anything so well rooted cannot possibly be a threat. Berlin, at least, offered something of a subculture sanctuary.

Next, Hirschfeld trod into murkier territory. The identity of the German nation drew from codes of honorable "masculine" behavior—as a sphere of male power, and with all the connotations of military prowess.[13] The idea of homosexuals in the military offered endless fodder for caricature in the press, and always threatened scandal. But that didn't mean it wasn't widespread. Hirschfeld referred to "situational" homosexuality, which allowed for a soldier to return in the evenings to a "friend" who cooked for him, fussed over him, packed his lunches. These liaisons could "make life in the metropolis more comfortable" when "lack of money, or of maidens" meant long and lonely hours. The soldier and his friend may or may not have had sexual relations, but the soldier generally provided monetarily for his partner before "return[ing] home [and] living as a married farmer far from his Berlin garrison."[14] The fact that the military was, at least, an extremely homo-*social* structure wasn't lost on other theorists, including a young man we will meet later named Hans Blüher. Hirschfeld's point stood firm: outside of the law (and in spite of it), many were willing to accept the "third sex."

Unlike the father who rejected his son at Christmas, there were plenty of parents who chose radical support and approval. An aging doctor of Hirschfeld's acquaintance accepted his son's male lover into the family and referred to the couple as his "two lads," even settling a joint inheritance upon them at his death. At the other end of the social spectrum, a simple day laborer discovered that one of his sons loved a male dressmaker. The dressmaker then played matchmaker to the man's other son, fixing him up with a homosexual friend. The surprised and somewhat confused father agreed to both matches, because his boys seemed happy. "There are mothers," wrote Hirschfeld, "well aware of the circumstances, who exuberantly relate that their son, their daughter, has found such a wonderful friend" and prefer it to seeing them in trouble with those of the opposite sex.[15] (If we are surprised by this acceptance—and I admit, I was—it says a great deal more about our own perilous and divisive time than it does about the historical one.)

From here, Hirschfeld turned to "obviously homosexual princes, counts, and barons" and their gossip over which new duke would be the season's heartthrob. One story tells of an unsuspecting heterosexual prince who was invited to a hunting party by a homosexual magnate; rising early, he surprised the host wearing scarlet silk women's garments. If so many people across the classes have these natural incli nations, Hirschfeld asked, why have they been criminalized? And why should any law concern itself with what "adults in free agreement do with each other?"[16] Paragraph 175 made no one safer; it only opened up the widest possible avenue for blackmailers. What must be kept secret may become a weapon against you. It had already caused trouble among the highest echelons, where even friendship with the Kaiser did not save one from an ignoble end.

When Friedrich Alfred Krupp was laid to rest, Kaiser Wilhelm II gave the eulogy, doing his best to exonerate his friend and villainize the newly empowered press. But the story would not be reburied.[17] The government could neither contain nor control it; scandal provided both leverage and veto power. Hirschfeld's *Berlin's Third Sex* found an eager readership abroad, too. At the back of the book Hirschfeld printed a short "What People Should Know" section, asserting that homosexuality as an identity was natural, innate and inborn,* and ubiquitous. Feeling sanguine about science's role in broadening perspectives, Hirschfeld asked that such identities be accepted, if not celebrated. The SHC followed in good faith, with 1,000 homosexual members coming out publicly in 1905.[18]

This did not lead to the hoped-for swell of self-outings proposed by Adolf Brand. As scandals mounted, another threat loomed. The masculinist principles that had attracted Brand also undergirded the Wilhelmine empire: a man must present as an unassailable masculine figure. The new visibility of homosexuality, whether treated by science or excoriated in the press, had power to destabilize. If a high-ranking figure were suspected of homosexuality, it not only shook his authority as a man, it meant he could be blackmailed to the detriment of the nation. The scenario was not only likely; it was imminent, treacherous, and struck at the heart of the Kaiser's inner circle.

---

* Though sometimes used interchangeably, "innate" means "native" or natural, derived from within, while "inborn" here means congenital. Hirschfeld wanted to demonstrate how both the person's nature (their state of mind, psychology, predilections) *and* their body's physical makeup at birth influenced sexuality.

THE FALL OF THE ROUND TABLE

On November 7, 1906, Kaiser Wilhelm II rode a short distance north of Berlin to Liebenberg Castle. A knight's estate in the sixteenth century, it had been transformed into a landscape park with a *schloss*, or castle, whose butter-toned walls were reflected in a lake, the whole nestled against a woodland well stocked with game: the private paradise of the wealthy aristocrat Philipp Fürst zu Eulenburg, recently elevated to the rank of prince. Wilhelm planned to join him for a three-day hunting trip.

The Kaiser had met the (older, arguably wiser) Eulenburg before taking the throne at the age of twenty-nine, a surprise elevation following the death of his grandfather and father within a few months of each other. Willful, autocratic, and subject to whims and vanity, Wilhelm surrounded himself with those eager to please him—and please they did. By the turn of the century, Eulenburg had established himself as chief confidant, the man in charge of creating and supervising Wilhelm's inner circle, which was dubbed by its detractors the Liebenberg Round Table. The coterie functioned almost as a second seat of government, much to the Reichstag's dismay.[19] This privileged inner ring included Eulenburg's closest friend, Lieutenant General Kuno von Moltke, municipal commandant of Berlin. To its critics, even to chancellor Bernhard von Bülow, the Round Table was a byzantine "camarilla," a group of irresponsible and self-serving advisors. They held seances; they wrote homoerotic poetry; they represented, in fact, just the kind of homosocial masculinist ideals Adolf Brand espoused.

There were rumors about Eulenburg's sexuality, too. Though married with children, he had left Vienna in a hurry, supposedly to avoid a scandal. Few dared speak it in plain terms, but many assumed that he and Moltke were lovers, especially after Moltke's messy divorce and rumors of his "abnormal" sexuality.[20] This might have remained mere gossip if not for stolen letters made public, revealing that Eulenburg and Moltke gave each other pet names, such as Phili and Tutu, "sweetie" and "old badger."[21] Pet names alone weren't enough to topple the government—not yet. But this was the end of 1906, a disastrous year for German foreign policy. The timing, for Wilhelm, could scarcely have been worse.

The Germany that emerged after the Franco-Prussian War, under Imperial Chancellor of the German Empire Otto von Bismarck, was heavily invested in a bullish, virile masculinity. Though Wilhelm II replaced Bismarck in an ugly split after he ascended the throne, he retained the same martial–masculinist values. Strength, honor, courage, self-restraint, and "respectability" not only safeguarded Wilhelmine traditionalists from "modernity," they agreed with Germany's sense of political identity and national "spiritual and material vitality."[22] Femininity would not be countenanced.

The unification of Germany under the previous kaiser and his successful exploits of military conquest had gained an almost mythic status. Military might was also seen as the principal guarantor of Germany's importance on the European stage in the midst of massive upheaval. Much of Europe had spent the last half of the nineteenth century preparing for—and fearing—a continent-wide war. The dread spilled from newspaper headlines into literature, so that even the mysteries of Sherlock Holmes printed in the *Evening Standard* featured regular plots that threatened to send Europe into chaos.

Back in 1898, as Berlin began building its navy, Chancellor von Bülow had been optimistic about his nation's chances of becoming a world power, but as the Western Powers united, Germany found itself increasingly isolated. Left with no real allies beyond Austria, Bülow, Wilhelm II, and foreign minister Friedrich von Holstein debated possible solutions. The Kaiser favored a Triple Alliance between Germany, Austria-Hungary, and Italy, but Bülow warned that the Italians could not be trusted. By 1903, his fears proved correct; France, Great Britain, Spain, and Italy signed interlocking agreements, cutting off any chance for German affiliation. France, still considered Germany's chief rival, also controlled territory in North Africa, having colonized the Moroccan port of Casablanca.

The situation seemed increasingly desperate; Germany needed a show of strength. The Kaiser proposed an alliance with Russia, but Holstein and Bülow balked; it was neither "wise" nor "possible," because France and Russia were already allies.[23] Granted, that alliance dated back to 1894, at the end of the Franco-Prussian War, when both countries had been humiliated by a rising Germany and the ambitions of Otto von Bismarck. It was Bismarck's victory that had ultimately united Germany; surely friendship with Russia could be nothing but trouble. But the Kaiser was keen to assert his authority, to make a name for himself as his forebears had done and silence those who worried that Germany was growing weak and effeminate. As usual, he determined to follow his own advice.

Wilhelm made several overtures of friendship toward the tsar, but the Russian ruler refused to sign a treaty unless France was notified. Unfortunately, doing so would also alert Great Britain, and that was a conflict Germany wanted to avoid. Talks stalled, and the window of opportunity threatened to close indefinitely. In an attempt to redirect Wilhelm, Holstein and Bülow turned their attention to the African continent. They convinced the Kaiser to visit Tangier, court the sultan, and woo a Moroccan alliance of their own. This new tactic trod upon France's preexisting claims in Morocco, putting Germany in direct conflict with France (and Great Britain)—exactly what Wilhelm had wanted to avoid.

The Kaiser needed to back out, but also to save face. First, he issued a non-public declaration of war to the French Foreign Ministry as a warning shot. Then, he insisted on an international conference of fourteen nations as a tribunal for France's Moroccan policy, which, Germany claimed, went against international interests in the region. The nations agreed to meet, which seemed to be a step in the right direction; unfortunately for the Kaiser, France called his war bluff and the conference ruled against Germany. Meanwhile, the Russian tsar withdrew his suggestion of friendship entirely, and Germany found itself even more isolated than before. With enemies on all sides, no action could be taken that wouldn't pull the strings of the wider web. Wilhelm complained bitterly about a future of constant bargaining "with the Franco-Russian

Alliance, the Anglo-French Entente [agreement], and an Anglo-Russian Entente, with Spain, Italy, and Portugal as secondary satellites."[24] How had it all gone so badly wrong?

When Wilhelm went on his hunting expedition to Liebenberg, his foreign policy lay in tatters. Perhaps he thought the crisp air of Eulenburg's estate would clear his head. Maybe he was looking for an escape from the business of politics. Alas for Wilhelm, he hadn't seen the guest list.

Raymond Lecomte, the French ambassador to Berlin, had a reputation among the city's social elite. Sporting a curled mustache over a strong jaw and under a fine, aquiline nose, the flamboyant Lecomte could often be found at the city's homosexual bars and other entertainments. He was an example of the sort of feminized man lampooned in the press as ruining the nation, and he made no secret of his conquests. Commissioner Tresckow (who had replaced Hüllessem) called him "king of the pederasts."[25] Lecomte had made fast friends with Eulenburg, and it just so happened that Lecomte had visited Liebenberg during the Morocco crisis, when everything hung upon whether Germany would "really" declare war on France over a stake in North Africa. No one wanted that, and both France and Great Britain had been on tenterhooks, which gave Germany bargaining power. Under the leafy canopy of the park at Liebenberg, however, Lecomte had learned that the Kaiser was bluffing. He carried that information back to his masters in France, destroying Germany's hopes for expanding its international reach.

Was it true that German foreign policy had been routed by an unguarded chat on a bucolic afternoon? Had Eulenburg really given up state secrets? The rumors flew. *Vorwärts* journalist Maximilian Harden believed he had—and he was willing to put the accusation in print. Harden had already broken two scandals, outing "Count H" (a relative and close friend of the Kaiser) and Friedrich Alfred Krupp as homosexuals. He claimed that he wasn't against homosexuals in general, only that they should not be in positions of power where they could undermine the masculine character of the country. Harden identified as a nationalist, someone who privileged Germany and German power. Homosexuals, he claimed, were a "pink" international group—like the "red" socialists or the "golden" Zionists (a deeply anti-Semitic notion). Their sexuality "provide[d] a unifying band beyond all walls of faith, states, and social class" and, Harden warned, united them "in a brotherhood of protection and defense" uninterested in Germany's foreign ambitions.[26] The connection between homosexuals and Jews was tacit; it would grow more explicit with time. For Harden, same-sex desire threatened the nation, and the cheeky French diplomat and Prince Eulenburg were pink insurgents.[27] Not satisfied with the damage already caused to the empire, Eulenburg had invited Lecomte once again to Liebenberg, this time to rub shoulders, share wine, and sit at the same table as the Kaiser. How dare he?

For his part, Lecomte protested that only the merest of banalities passed between him and the Kaiser, but for the first time, those who opposed Eulenburg's influence had real ammunition to use against him. Harden wasn't about to lose his chance.

Harden launched his first attack ten days after the Liebenberg hunt, following it with two more contemptuous pieces in January directly naming Lecomte. Then, in April 1907, Harden openly accused Eulenburg of treason: "That [the French Ambassador] was able to report to Paris with such exactitude on the feeling at the court was certainly not his own doing," he wrote. "Lecomte . . . has been an intimate friend of Prince Philipp Eulenburg since his Munich days, and without being overzealous or requiring indiscretion from his romantic friend he can learn many things that are otherwise unobtainable."[28] It's important to see the careful rhetoric here; words like "intimate" and "romantic" and "indiscretion" combine with a serious warning about German security. For the first time, Harden effectively tied fears of German emasculation to a clear and present threat to national security.

The Kaiser's handlers originally tried to prevent the scandal from reaching his ears (he did not read the papers), but it seemed plain that he would be dragged into it as well. Wilhelm's nephew was given the unpopular job of breaking the news, and such was Wilhelm's fury that he banned both Eulenburg and Moltke from court and demanded that

they legally clear themselves. Only thus might they save their own repu-
tations and his as Kaiser. Eulenburg duly began a libel suit. Moltke took
a different strategy; he challenged Harden to a duel. This, too, became
news, and things promised to get very ugly indeed.

In the past, blackmail cases against homosexuals (like Krupp) had
stirred sympathy, and Hirschfeld's *Berlin's Third Sex*, with its portrayal
of wrecked lives, had driven the point home: something must be done to
protect the vulnerable. For a brief moment, it seemed that a change had
come, and scientific and political organizations had asked Hirschfeld
and the SHC for educational lectures about homosexuality.[29] No more.
The Liebenberg Affair (also known as the Eulenburg scandal) had taken
the matter from personal and private to national and public. At stake
was nothing less than German national identity.

With such a looming threat, the general public withdrew its sympathy for homosexuals and united against Eulenburg and anyone else
suspected of deviating from the sexual norm. Public and global reaction, pushed by Harden and the scandal press, resulted in something
like hysteria—a panic over homosexuality, a serious masculinity crisis.
By the end of it, the Kaiser and his inner circle had suffered humiliation
on the national and world stage as Moltke, Eulenburg, and a long list
of aristocrats and military leaders were accused of violating Paragraph
175—and, worse, of being unmanly. The Prussian leadership lost its
legitimacy, the popular press proved its political power, and the science
of sexology entered the everyday lexicon. The world—and Germany—
would never be the same. Neither would Magnus Hirschfeld, who found
himself in the middle of it.

THE PROCEEDINGS REQUIRE SOME parsing. Harden accused Eulenburg
and Moltke in the press, not in court. To clear their names, they would
have to sue for libel, but cases compounded and countersuits were filed.
Moltke's case against Harden cited eight articles containing accusations
of homosexuality. Harden's defense rested on something that wasn't
there, rather than something that was. Since Moltke did not pursue

women, Harden argued, he *might* pursue men: "in this trait one must distinguish between a tendency to unnatural activity and the mere existence of impulses of an unhealthy and abnormal nature."[30]

The concept of sexual inversion had been around since the nineteenth century; Freud had popularized the term, applying it to those who felt desires or performed behaviors usually expected of the opposite sex. Harden had to prove two things: first, that Moltke had abnormal inclinations—not that he acted upon them, but that he *possessed* them—and second, that Moltke was a politically dangerous person because of those inclinations. Harden was essentially suggesting that, even in the absence of evidence, Moltke could still be guilty of inversion on the inside. It would be difficult to prove; he'd have to choose his witnesses carefully. He began with Moltke's ex-wife, Lilly, and her adult son from a previous marriage.

Lilly supported Harden's defense. She claimed that Prince Eulenburg had interfered in the marriage and demanded that she give Moltke a divorce, saying, "Release my friend, give me back my friend." Lilly also stated that immediately after their wedding, Moltke had tried to leave her behind; she also claimed that the marriage had never been consummated. But was Moltke "abnormal" in his sexuality? Lilly affirmed the charge, saying that Moltke had told her, "I don't find you revolting as a human being, but rather as a woman." Her son, a young army lieutenant named Wolf von Kruse, gave his statement next. He testified that Eulenburg had once left behind his glove and that Moltke picked it up and kissed it, whispering, "My soul, my love." Technically, none of this proved that Moltke had violated Paragraph 175 or that his relations with Eulenburg were necessarily sexual—but it did not need to.

"I claim that [Moltke] has such an inner emotional orientation," Harden said in court, as to be considered homosexual. They needn't take his word for it; he'd invited a well-published sexologist, whose most recent book took pains to show that homosexuality wasn't about acts as much as nature and identity. Magnus Hirschfeld was about to go under oath.

Harden had invited Hirschfeld under false pretenses. Hirschfeld thought he would be testifying on Moltke's behalf and clear him of criminal charges of sodomy; he also saw the case as a way of speaking about his mission. Harden expected Hirschfeld to say there was nothing shameful about homosexuality. He welcomed it, in fact, so long as Hirschfeld inadvertently proved Moltke's homosexual leanings. Though well-intentioned, Hirschfeld walked right into a trap.

The stakes were enormous. Already, the trial had provided fuel for newspaper articles all over Berlin, and also in New York and London. German and foreign journalists clamored for seats and squabbled over press tickets; crowds formed to shout, cajole, or cheer the various players as they entered the court. Demand for seats rivaled that for virtuoso concerts at the opera.

Hirschfeld took the stand in a rowdy and boisterous courtroom. The delivery needed careful handling, so he began by explaining the difference between friendship and love. The homosexual feels a genuine "love attraction" for someone of his own sex, he explained. But "whether that person engages in homosexual behaviors is irrelevant from a scientific perspective." Homosexuals and heterosexuals could be celibate, platonic, interested only in love as an ideal. One could be a homosexual and yet never engage in homosexual acts. That, on its own, might have cleared Moltke of any future criminal proceedings. But criminal proceedings had never been Harden's aim. Harden knew Hirschfeld's work on innate and inborn homosexual nature. He coached his lawyer to cross-examine, getting Hirschfeld to explain further; if Moltke denied being homosexual, then how did one explain his abnormal behavior toward the prince? That is, might his nature be different from his public presentation—entirely apart from whether or not he had violated the sodomy law? All acts aside, might there be something about Moltke's nature that even he himself was unaware of?

Hirschfeld took the bait. Yes, it was possible for someone to be unaware of their own nature, he explained. Moltke might be unconsciously homosexual; homosexuality might live deep within him, at the core of his being. But he'd been born that way and could not help it, even if he himself did not acknowledge it. One can almost hear the gasps in the courtroom. Hirschfeld quickly followed by saying that a homosexual disposition was neither criminal nor uncommon, but the damage had already been done. By divorcing identity from act, he had made an accusation of homosexuality much more difficult to disprove.

The idea of effete homosexual men had strong roots, and it corresponded with a disdain for women generally. When Moltke's lawyers attempted to discredit Lilly, they leaned heavily on witnesses who had seen her attack and beat her husband. She'd left him with bruises, sometimes more substantial injuries; he had locked himself in the bedroom for fear of her and even kept buckets of cold water by his bed to throw at her to fend off sexual advances.[31] On one hand, this damaged Lilly's credibility; on the other, it further emasculated Moltke and, by association, the military he represented. Everything seemed to play directly into Harden's hands.

Harden preferred the stereotype of homosexuals as effeminate and weak, and in his newspaper during (and after) the trial, he added to this various sexist stereotypes of women: they could not make important decisions, they did not have powers of objective judgment, they had a distorted view of reality. According to Harden, it was little wonder that Germany's foreign policy was failing; the governing officials lacked the masculine drive for decisiveness—for war. "In Germany, our politics are too sweet and soft . . . if we show that in an emergency, the sword will be drawn as soon as the honor and the future of our nation requires it, then our position in the world would be much improved," he wrote.[32] This last tactic achieved Harden's second goal: Moltke was politically dangerous simply because he was homosexual, since being homosexual made him, in effect, like a woman.

Harden was defending himself against a charge of libel, but the trial soon became his personal assault against the Liebenberg Round Table, the trial (and its coverage in the news) merely a means to that end. Hirschfeld had served Harden's purpose; now Harden distanced himself from Hirschfeld's assertion of equality between homosexuals and heterosexuals. He returned to earlier experts who had testified that homosexuals were both abnormal and pathological. He argued that homosexuals followed a principle of the "individual" and of self-preservation, that they recognized no authority and no national boundaries. That didn't align with Hirschfeld's views in the slightest, though it might almost be quoted from Adolf Brand's *Der Eigene*. To drive home the point, Harden claimed that by placing homosexuals in positions of power, Germany left itself open to spies like Lecomte, and the prosecutor agreed, asserting that homosexuals had the "morals of dogs."

Harden had won. The judge awarded him the victory, and Moltke's sexuality became a matter of public record in the judge's written decision: "He has an aversion to the female sex, he has an attraction to the male sex, and he has certain feminine features. These are all characteristics of homosexuality." The trial no longer concerned libel at all; the "third sex" itself was on trial, and not just within the courtroom. Following the Moltke trial, the new charge of "dangerous" homosexual could be leveled at all other members of the Round Table, including Prince Eulenburg himself.

Somehow, the trial's focus had shifted from the exoneration of one man from a charge of libel to an ambiguous but universally embraced idea of "manliness." The satirical press presented caricatures of Eulenburg and Moltke as effeminate cherubs, or displayed military men in scandalous circumstances. Additionally, the aristocracy came under fire, as middle-class publications accused them of being over-refined, homosexual, and pacifist, a combination equated with being unmanly and unfit for office. What had begun as a seemingly inconsequential libel case now threatened the Kaiser's own masculinity; in response, he enacted a purge of state, removing all officials who were thought to be homosexual. He is also rumored to have suffered a nervous breakdown.[33]

THIS WAS ONLY THE beginning. Two days later, the verdict was appealed and a retrial announced. A few days after that, Chancellor Bülow brought his own libel suit—not against Harden but against Adolf Brand.

The Harden trial had annoyed Brand on two grounds. To begin with, he was jealous of the attention. Here was a chance, at last, to perform the mass outing he'd always desired—but Harden hadn't gone far enough. Secondly, he seethed at Hirschfeld's claims of "unconscious homosexuality," as for Brand everything came down to conscious choice—and an *Übermensch* choice at that. He published a special issue of *Der Eigene* asserting that yes, Eulenburg was homosexual, as was Moltke, but they were strong, manly homosexuals—nothing like Hirschfeld's effeminates. In fact, Brand went on, Chancellor Bülow was a homosexual too, and lived with his private secretary as his lover. Still not content, Brand outed Bülow's nephew and Eulenburg's son-in-law, all of them manly men. If there was going to be a bid for masculinity, then by God, Brand wanted homosexual *Übermenschen* on the ticket.

Surprising no one but Brand himself, this quickly landed him in court.[34] The trial commenced a week after the Harden trial ended, and now it was Brand's turn to be quoted by a rabid press. The *Berliner Neueste Nachrichten* carried the story on November 6, 1907: "I described the chancellor as homosexual in my article," Brand said under oath. "But in doing so I have not reproached him. Since I strive for the elimination of Paragraph 175 and for the social rebirth of friend-love, the last thing I wanted was to insult Prince Bülow." If Hirschfeld's testimony had been foolishly optimistic, Brand's was disastrously so. The court found him guilty of libel. It did not help matters that Hirschfeld, who was called in this trial as well, failed to corroborate the rumors about Bülow, saying he'd never heard anything about it. (Brand claimed that Hirschfeld possessed evidence given to him by Count Günther von der Schulenburg; Hirschfeld denied it.)

Eulenburg himself came to Bülow's aid as a character witness, but used the opportunity to excoriate Hirschfeld: "All the fine nuances that he has constructed in his system result ultimately in the reality that no person can any longer feel secure not to be viewed as homosexual." This conclusion hadn't been lost on the press, either; Hirschfeld had already been attacked as pushing pseudoscience, with *Die Münchener Neuesten Nachrichten* calling him a propagandist "poisoning" the people. "Real science should fight against this," fulminated the writer. Psychiatrists, notably the Russian Marc-André Raffalovich, blamed Hirschfeld's Scientific Humanitarian Committee for spreading homosexuality, as though it were a contagion.[35]

The court served Brand the maximum penalty of eighteen months in prison and required him to write a statement retracting his charges, in which he remarked that the only bright spot was seeing Eulenburg (whom he admired) at the trial.[36] Unfortunately for Eulenburg, Harden would use the Moltke retrial to set his next snare.

The retrial began on December 16, 1907, and would continue well into 1908. Once again both Moltke's ex-wife and Hirschfeld took the stand. So, too, did the prince of the Round Table. Eulenburg denounced Lilly, calling her jealous, unstable, hysterical, and violent. Bullied and distracted, she "melted in tears" and gave conflicting testimony. By the end, she had retracted her most serious accusation, that she had seen her ex-husband and Eulenburg in compromising circumstances, and the court discounted the rest of her testimony as a result.[37] Hirschfeld's diagnosis of Moltke's subconsciously homosexual nature fell into question, too, and he withdrew it. Harden's defense faltered as a parade of witnesses defended Moltke's character—and once again, Eulenburg was among them.

That was what Harden had been waiting for. Max Bernstein, Harden's lawyer, knew that in the Brand trial, Eulenburg had denied accusations of homosexuality while on the witness stand, under oath. Bernstein wanted him to do so again. He began his cross-examination with a seemingly simple question: were any of Eulenburg's actions, even if not punishable by Paragraph 175, evidence of "abnormal" inclinations? Was he, like Moltke, an unconscious homosexual with a disposition beyond his control? Bernstein—on Harden's behalf—was happy to repeat Hirschfeld's testimony that homosexuals were born and not made, but with a difference. Such men as Moltke were born (he claimed) indecent and amoral. They should not be granted power of any kind, and should be thought of as pathological (if pitiable) creatures.

Eulenburg responded exactly as predicted. If homosexuality—

and indeed, anything remotely approaching it—were going to be used against him, he would declare himself entirely innocent of any "obscenity."[38] That was a mistake. Unknown to Eulenburg, Harden had already hired a private detective to dig up evidence, and 144 allegations of improper or illegal acts were presented to the court. None of them would convict Eulenburg under Paragraph 175, but it didn't matter. He was guilty of a different crime: he'd lied on the stand and would fall to the charge of perjury. His castle would be searched, producing books published by Max Spohr and the SHC related to the homosexual rights movement.

Harden lost the retrial, but he had won a much bigger prize. The prince had been, it seemed, a silent supporter of the homosexual cause. Now, it was his undoing. Hirschfeld had previously left the courtroom with his nerves in tatters; Eulenburg had to be carried out. During the next trial, for perjury, he collapsed again. Further prosecution was delayed due to his ill health, but he was effectively exiled from public and political life. The final trial closed in 1909 without a decision.

The Eulenburg scandal erupted in newspapers across Europe just as Germany entered a period of deep isolation. Harden had aligned homosexuals with weak aristocrats, traitors, pacifists, and women; the media onslaught popularized a new bourgeois masculinity of "honorable belligerence" bent on misogyny and nation-building through combat. Historian Norman Domeier suggests that "professional warmongers" eagerly "seized" upon homosexuality as a political–moral construct not just to reinterpret past failures but also as a means of aggravating current conflicts. The ultra-conservative, imperialist *Leipziger Neueste Nachrichten* went so far as to call Eulenburg's "camarilla" a homosexual disease-carrier of "unmanly" reconciliation and distasteful peace. The *Deutsche Tageszeitung* called for a "fresh and merry war" to restore the nation's "health, its strength, its juices."[39] (The allusion to virile sexual secretions is no accident; the desire for "re-masculinization" had only just begun and would cross over into sexual science and endocrinology in the coming decade.)

Germany's national identity was not only masculine, it was pointedly anti-feminine.[40] The *Neue bayerische Landeszeitung* described Eulenburg as "unmanly, effeminate, indecisive soft-soap" and called German policy a "eunuch" without backbone, without "juice and strength."[41] Only a "strong, re-masculinization" of the state would save Germany from threats of degeneracy and effeminacy.[42]

Rapid industrial growth, immigration, and the budding women's movement were changing the relationships among and between men and women. New roles threatened what many men considered their solemn and exclusive rights, and societies like the German League for the Battle against Women's Emancipation intended to claw back any independence women might gain.[43] The more securely each men's association defined its inclusion, the more it repudiated outsiders. The hatred of homosexuals began, in many ways, with a hatred of women, but it didn't end there.

Meanwhile, homosexuality—still a new term—was now known in Italy as *la Berlinese* and in France as *le vice allemand* (the German vice), and Hirschfeld was seen as somehow responsible for its continuance. "Homosexuality is contagious," wrote French military doctor Georges Saint-Paul under the pseudonym Dr. Laupts. "[It] spreads in France and Germany the moment when it is studied, discussed, and written about."[44] Hirschfeld countered that the only thing "catching" was a phobia of the third sex, "delusions" that "cropped up like mushrooms."[45]

The scientific interpretation of the "nature of homosexuality" remained as clear as ever: same-sex desire was a natural and historically constant biological variant.[46] Yet the uninformed and misinformed were ready to believe utter nonsense instead. Scandal became paranoia, and paranoia led to violence. "The terrible aggression homosexuals were exposed to during the last year was transferred unto me," Hirschfeld wrote, leaving him "exposed to poisonous invectives of such a kind I had not thought possible after my long period of scientific research." Worst of all, not a single member of the Reichstag rebuffed the claims that homosexuals were "sick people . . . not worthy of esteem or sympathy."[47]

Dismayed, discouraged, and exhausted, Hirschfeld nevertheless submitted a new petition against Paragraph 175, with 5,000 signatories, to the Reichstag commission. He did so in vain; they refused to read or even discuss it. The trials against Harden, Brand, and Eulenburg had deeply damaged the cause. Brand blamed Hirschfeld for "feminizing" homosexuals, but Hirschfeld's own insistence upon the inborn, biological nature of homosexuality had likewise been used against him. Happy to agree that a person might be born homosexual, members of the Reichstag now perceived them as "degenerates" (a word still weaponized against transgender and homosexual people), a threat to the nation, and something to be eradicated.[48] "It seems to me," Hirschfeld wrote, "that all my efforts to lift the heavy weight of prejudice, which had already had positive results, were pushed into an abyss—with one body blow."[49]

When Hirschfeld and Spohr established the Scientific Humanitarian Committee in 1897, it seemed they were on the cusp of overturning Paragraph 175. With the support of key Social Democrats, their first petition went straight to the Reichstag, and success was tantalizingly close. Now, Hirschfeld was facing violent aggression, fear, and prejudice. Soon after the trials, a political caricature circulated that sneeringly exaggerated his Jewish features: a dark, squat man in spectacles banging a drum through the streets. The caption read, "Foremost champion of the Third Sex!" It was not meant as a compliment.[50] Soon came character assassinations in German, French, and British newspapers, most of them couched in increasingly anti-Semitic terms.

In the backlash of the affair, right-wing papers declared that Hirschfeld's ethnicity (rather than his still closeted sexuality) made him "unfit for citizenship."[51] The same papers that demanded a cull of homosexual soldiers now cried out for all Jewish officers to be removed, too. Then came the leaflets dropped in front of Hirschfeld's house: "Dr. Hirschfeld: A Public Danger: The Jews are our Undoing."[52] And finally, the first threat to his life: the newspaper *Germania* published a call to all "true" Germans to "make an end of people like Dr. Hirschfeld."[53]

It seems incredible that the Harden proceedings alone created so drastic a change. Hirschfeld referred to it as a panic, a "hysteria" over homosexuality that brought all his work for homosexual rights into question.[54] How had homophobia become intrinsically linked to both misogyny and anti-Semitism? Who—or what—had watered the seeds of hatred? And was there time to stop it?

4

UNBRIDGEABLE DISTANCE

There seems no end in sight to all these tragic events.

—MAGNUS HIRSCHFELD,
*SEXUALPSYCHOLOGIE UND
VOLKSPSYCHOLOGIE*

HIRSCHFELD LOOKED UPON THE WARM, WEATHERED STONE OF THE cathedral of Trieste, Italy, dedicated to San Giusto Martire, St. Justus the Martyr. From the hill behind, a wide vista allowed the briefest glimpse of the Mediterranean Sea, but he had come to view the medieval churchyard instead. Tufts of green crept through the stone and around the weathered columns. Among them, a grave.

Hirschfeld knelt to place flowers upon it and from his jacket withdrew Goethe's *Italian Journey.* He'd marked several passages praising the genius of Johann Winckelmann, an eighteenth-century German archaeologist and art historian. Winckelmann was the first to define ancient art periods, and famously wrote, "The only way for us to become great, or even inimitable if possible, is to imitate the Greeks." He was partly responsible for Germany's new appreciation for—and emulation of—Hellenic ideals, and his *Reflections on the Painting and Sculpture of the Greeks* (1765) became a "manifesto of the Greek ideal in education and art."[1] He was also homosexual and—like Karl Ulrichs a century later—traded the persecution of Germany for the more welcoming climate of Italy.

In some ways, that's what Hirschfeld was doing, too. Shaken by vicious attacks in the press and eviscerating articles by fellow sexologists, he felt alone and defeated. Not one member of the Reichstag law reform commission, even those who claimed to support the cause, had stood up for Hirschfeld or for the rights of homosexuals. The assessor of the SHC's 1907 petition stated that they were "sick people not worthy of our esteem or sympathy."[2] Harden had used Hirschfeld's own science to link congenital homosexuality to "moral degeneration" in a climate ripe for arguments about genetic purity. The "trials of insults, cases of abuse of military authority, [and] of slander" had been sufficient to destroy the "scientific work of . . . many years."[3] Perhaps it was best that Max Spohr had died in 1905; he didn't live to see how little enlightenment their ceaseless campaigns had brought, or how easily their triumphs had been overturned. It seemed they had enemies everywhere. Hirschfeld was seriously considering resigning from the SHC entirely. Frayed nerves had weakened him physically, too; unwell and troubled, he had come to pay tribute to an inspired forebear.

Winckelmann rose to be librarian at the Vatican, his work admired by Goethe and influential on criticism of Greco-Roman art. Yet despite all, he had been murdered in a hotel not far from where Hirschfeld now stood by a fellow traveler, one Francesco Arcangeli. A cook by trade and a petty thief by inclination, Arcangeli claimed he thought Winckelmann a Jew and a spy. The authorities charged him with attempted robbery—though even contemporaries suspected it might have been a sexual assignation gone wrong, or that Winckelmann had been killed for making homosexual advances.[4] Arcangeli had attacked Winckelmann in his bed, stabbed him seven times, and left him for dead.

In the shade of cedars, Hirschfeld could feel the wind, could perhaps just catch the scent of salt sea air. Beauty always helped him see things, as he put it, in proportion. Calmed in spirit, he asked himself: Have I deserved such frightful reproaches? The answer must assuredly be no. To believe otherwise would mean that Winckelmann, too, had deserved the abuse of a biased and hostile world. "I lingered in solitude in the old impressive cemetery," Hirschfeld later wrote, "reading Goethe." When he descended the hill, reabsorbed into the picturesque city, his heart lifted: "I couldn't believe that my painstaking work had been devoted to a wrong cause." And as for Winckelmann: "Your feelings were at the root of your many fears, but there was nothing bad about them. Not you, not nature, but the law is wrong."[5]

Hirschfeld returned from Italy ready to continue the fight; he and the SHC would "confine ourselves to a calm, objective defense through scientific work," and keep doing so as long as anyone "may still be suffering from erroneous assumptions and ideas."[6] But his very first task was to write his own defense, published as *Sexualpsychologie und Volkspsychologie*: roughly, the psychology of sex and of the public's response to it. Like Freud, Hirschfeld considered sexuality to be part of psychic identity. Even so, he disagreed with Freud's conception of same-sex desire in adults as pathological, that is, as a disease or sickness. In fact, he used his "sexual psychology" to query a different kind of sickness. Hirschfeld's overriding question still resonates here and now, over one hundred years later: How do we first begin to hate?

Prejudice against homosexuals had been artfully employed by Harden to ruin Eulenburg and Moltke, but after 1909 it took on new and even more damaging dimensions. The word *Homosexualität* had scarcely been mentioned in the wider public German lexicon before the trial; after it, the word appeared internationally, but always with monstrous connotations of pederasty (pedophilia) and degeneracy. The power of print that had helped establish the SHC now threatened to destroy its work, and Hirschfeld's assessment of the danger sounds uncannily modern: "There are the most intimate interrelations between the press and the public, and what we call public opinion is for the most part based on oral, written, and above all on printed suggestions." The more impressive or famous the person, "the more self-confident he appears and the more forcefully he speaks," the greater the effect—even when (especially when) he is wrong. Above all, Hirschfeld wrote, the "suggestion of tradition proves particularly disastrous."[7] We know it all too well. Calls to an imaginary past, the bluster of talking heads, the use of fame to eclipse reason: if Hirschfeld were speaking figuratively, he was also speaking prophetically.

Hirschfeld had already experienced anti-Semitism, but now the "Jewish science" of sexology, and the associated acceptance of homosexuals, was accused of targeting and grooming young men. Jews were a threat to German boys; Jews would make them effeminate; Jews would make them homosexual—and prominent homosexual men were at pains to limit the damage. It also ultimately shaped the work of Sigmund Freud.

Freud and Hirschfeld did not unite against these attacks. Despite their early association, the two men fell out over Hirschfeld's use of the questionnaire to assess homosexual life. By 1908, the rupture was such that some of Freud's work, originally written for the SHC *Yearbook*, was published instead in the *Journal of Sexual Science*. In a letter to Carl Jung, Freud accused Hirschfeld's editors and the SHC of "skullduggery," claiming that he wasn't informed of the change until months later.[8] The rift would continue for the rest of their lives. Freud discounted Hirschfeld's concept of "born" (that is, biological) homosexuals and remained uninterested in legal reform.[9]

Freud had, until 1900, been in a close friendship with Dr. Wilhelm Fliess, a relationship with homoerotic dimensions wherein Freud played the "passive" and feminine role. As part of overcoming his "unruly homosexual investment" (Freud's words), he produced the heterosexual and heterosexist Oedipal complex, that is, a theory which promoted heterosexuality as the only normal and natural expression of sexuality. Historian Daniel Boyarin describes the theory of psychoanalysis itself as an act of "repression/overcoming," and the Oedipus model as a repudiation of passivity and femininity, the specific repression of homoerotic desire. The Jewish psychoanalyst needed to distance himself from the shadow of homosexuality; he likewise ceased writing about male hysteria, fearing that it fed into the already long-standing (at least as far back as the thirteenth century) trope of Jewish men being a "sort of woman." Freud hoped that his Oedipal complex could explain away homosexual impulse, and (since it championed heterosexuality) save him from the worst barbs of an increasing anti-Semitism.[10]

The combined power of racism against Jews and the fear of losing masculine power cemented under German nationalism. It became of national importance to indoctrinate boys into ideal white, German, heterosexual male society, which led to the formation of dedicated youth groups: get them while they're young, protect them from the influence of women. The first of many was called the Wandervögel, established in 1901, and it would one day provide the blueprint for the Nazi Brownshirts, just as "belligerent" manliness would set Germany on a course for two wars and the Third Reich.

This is the story of how hatred begins: small, discreet, and in service of the "future." But it's also a story about those who must live within that society—and without the benefit of Hirschfeld's scientific background. Hirschfeld believed that sexology owed a debt to present and future intermediaries, wherever they were. He didn't yet know that one of them was in Saxony, in the midst of a sexual awakening.

BEING DORA RICHTER

Dora waited in the broad-leafed wood, not far from the training school. Spring twilight promised darkness and cover. Would he come?[11]

The boy had a lovely form and a beautiful face: a manly jaw and a strong chin. But Dora had fallen in love with his emotional qualities. Such intelligence! Such character! Her heart leapt whenever she saw him, and she saw him nearly every day, but she didn't dare confess her feelings in person. She'd decided to send him an anonymous letter asking to meet, with the time and place for a lovers' tryst. Of course, once sent, she couldn't recall it. Had he even received it? Anxious and doubting, she smoothed the skirts of a brand-new dress. All her pocket money had gone toward its purchase, along with soft underclothes and a wig to disguise her real hair, which was cut short as befitted a boy. Would he notice? Would he care for her at all?

It wasn't her first crush. That had happened back in grammar school, when she fell for her twenty-six-year-old teacher. She'd been too young for him, of course; it wasn't a possibility—not in her waking life. In her dreams, though, he "embraced [her] like a woman, hugged and kissed [her]." Idealized and rapturous, the infatuation awakened her sexuality, but left her pining with unrequited longing. It was mere fantasy, then, but Dora wasn't a child anymore, and the boy who made her heart race was a schoolfellow, seventeen like herself. A shudder of arousal ran through her; tonight, she would make love for the first time.

The light had slipped away before she heard his approach in the sheltering darkness. The boy looked surprised. How did she know of him? Had they met? Dora told him she'd seen him before and had "taken such a deep liking," but could think of no other way to meet him. Flattered and enchanted, the boy offered her his arm. You're such a pretty girl, he said; would she care to walk with him? The leafy lane beckoned, and Dora went willingly. She had pleased him! Once within the shadow of boughs, he proved it by kissing her eagerly. Then, he reached beneath her skirt.

"Not there," she told him.

"Are you ill?" he asked. Dora trembled and blushed.

"I am modest," she said. Her suitor took her by the shoulders and pushed her to the ground beneath him. She could feel his weight pressing against her thighs.

"You put it in, then," he panted. "I must have you!"

Dora had been waiting for this moment; she'd thought of nothing else since getting ready hours before. Like a ritual, sacred to her, she cleansed herself with an enema, lubricated herself with petroleum jelly, and then bound up the genitals she hated so they could be neither seen nor felt.

"Yes," she agreed, reaching between her legs and guiding her lover inside. Yes to be wanted, to be fulfilled like this. To the youth, she was a strange and lovely girl from the village. He didn't know that Dorchen, as she called herself, was also known as Rudolf, or that they were classmates and even acquaintances. She wanted him never to know. That she had been born and christened a boy in a strict Catholic family, sent away to train for the life of a man, expected to marry and produce heirs as a son—these were her private shames. To keep him in ignorance, she could not risk seeing him often. This moment of delight would be fleeting, but that night, in his arms, she was Dora: Dora Richter.

Dora no longer lived at home; she was now a baker's apprentice, working in the mornings and going to a vocational school for additional training in the afternoons. At seventeen, Dora looked particularly girlish, even in men's clothing. The usual attire for a baker's apprentice in Saxony comprised high-waisted trousers, a stiff cotton shirt, and a short toque; Dora found it ill-fitting and awkward, and never felt at home in such clothing. Her cherubic features and bright blue eyes hadn't gone unnoticed at school; in her first days two boys made sexual advances. She didn't like them; they weren't like *her* boy. And anyway, she wanted to be loved as a woman, not a man. To be loved as herself. When Dora put on her women's underclothes of lace and satin, when she robed herself in the beautiful dress and donned her luxuriant wig, she felt whole. There was something about dressing as a woman, about changing the outward character, that made Dora feel at peace.

VESTIS VIRUM FACIT—CLOTHING MAKES the man. The proverb can be traced to an early Greek expression, and later to Erasmus's *Adages*. Fashion has long been part of the identity-forming process, but the details of clothing themselves don't signify identity. Trousers, after all, were a late invention for horseback riding; the beloved Greeks wore robes and togas; aristocratic men a few centuries earlier dressed in hose and heels, wigs and lace.

But what was happening to Dora and others who preferred to dress in clothing that crossed gender expectations? In Hirschfeld's tours of establishments throughout Berlin, he encountered many with this drive. Much to his surprise, most of them were not homosexual. He had followed Ulrichs's original understanding of urnings as having a male body and a female soul (or a female body and a male soul), but now he observed a practice that did not seem to stem from sexual preference.

In October 1911, Hirschfeld invited several sexologists, including Paul Näcke, Dr. Ernst Burchard, and a Dr. Merzbach, to his apartment. Waiting for them were six people assigned male at birth and who largely still regarded themselves as male, dressed in elegant women's clothing.[12] To describe them, Hirschfeld coined the word *Transvestiten*, and they weren't there just for show. He initiated a dialogue between the scientists and the "transvestites" about their aims, their sexuality, and their practices. He intended to write a book of case histories and wanted the input and approval of his colleagues, but he also wanted the input of the cross-dressers themselves. It would be his first project upon returning from Italy.

Like the word "hermaphrodite," "transvestite" (*Transvestit* in German) comes with baggage. It means, literally, to "dress across" (or cross-dress), but for Hirschfeld it offered a broader umbrella. Of his guests, five were heterosexual and one homosexual, and, despite overlapping desires, they approached their transvestism in unique ways. The book Hirschfeld wrote with their help, *The Transvestites* offers the first glimpse into the lives of those we now refer to as trans or transgender.*

The Transvestites required Hirschfeld to dismantle his earlier theories and reform them. A majority of the case studies included were heterosexual (that is, the subjects considered themselves male in sexual terms, and desired women sexually); as a result, Hirschfeld separates *Transvestiten* from homosexuals for the first time. If cross-dressing was unrelated to sexual preference, then sex and gender must be differentiated, too. During and after the Eulenburg affair, Hirschfeld had come under fire for linking homosexuality to femininity; he responded by explaining that discrete, tidy genders didn't exist. "Each new truth destroys the one held before it. The deeper we are forced into the countless forms of . . . nature," the more we have to "learn afresh." Hirschfeld wasn't just willing to tear his own work down for rebuilding, he wanted society to do the same—to see the deeply held biases and presuppositions that undergirded "the foundations of government, society, and religion." The separation of humanity into male and female halves was a myth and, worse, a cage. If humans can join such opposites as "energy and matter, God and nature, body and soul," he asked, then why "hold fast to the dualism of the sexes"?[13] Imagine so bold a claim landing in the public arena in 1910!

---

* At this point, the term "transvestite" includes those who are heterosexual and cis as well as those who are homosexual and those who are trans. The groups would not be differentiated until much later in our story.

Dual, divided gender simply did not exist, and it was up to the scientist, Hirschfeld explained, to adjust when new information presented itself. That's the point of science: to ask questions and to expect "new mixtures, new types" the further we look.[14] Like many of his peers in sexology, Hirschfeld had originally thought the drive to cross-dress must be pathological, an obsession, a "self-deception." Now he knew better. The remedy for errant thinking is data; look at the cases themselves, he insisted, cases who willingly and happily submitted themselves to be studied, proud and courageous if that meant being better understood. "I have," he wrote in the opening of *The Transvestites*, "followed up most of them for many years." Some as patients; some, undoubtedly, as friends.

The *Transvestiten* told Hirschfeld their origin stories; most had had an early understanding of their situation, usually a feeling of being different and of being trapped. Case 3 spoke of horror and confinement when forced into the clothes of their assigned gender: "I feel as if I have been violated and subjugated, and as if I were taking flight on all sides . . . to escape the circumstances. However, when I see myself in a woman's costume, I become completely peaceful . . . like coming home to the entire individuality." Case 11 described the urge to wear the clothing of women as "hunger and thirst." Case 15, a person assigned female at birth, spoke of being "light, well and able"—of being "free" in men's clothing. "Why," she asked, "was I not born a boy?" In most cases, the feeling that identity and gender were at odds came early, at the age of four or five. The sense of dislocation grew stronger through puberty. Hirschfeld's realization speaks to the "making" part of *vestis virum facit*, clothing's power of making, informing, and representing identity. Cross-dressing, he wrote, "is a form of expression of the inner personality." Meanwhile, taking off gender-enforced clothing felt like letting a "burdensome mask fall."[15]

Unfortunately, Hirschfeld's bold claims about ending the gender binary aren't entirely borne out in his book. Most of his patients thought in terms of being one gender or the other, as the cultural context of the time didn't allow for any other interpretation. Those assigned male at birth dreamed of getting pregnant, of suckling infants, of being surrounded by handicrafts or objects presumed to be feminine. As Dora would put it in her intake interview, "I have always lived for spending time with sweet nothings, for tidying, and cleaning up rooms, and making things pretty."[16] This aligns with then-current cultural expectations for women, a period-driven understanding of femininity that even Hirschfeld didn't quite get away from. Doctor and patient alike worked from within a framework and even a language that doesn't allow much variation, but they broke other boundaries as they went along. The division between "transvestite" and 'homosexual," for instance, would become increasingly important to the formation of a transgender community, since "not all homosexuals are effeminate" and "not all effeminate men are homosexual."[17]

In this first book about *Transvestiten*, Hirschfeld's cases were generally assigned male at birth and married to a woman. In one case, the wife happily shared clothes with her husband and gifted him earrings; another's daughter referred to her father as "Papa-Lady."[18] Hirschfeld took pains to provide the degrees and titles of each, the jobs they held, and their social standing as proof against claims of pathology; "transvestites . . . are intelligent, conscientious people who have diverse interests and a broad education."[19] But most important, Hirschfeld took them at their word. In the case of T., assigned female at birth but requesting a name change and to live as a man, he wrote, "there is no reason not to believe the patient's statements," and to deny her request would leave her subject to depression and suicide; "T. is irreproachable" and the "issue of her petition is, frankly, a matter of existence."[20]

To be a *Transvestit*, then, was not to be pathological, nor ill, nor mentally suspect. Hirschfeld went on to contradict other sexologists, particularly Havelock Ellis and Richard von Krafft-Ebing, by explaining that neither does cross-dressing equate to homosexuality, auto-eroticism, or fetish. Instead, inclinations like these justify "assuming that there is a feminine [or masculine] characteristic in [the] psyche, which, however, in no way deserves mockery and scorn."[21] Clothing, he wrote, is an "unconscious projection of the soul," evidence of male and female psyches expressing themselves in contrary physical bodies. So powerful were these feelings that the people he wrote about "withstand very great resistance and inhibitions, not the least of which is the contrast between body and soul."[22]

For once, there were victories to hand. Hirschfeld had not been able to overturn Paragraph 175 for the homosexual population, but there was no law against cross-dressing. In 1909, he successfully petitioned for a "transvestite certificate," the *Transvestitenschein*. While there was no specific law against cross-dressing, it frequently fell under the heading of "public indecency" and police used this broad definition to put those who practiced transvestism behind bars. Now, those carrying the pass, which offered proof of professional (medical) permission, could not be arrested.[25] The pass did not allow a person to change their name, nor did it confer a change in assigned sex—or rather, not yet. (Hirschfeld would have a hand in getting around that sticking point as well.)

In *Sappho and Socrates*, Hirschfeld had branded homosexual men effeminate. He realized his error, and on the heels of *Berlin's Third Sex* wrote a pamphlet titled *Geschlechtsübergänge* (roughly, Sexual Transitions), in which he attempted to make amends. The "absolute man" and "absolute woman," he explained, were fantasies, abstractions. All human beings existed on a continuum.

THE SPACE BETWEEN

In 1910, sex chromosomes had already been discovered, by Nettie Maria Stevens and her mealworms. Hirschfeld understood the role chromosomes played in determining sex characteristics, but he also understood that human gender, sex, and sexuality spanned enormous territory. Still struggling to free himself from the same binary thinking that undergirded everything, Hirschfeld was increasingly certain that gendered identity, itself, was a spectrum and not an immutable fact. Among the first to describe such a spectrum, Hirschfeld included man and woman, hetero- and homosexual, and also the variations between. Multiple combinations of genitalia, secondary sex characteristics, sex drive (desire), and emotional characteristics could be blended in many different ways.

He'd first called those in between the third sex, but now he felt that was far too unambitious. In his new formulation, Hirschfeld suggested that there might be, mathematically speaking, 43 million possible combinations![24] That's a far few more than three. Hirschfeld needed a greatly expanded theory. He would call it *sexuelle Zwischenstufenlehre*, or sexual intermediacy.

"What, then, is womanly, what is manly?" Hirschfeld asked. Chromosomes might be responsible for an egg's development, but many physical traits arrive during puberty at the behest of those inner messengers, the hormones. Hirschfeld also suggested that there were "very probably also manly and womanly" egg and sperm cells—cells with a predilection even before their union. He wasn't far off the mark. Cell physiology now reveals that XX and XY cells can and do behave independently of their respective sex hormones; these cells even have their own "sex," so to speak, which can drive molecular and genetic changes.

In 1910, however, Hirschfeld had to rely upon macroscopic observations of bodies, behaviors, and psychology. "Many persons exist," he explained, "who, in spite of carrying egg cells, exhibit characteristics that in general belong to the male sex." The reverse was also true. He agrees that in common parlance we refer to "bearers of semen cells simply as men, the possessors of egg cells flatly as women"—but this is mere shorthand. There are, he wrote, women with "manly characteristics" and men with "womanly" ones—and he wasn't speaking only of the body but also of the personality. Such things combined to make an individual's gender identity, so Hirschfeld suggested four categories for parsing it: 1) the sex organs themselves, 2) secondary physical characteristics, 3) sex drive (which sex the person is attracted to, and to what degree), and 4) what Hirschfeld referred to as "emotional characteristics."[25] Already he had begun to recognize the limitations of calling such persons "transvestites," since that refers only to clothing; he needed something far broader. These people suffered a "gap between body and soul . . . painful to be felt," for which clothing served as "not a veil, but a disclosure of one's true sex."[26]

"There are women," Hirschfeld writes, "who are more suited to a

public life; men more to a domestic life"; moreover, there is "not one specific characteristic of a woman that you would not also occasionally find
in a man, no manly characteristic not also [found] in a woman."[27] Many
nevertheless will align themselves with one side of the binary or the
other. For those who did not—who existed between the "male" and the
"female"—he chose the term "intermediary." By joining those whom
we would today consider transgender with homosexuals and other gender nonconformists, Hirschfeld does away with divisions between, for
instance, masculinist and feminist ideals. As an umbrella group, he
wrote, the intermediaries made up "a third of the total . . . world population"—an estimate he considered conservative rather than overstated.
No longer a scattering of rare minorities, intermediacy should be seen
as a "widespread and natural phenomenon" present the world over since
ancient times; to prove it, the third volume of *The Transvestites* provides
one of the first transgender historiographies on record.[28]

As a term, "intermediary" suggests a transitional state, but also offers
an in-between state of being, the closest we come to nonbinary identity
in Hirschfeld's three-volume work on *Transvestiten*. Hirschfeld noted
that the term "described only the external side," while the "internal is
limitless." Intermediacy didn't deal with externals but with something
innate, natural and inborn, even when it wasn't specifically governed
by the genitals or hormones: "sexual individuality with respect to body
and mind is inborn, dependent upon the inherited mixture of manly
and womanly substances [and] independent of externals," he wrote.
Here again we see the divergence from Freud, for whom external factors (especially in childhood) are the bedrock of identity. Instead, for
Hirschfeld, sexuality and gender are "formed in advance by nature and
[are] dormant in the individual long before it is awakened." Hirschfeld
explains that a person of intermediate gender may be "subject to temporary, even periodic changes" but "develops consequently nevertheless"
and "maintains the same characteristic impressions in all essentials for
the entire lifetime."[29]

Hirschfeld had just developed a distinction between sex as physical—as
"sexed" organs, hormones, and externally visible markers—and gender

as identity. As Rainer Herrn, who has written the definitive book on early transgender surgery and hormone experimentation, points out, the theory offers a reconciliation in which cases formerly considered abnormal (homosexual, transgender, and intersex among them) become representatives (albeit particularly conspicuous representatives) of a normative gender spectrum.[30] The theory of intermediacy represents a turning point in sexology, and an impressive leap forward.

The practice of determining identity from physical characteristics already had a long and storied history. Physiognomy purported to divine a person's character from facial features in the eighteenth century, phrenology from the bumps on the head well into the nineteenth. Similarly, Italian criminologist Cesare Lombroso introduced the idea that a "born criminal" could be diagnosed by what he called "atavistic" (primitive) features. Each of these models presupposed a "normal" or "ideal" physical form, then linked that preferred set of features to preferred moral and cultural characteristics. And what was that preferred ideal? White, male, cis, heterosexual. Anyone who deviated in appearance or behavior (so went the theory) was necessarily a lower, less evolved being. Race hygiene and Galton's eugenics reinforced this ugly concept only too well.

By suggesting that a person assigned male at birth could have the sex organs and physical characteristics of a man but the emotional characteristics of a woman, Hirschfeld decoupled two aspects of being we still struggle to differentiate: what you look like does not determine your inner self, your sexuality, or your sexual identity (what we think of today as gender). That battle would not be easily won. Germany invested heavily in masculinity, and prejudice and patriarchy had the start of him.

In 1902, German anthropologist Heinrich Schurtz wrote a definitive study that would change all of anthropology—and also reinforce masculinist German identity. His book, *Altersklassen und Männerbünde*, overturned the then popular idea that early human societies were matriarchal (led by women). Basing his work on modern indigenous groups, Schurtz claimed that civilization owed itself to the power of male bonding and masculine rites of passage. From this, he concluded that the free association of "male bands" or *Männerbünde* (and not the woman-centric family) drove higher development among human ancestors.[31] Men were inherently superior, acting as the "masculine engine of all human culture and social evolution." By contrast, women wanted only to reproduce and had no higher aims. In his work, Schurtz rendered women mute and nearly unintelligent. Obviously, then, men could only converse usefully with other men. Between the sexes was not merely an uncrossable distance, but "unbridgeable opposition."[32]

This despicable and utterly incorrect theory would be embraced by a new movement of boys' clubs, and would capture the misogynist imagination of a writer named Hans Blüher. Blüher would become the principal proselytizer for *Männerbünde*, stirring up hatred against "impure" Germans (women, homosexuals, and Jews) and valorizing war, conquest, and violence.

A SOCIETY OF MEN

Hans Blüher grew up in the shadow of Berlin. His father owned a drugstore in Steglitz, a bourgeois suburb to the southwest, where Hans would attend the Gymnasium—advanced secondary school—in preparation for university. The school had set up a boys' study circle the year before, sponsoring youth activities such as hiking and camping in the "spirit of adventure." By 1901, their little group would be formalized as an official association: the Wandervögel, or "hiking bird." Chapters proliferated, and soon hundreds of young boys would hike into the countryside to be inducted into "men's" society. Like other counterindustrial movements, including nudism and vegetarianism, the Wandervögel emphasized health and hygiene as well as camaraderie. Boys met boys of a similar age and learned to balance the pressures of modern life through nature and physical exertion.[33]

Blüher would be inducted by a young man not much older than himself, Karl Fischer. A charismatic and domineering leader, Fischer developed a rigid club hierarchy with himself as Führer. Each boy had to pledge his loyalty in an initiation that included the Heil salute, long before Hitler made it infamous. Would Blüher swear his allegiance and obedience in exchange for a place among his peers? Blüher pledged fealty, attracted by friendship and a reprieve from the "stern discipline and rigid authoritarianism" of prewar Germany.[34] Largely unsupervised, these *Übermenschen*-in-training were free to do as they pleased, so long as they did it with members of their own sex. And boys, among boys, will love boys.

Blüher's first sexual experience occurred at the Gymnasium. Rooming together at night, the boys were, he wrote, "seized with a fully aroused Eros which swept through us in the darkness." Most of his classmates were sexually active, experimenting with and upon one another—but Blüher had fallen in love. The boy came from another Wandervögel troop. They had seen each other before, but in the knee-high grass of a weekend's trek, the boy appeared transformed: "I saw suddenly how beautiful he was, and from that moment I was in flames."[35] Blüher was fifteen, a few years younger than Dora was when she planned her tryst, and less careful. Another troop leader surprised Blüher and the boy in the act and demanded they be immediately dismissed for "moral transgressions." His secret had been dragged into daylight.

As a homosexual, Blüher could be cast out of the troop, suffer punishment, and perhaps face the law. He feared the worst as he awaited the verdict, but Führer Fischer took Blüher's side and declined to punish him. Heated arguments erupted, but still Fischer refused. The conflict ultimately split the wandering birds in two: the Wandervögel and the Alt-Wandervögel (where Blüher remained), though Fischer's fiery demeanor led to his own dismissal from the Alt-Wandervögel not long after. In his place, Wilhelm Jansen would take over the Alt group leadership and, as an openly homosexual man, he quickly took the young Blüher under his wing. A friend of the masculinists Benedict Friedländer and Adolf Brand, Jansen also belonged to Hirschfeld's SHC. For the first time, a youth organization had direct connections to homosexual rights. It seemed, at first, to bode well for both.

Through Jansen, Blüher met Friedländer and read his Greek-influenced *Renaissance des Eros Uranios*. The idea of a "hyper-virile homosexual" appealed to Blüher's ego, while helping him make sense of his homosexual leanings. In Friedländer, he had found an example of the self-proclaimed elite of manly men that the Wandervögel *Männerbünde* so cherished. Blüher attended SHC meetings with Jansen, met Hirschfeld, and even gave a lecture on the value of the youth movement to their cause. Despite being indirectly responsible for the split, Blüher quickly set himself up as the Wandervögel apologist, even planning to write a book about the movement's history. As encouragement, Hirschfeld offered to write the introduction, but their brief friendship already showed signs of schism.[36]

Blüher idolized the masculinists and was an ardent admirer of Schurtz's anthropology. He had no use for men with a bit of woman in them; he considered effeminate homosexuals an aberration to be stamped out. The "male" could not coexist with the "female"; there could be no feminine and masculine mixture of traits; it would violate the unbridgeable divide between the sexes. Blüher argued that women had no place in culture—and that men who identified themselves in feminine ways should be treated as suffering, at best, a terrible sickness. Misogyny had become its own kind of homophobia; Blüher considered Hirschfeld's transvestites a sign of German degeneracy. When the Liebenberg scandal unfolded, Blüher felt that his *Männerbund* ideas had been entirely vindicated. It was not Prince Eulenburg's homosexuality or the homosocial Round Table that led to disgrace, in Blüher's opinion, but their *femininity*. He saw women as weak, and so agreed with the view that Eulenburg and his ilk were too weak to rule, even that they threatened the nation.

After Eulenburg's fall from grace, the Kaiser's homosexual purge swept through the government and military, as well as social and civic institutions.* The term "witch hunt" is overused in modern parlance, but it is more than appropriate in this instance. As an organization with homosexual affiliation, the Alt-Wandervögel came swiftly under suspicion, and Jansen along with it. Jansen had spent a fortune building an

---

* "Purge" is a useful way of describing what is happening at present with bans and legislation.

expansive clubhouse, equipping the facility with a swimming pool and nude sunbathing area. He had also installed a studio for nude photography sessions and this, given his open homosexuality, led to rumors, and rumors to accusations. Newspapers suggested he had sexual relations with the boys in the Alt-Wandervögel. No evidence or witnesses came to light, but Jansen was forced to resign in 1908, and the Parent Council performed its own purge of any troop leaders or members suspected of homosexuality.[37] That same year, Blüher pursued his first relationship with a woman and publicly denied that he was homosexual. The timing is, let's say, suggestive. He might have believed that the highest passion could only be between men, but it was no longer safe to explore male love—not now that it had been "sullied" (in his mind) by the feminizing influences of Eulenburg and Hirschfeld.

Hirschfeld pressed on; *The Transvestites* appeared in 1910 (and an addendum with photographs in 1912). In it, he produced a timeline of sexual intermediacy, scrolling through history to point out homosexuals and transgender people in every age. Blüher was about to release his own history, however, also in three volumes: not just the story of the Wandervögel, but of the *Männerbund* movement itself. Like Hirschfeld, Blüher linked his history to the ancient Greeks; unlike him, he valorized war bands, conquest, an ideal of masculinity that must dominate the weak. He sexualized Schurtz's theories, explaining that homoerotic possibility was essential to male bonding—not the act of sex, but the desire. Otherwise, men could not break away from women and "smash" the family as "social determinant." Germans, he writes, are the inheritors of this glorious history, and the *Männerbünde* would ensure their future. A true German could not be, in Blüher's assessment, effeminate, weak-willed, Catholic—or a Jew.

Why advance anti-Semitic views in a multivolume work originally introduced by Hirschfeld? Partly because he had changed his allegiance; he wanted to distance himself from Hirschfeld and the SHC with their support of women and "feminine" gay men. His first two volumes were received enthusiastically amid an explosion of new Wandervögel chapters many thousands strong. But the third volume, *Die deutsche Wan-*

dervögel bewegung als erotisches Phänomen (The German Wandervögel Movement as an Erotic Phenomenon), which claimed that homoeroticism was the "binding and creative" force of the *Männerbund*, drew fire from the association and from conservative groups, who attacked him as un-German. One of the Wandervögel's own publications asked if Blüher were—like Hirschfeld—a Jew, even as the Wandervögel umbrella association rebuked him for "glorifying homosexual inclination."[38] Against these twin claims, Blüher defended himself by claiming racial purity and returning to the years-old rift that first split the SHC. His version of "masculine friend-love," he claimed, was pure, German, and healthy— unlike the Jewish science of sexology and Hirschfeld's perverse ideas about homosexual rights. "My racial heritage gives me the security," he wrote, and besides, "I love German girls with blond hair and plan to procreate my race."[39]

Journalist Max Harden had prepared the soil, his case against Eulenburg strengthening ties of prejudice between and among homosexuals, Jews, and women. Blüher further connected the idea of homosexuality to German Jews who "suffer at one and the same time from a weakness in male-bonding [*Männerbundschwäche*]" and excessive relations with family, a "feminizing" social sphere. He wasn't the first to make the connection; in 1903, Otto Weininger had argued that "the congruence between Jewishness and femininity is complete" in a supremely anti-Semitic and misogynist work, *Geschlecht und Charakter* (Gender and Character). (He also suggested that women did not think and were fit only to be mothers or prostitutes.)[40] Weininger's work would influence Hermann Broch, James Joyce, Elias Canetti, Ford Madox Ford, and Franz Kafka. Blüher's name could now be listed among the bestsellers, too; his books were all over Germany. The *Männerbund*, even in its earliest formation, catered to insiders. Women, Jews, and homosexuals were outsiders and did not belong, and thanks to Harden and the Eulenburg trials, Hirschfeld now represented all three.

Blüher turned his back on Hirschfeld and the homosexual emancipation movement and instead championed the "conservative revolution"—a phrase Blüher coined, and one that would become synonymous with right-wing responses to progressive ideals.[41] That phrase would be dragged in and out of the media over the next decades, until it was adopted by Nazi forces against the democratic Weimar Republic. Blüher would become one of the most important right-wing ideologues, "propagating a purification of German society,"[42] such that even Heinrich Himmler, architect of the Holocaust, cited Blüher's work in his speeches.[43] Blüher himself would later condemn Hitler and repent his own virulent anti-Semitism, but the fact remains: to cover his own deep-seated fears and to screen his reputation, he helped lay the foundation of hate through misogyny, anti-Semitism, and homophobia upon which others would build.*

THE LIFE OF A WOMAN

Like Blüher, Dora suffered exposure, though of a different kind.[44] Shortly after her first meeting with her amorous boy, the school held a costume party. She couldn't resist the opportunity to dress again in women's clothes, so she purchased a traditional Bavarian dirndl for the occasion: laced bodice, low neckline, and a wide, high-waisted skirt and apron. Apple-cheeked and blushing, she proudly joined the party with friends—only to encounter her lover there. There wasn't time to react, nowhere to hide, and no way to warn her friends to be silent about her identity. "Doesn't Rudolf look strikingly genuine in girls' clothes?" one of them asked—and Dora's lover stood open-mouthed in shock. Ashamed and angry, he stormed out of the room with Dora close on her heels. Please forgive me, she begged him, "I acted out of genuine and passionate love!" The boy promised to forgive her, he said, because he took pity on her—pity for being what she was! No longer seeing her as a girl, he labeled her a homosexual.

Outed among her peers and chastised by her apprentice master, Dora

* American journalist and transgender rights activist Erin Reed suggests this has echoes of the current Gays Against Groomers, a right-wing anti-trans group.

determined to make a new life—as a woman—at a dining house.* It buzzed with constant activity, the clatter of dishes, the sound of voices. One of the larger establishments in a university town, the Speisesaal offered traditional fare, plenty of company, and regular employment for the hardworking waitress. It offered its share of adventure, too.

They called her *hübschen Kellnerin*, "pretty waitress," and courted her with flattery. Dora blushed and fussed; she enjoyed flirting and learned to be coy. Another waiter had helped her get the job. That was down to flirting, too, in some ways; Dora had been out in her wig and false breasts, allowing herself the peace of proper clothing, when she'd happened upon him. Oh yes, there were always jobs for pretty waitresses! Dora could scarcely believe her luck; now she went about both day and night as a sweet young maid. For two full years she never had to wear men's clothes and, using her previous ingenuity, she'd managed even to have a few boyfriends among the "young and beautiful" students— almost always brief, transient affairs.

But the life of a woman came with risks. One night after work, a man asked her to walk with him. He led her down an alley where the light scarcely reached, and in the dark demanded that she perform oral sex. Dora had never even considered this; to put a penis in her mouth seemed horrific. It's a perversion, she said; she didn't know anything about perversity. He insisted, and she did as she was told. Lesson one of womanhood: there were things that might be done to her against her will. She meant to be ever so careful, but there was much she still didn't know about the world. And working as a waitress wouldn't do forever. Dora had a plan.

The *Deutsche Wanderbühne*, German traveling theaters, were roving troupes of professionals without a set stage. By 1912, they had been largely displaced by permanent theaters in the cities, leaving the remaining *Wanderbühne* to frequent smaller towns with appreciable

---

* As Erin Reed remarks, the practice of leaving your home and everyone you know in order to be "out" full-time would continue to be the standard practice at least through the 1970s and 1980s.

audiences. When one troupe visited her dining house, Dora watched them perform and applied to the leader as a female impersonator. As she was already successfully embodying the role, why not do so on stage and be paid for the trouble? The leader agreed, and Dora packed her things, giddy with all that the stage promised. There would be dancing, the leader explained, after every performance. She could discard her masculine persona, live fully as a woman, and delight in the role of actress! There would be men, and lovers, and applause, and Dora would never stay long enough for her lovers to make an unfortunate discovery. It wasn't fraud, in Dora's eyes; it wasn't even impersonation. She was not a man pretending to be a woman; she was a woman indeed, inside if not outside. These were, she would later reflect, her happiest years. Unfortunately, they weren't to last; those giddy days would end in war.

The hatred and division fueled by foreign policy, the threat of war and fear of traitors, presaged something else—something bigger. The web that connected one nation to the next for decades had been strung on tenterhooks; it couldn't hold against additional crises. Germany's biggest mistake had been a mishandling of the Moroccan affair, but a far greater threat rumbled closer to home. The storm would break all over the world.

5

POWDER KEG AND PLUCKED STRING

JUNE 28, 1914, BEGAN BRIGHT AND FULL OF PROMISE. SUMMER IN Sarajevo offered warm winds and sunny skies above the Miljacka River. Sophia, Duchess of Hohenberg, and Austrian archduke Ferdinand traveled in a convertible Double Phaeton motorcar, the height of luxury limousines with a high, open back and curved fenders.[1] It provided no cover, as was best for taking in the view. Crowds gathered along the arched bridges and all through the streets to catch a glimpse of the famous love match. Sophia in her sun hat, Ferdinand with his grand mustache: they had wed despite Sophia's unequal standing and the disdain of Ferdinand's uncle the emperor. But the strictures of court seemed far behind them, here in warm sunshine. Today was their wedding anniversary. It would be their last.

The visit was more than a holiday, and tensions were running high. Despite the crowds and fine speeches, the archduke was not a welcome guest. He represented the colonizer. In 1908, Austria-Hungary had annexed Bosnia and Herzegovina, territories once controlled by the Ottoman Empire. Serbia declared war and fought to regain land along the Miljacka by joining forces with other Balkan nations: Greece, Bulgaria, and Montenegro. The Balkan League regained a significant amount of territory in 1912, but a year later, Serbia and Greece declared war on Bulgaria, their former ally. Factions formed and reformed, and a terrorist group known as the Black Hand began supplying weapons to militant Serbian nationalists. The region had become *Pulverfass Balkan*, the Balkan Powder Keg; it was ripe for violent upheaval.[2]

Ferdinand wasn't oblivious to the risks involved in a visit to Sarajevo, the Bosnian capital. The Black Hand had attempted to assassinate Emperor Franz Josef three years before. And yet Ferdinand had taken few precautions, even publicizing his visit to Sarajevo months ahead of time. Perhaps it was a show of strength, perhaps overconfidence—or perhaps, buoyed by their own happiness, the royal couple simply couldn't perceive the danger that dogged their steps. Meanwhile, members of the Black Hand had already infiltrated the crowd along the parade route, armed with semi-automatic pistols and explosives.

The first strike came when nineteen-year-old Nedeljko Čabrinović tossed a grenade at the motorcade. The chauffeur spotted it just in time and accelerated; the explosion missed the car but sent shrapnel flying into the crowd and other vehicles. Some members of Ferdinand's entourage were wounded, and this should have been enough to stop the parade. It didn't. Ferdinand was furious when he arrived at Sarajevo's city hall but gave his planned speech anyway. Then he and Sophia left the cover of the hall and returned to their motorcar; Ferdinand wanted to visit the hospital where his injured officers were being treated. They chose a different route, making speed down the Appel Quay. Then, suddenly, everything came to a stop. The details remain unclear, but somehow the leading car made a wrong turn, and the Double Phaeton turned down the wrong street. Realizing the mistake, the chauffeur put the car in reverse and tried to back out of the alley, but it was already too late. Pistol reports were heard; Sophia crumpled forward, and Ferdinand clutched at his neck. Blood pooled in the Double Phaeton, and Ferdinand was heard to say, "Sophie, Sophie! Don't die! Live for our children!" They would be among his last words. The archduke and his wife were dead by eleven in the morning, only hours after their arrival.

Franz Josef had just lost his heir, and Austrian newspapers carried his declaration. "To my peoples!," it read, the "flame of [Serbia's] hatred for myself and my house has blazed always higher." After these "murderous attacks" it was time to "raise the sword."[3] On July 28, Austria-Hungary declared war.

For decades, the careful web of nations had pulled taut, with every country holding its breath. Now, a vital thread had just been plucked, and tremors vibrated in all directions. Russia, treaty-bound to defend Serbia, mobilized and declared war against Austria-Hungary. And Austria-Hungary leaned on Germany, which, despite reservations, declared war on Russia, the nation it had recently sought to court. In turn, Russia called upon France. Germany determined to deploy troops in Belgium as a portal from which to attack France, in violation of Belgium's neutrality treaty. When challenged, Chancellor Bethmann Hollweg (who had replaced Bülow) called the treaty a mere "scrap of paper" to be dispensed with.[4] Unfortunately for him, that scrap had been signed by Belgium and Great Britain. Within hours, Britain declared war against Germany, and so also against Austria-Hungary. The web of alliances fell a-tangle: all of Europe was at war.

NO MAN'S LAND

Hirschfeld didn't begin as a pacifist, though he would become one. He'd caught the nationalist sentiment and even wrote two pamphlets: *Warum hassen uns die Völker* (Why Do Nations Hate Us) and *Kriegspsychologisches* (War Psychology). Like many Germans, he was swept up in the injustice of the assassination and the hope of a swift and favorable conclusion. The war, he thought, might also offer an opportunity.

The crisis of masculinity in Germany had vilified homosexuals, even using homophobia as a provocation for entering the war in the first place. Thanks in part to Maximilian Harden, public opinion deemed homosexuals unfit to be officers, who "should be an example to the men in arms, who follow [their] commands and [their] moral way of life."[5] Harden said homosexual men had no sense of nationalism; Hans Blüher insisted that they were weak and effeminate. These sentiments meant that many were barred even from entering military service. But if war was unavoidable, thought Hirschfeld, then it could allow homosexual men to prove their valor and courage and to break the stereotypes he had (accidentally) helped to create.

As a result, Hirschfeld spent hours counseling young men on how to pass as heterosexual, and both cis women and *Transvestiten* (trans men) on how to pass as cisgender men.[6] They promised to write him letters in return, so that he could publish accounts of their bravery in service to the nation. He would be as good as his word, but, sadly, many of his correspondents would never return home. There is no such thing as a "fresh and merry" war. There is only death and mangled bodies. War didn't make men; it massacred them. In 1916, Hirschfeld joined up as a Red Cross inspector and saw the horrors for himself.

They called it no man's land: the strip of scorched earth, shrapnel, stinking mud, and rotting bodies that stretched between the lines of trenches. Bombs fell from above. Poison gas, first unleashed by German forces in the Second Battle of Ypres, would be revisited upon them by the British shortly after. Clouds of it seeped into tunnels and strongholds, killing, blinding, maiming. There were tanks. There were flamethrowers. And then came the rain. Everything sank in the churned mud, from horses to weapons to people. The wounded who made it to shell holes couldn't get out of them again and slowly choked and drowned. Rats took up residence inside corpses; bodies were eaten by maggots and bacteria from the disturbed soil. The First World War offered a wasteland of barbed wire, the thunder of shells, and the horror of disfigured soldiers as far as the eye could see.

Losses were heavy on every side, but the tide turned against Germany on July 24, 1917, when American forces arrived in France. By then, German nationalism had dissolved in the wake of 2 million dead soldiers. The total loss of life in Europe was 9 million soldiers and 5 million civilians who died from disease, starvation, or exposure.[7] Of those who survived, 21 million were wounded, many of them permanently disabled. In Germany, this was a demographic catastrophe; an entire generation was lost in the space of a few years. In place of a once-healthy workforce, the nation possessed 2.7 million disabled veterans, over a million war orphans, and half a million widows—most of them (and most of the deceased) under thirty.[8] As a nation, Germany ended the war broken, hobbled, on the edge of economic crisis and civil war. The feeling of hopelessness, and of meaninglessness, descended on survivors, many of whom struggled even to locate and bury their dead.

Hirschfeld's published work, *The Sexual History of the World War*, was a memorial rather than a celebration. Many of the homosexual men who joined the fight did so because they were alone and unmoored, abandoned by family. "Better that my mother should say, 'My Fritz died a heroic death in the fatherland,'" wrote a German pilot, "than that people should say 'So, a [homosexual] suicide, eh?'" In another case, a lieutenant exposed by blackmail for homosexuality and subsequently dismissed begged to be allowed to reenlist. Send me where the fighting is heaviest, he asked, so that it might end his life. The war was not a hoped-for "opportunity" so much as a "wish or hope . . . that a bullet might put an end to their lives."[9] The trans men felt less hopelessness but were no less committed to death on the front. For those assigned female at birth, a soldier's life was a "masculine occupation, *par excellence*." Erna B. tried repeatedly to join the German army, and Hirschfeld supported Erna's case; since Erna had "always felt and acted like a boy," why shouldn't Erna be permitted to join up as a man? Erna became Ernest and left for the front line. Cisgender lesbians and heterosexual women alike made similar sacrifices. One young girl from Budapest disguised herself as a boy, joined the Austro-Hungarian army, and went in search of her lost brother. She found him dead in a muddy trench and fought in his place until she too was wounded. Cis women and transgender men "took their places in the field and fought for their newly achieved freedom in magnificent disregard for death."[10] The Wilhelmine ideal, backed by law, refused to allow intermediaries to serve, refused to even acknowledge their identities, but in the end was willing enough for them to die in battle.

The war years changed Hirschfeld into an ardent pacifist. Working with the International Red Cross, he'd glimpsed artillery-mangled faces, bodies ripped apart, and infections from fetid trenches that ravaged survivors. Such was the waste of human beings in a war no one had wanted. The work had, however, lifted his own reputation. At the war's end, Hirschfeld would travel to Switzerland to negotiate the exchange of prisoners; they were not enemies anymore, just men—boys, even. War, Hirschfeld wrote, came of ambition, the drive for conquest, and the need for camaraderie.[11] He laid the blame, in other words, on the *Männerbund* impulses cherished by Blüher. "Without the economic competition of the great capitalist states," he wrote, "without the imperialism unleashed by their industrial and colonial policies, without the armaments of the great European powers which had been piled up for decades," the war could never have happened.[12] Hirschfeld had had enough of nationalism and the pain it wrought, and, for once, so had most of the nation.

On the eleventh hour of the eleventh day of the eleventh month, 1918, Germany signed the Armistice. The ink dried in a French railroad car, hidden away in the Forest of Compiègne, while a disillusioned and grief-stricken Germany edged into civil war. Even as the Armistice was being prepared, the monarchy had assuredly fallen; fearful for his life, Kaiser Wilhelm II was forced to abdicate. He would claim, from exile, that he had never wanted war—never meant any of it to happen—certainly never meant to be chased out of his own homeland. His intentions didn't matter anymore.

THE COLD SWEPT IN with nights of freezing temperatures, but Sunday, November 10—the eve of the Armistice—dawned warmer. Five thousand people gathered in protest and in solidarity before the Reichstag to demand its immediate dissolution and the election of a democratic government. Germany was preparing to take its first steps as a republic—though, as Peter Gay writes in the classic *Weimar Culture*, what became known as the Weimar Republic was "an idea seeking to become a reality" long before the war ended.[13] Now it had its first opportunity to draw breath, and there to give it voice was Magnus Hirschfeld.

Under the auspices of the provisional government led by the Social Democrats, the League of the New Fatherland had invited Hirschfeld to speak about a future of peace and demilitarization. Pacifism, it seemed, had been restored to favor, along with a new interest in scientific progress. The democratically minded left were in power, and Hirschfeld was now treated with respect as a leading sexologist. Fifty years old and sporting what became his signature mustache and small round glasses, Hirschfeld stepped up to address the people. Like Karl Ulrichs before the Munich Odeon, he ascended the podium in a charged atmosphere. Above him, a new flag was buffeted by a stiff wind.

"Citizens of the new German republic," Hirschfeld began—and then came gunfire.

The Reichstagplatz erupted in chaos in a strange shadow-replay of Archduke Ferdinand's assassination. Monarchists had infiltrated the crowd, hiding weapons beneath layers of clothing and targeting those they saw as traitors. Terrified, the masses pushed into side streets as ceremony guards returned fire. The monarchists were overcome, but not before they killed several soldiers and wounded many more. Ambulances raced up the Simonstrasse, and Hirschfeld rose shakily to his feet.

Steeling his resolve, he began again. The abdicated Kaiser, he told the crowd, had hoped to march victorious through the Brandenburg Gate. Built on the orders of Prussian king Frederick William II, the gate symbolized empire. But on this, "the most memorable day of our history," Hirschfeld said, his voice rising, "another victor marched through the Brandenburger. This victor was the liberated German people."

The crowd reassembled at the sound of his voice. They were silent, rapt. A powerful orator, Hirschfeld gathered momentum, his words condensing in clouds of breath. It would be the most charismatic speech of his career, delivered over a square painted in new blood, to a people ready for change. Never again, he proclaimed, "Never again in all future should the will of a king be the law of the land. The only law will be: 'Everything decided by the people for the people.'" The words echoed American statesmanship, but though Hirschfeld called for a "true state" built on "democratic rules," he made the difference absolutely clear: "we want a *socialist* republic [my italics], the union of all citizens of Germany, mutual care for one another, the evolution of society into one organism, equality for all." They would aim for "the unity of all nations on earth" with an end of "economic and personal barriers," and a proletariat with a "right to choose." Then, and only then, could all people live a "life of human dignity and pride."[14] Hirschfeld lifted his hands to the people surrounding him: Long live the free German republic! Hurrah! Applause thundered like cannons.

In Hirschfeld's words were the seeds of social, sexual, and gender justice, a new Germany that would lead the way through tolerance and peace. Two days later, the new government made good on its first promise: on November 12, women received the right to vote,* and the Minister of Internal Affairs permitted Hirschfeld to organize the Foundation for Scientific Sexual Research. No longer an empire, Germany would begin the next year as a republic, with a constitution ratified by Social Democrats in the city of Weimar.

To supporters of the republic, the day felt monumental, like the rebirth of the world. Hirschfeld's speech, full of hope, acted as a clarion call to the Social Democrats and all who had rebelled against the monarchy in favor of a more equal union. But the Weimar Republic began as it would go on: divisively. Hirschfeld spoke, at best, to a slim majority. The rift remained between right and left, a divide that would ultimately settle along geographic lines, with the south of Germany resisting republican rule. The ceremony was split between the violence of a conservative, reactionary, prejudiced past and the hope of an inclusive, international, and just future.

THE POWER OF FILM

The palatial residence of Joseph Joachim, collaborator of Brahms and one of the most significant violinists of the nineteenth century, stood empty. Once the residence of an ambassador, it belonged now to Prince Victor Salvator von Isenburg. The building rose up in pale stone, four stories high with dormers and a recessed upper floor that permitted a small terrace and garden.[15] Hirschfeld could think of no better place for his Institut für Sexualwissenschaft, the Institute for Sexual Science. He

---

* Women were granted the vote in Germany before the United States, which did not enact women's suffrage until 1920.

just needed to convince the government, which had its own designs on the building. While negotiations dragged on, the SHC continued to meet in various rooms and apartments across Berlin, including Hirschfeld's own apartment at 14 In den Zelten, a few doors away.

The committee included luminaries such as dermatologist, psychiatrist, and psychoanalyst Dr. Iwan Bloch, sometimes called the first sexologist, as well as Dr. Numa Praetorius. A lawyer, Praetorius had lost his position due to his homosexuality and became an advocate for rights even before the SHC had formed. Born Eugène Wilhelm, he took the pseudonym as an homage to Ulrichs, who often wrote under the name Numa Numantius. Joining them were Helene Stöcker and radical feminist Hedwig Dohm, architects of what Hirschfeld called "the successful rebellion" against the "centuries-old enslavement" of women.[16] With luck, he hoped to celebrate the occasion of women's suffrage more formally within the elegant confines of 10 In den Zelten—but today, February 10, 1919, he was on his way to a more modest meeting of Scientific Humanitarian minds. He had incredible news, and it wasn't about real estate.

Earlier that afternoon, Hirschfeld had had an unexpected visitor: thirty-nine-year-old Jewish filmmaker Richard Oswald. He'd been born in Vienna as Richard W. Ornstein but changed his name when he took up an acting career in 1914. In 1916, he'd formed his own production company, and now—with short hair brushed straight back and tiny spectacles perched upon his nose—he'd come to Hirschfeld with a proposal. Fresh from the success of his adaptation of *The Picture of Dorian Gray* by homosexual icon Oscar Wilde, Oswald felt it was time to make a film about homosexuality itself.[17]

Hirschfeld had been accused before of making "public propaganda under the cover of science" and even of being a "freak who acted for freaks," but propaganda had largely been the tool of his enemies.[18] The war hadn't slowed the rise of *Männerbund* philosophy or "German purity," and the process of ratifying the new national constitution had been waylaid by factionalism. All the same, the Weimar Reichstag intended to reform the penal code, and perhaps the hated Paragraph 175 would finally fall. An educational film could drum up public support, popularizing Hirschfeld's ideas about intermediaries and making allies. The SHC had been taught a costly lesson about the power of public opinion during the Eulenburg affair; it was time to use it for their benefit.[19] Hirschfeld arrived at the meeting cold and late but excited about the possibilities. He presented Oswald's proposal for counterpropaganda; surely the time was now.

Film (still silent) was having a moment in Germany. Weimar cinema is best known for its Expressionist films, such as *Metropolis, Nosferatu,* and *The Cabinet of Dr. Caligari.* Expressionists offered monsters and shadows—"nightmare visions and psycho-horrors," as described in film historian Thomas Elsasser's classic analysis. For many, the genre either testifies "to the troubled political reality of post-First-World-War Germany" or foreshadows "the ideological turmoil to come."[20] Meanwhile, less avant-garde, more mainstream cinema aimed to enlighten and entertain the general public. Elsasser suggests that the division might best be thought of as internal and external; expressionists facing in toward the artist, educational films out toward society.

Hirschfeld chose the latter, but there were additional considerations. Should we, he asked, "limit ourselves to a purely scientific lecture about sexual intermediaries" or tell a story about an individual's personal fate?[21] Working closely with Oswald, Hirschfeld decided to do both. For the educational part, he would appear in the film, giving lectures. Of course, in the silent film era, a lecture was difficult to sustain—that's a lot of text on black flashcards, and much more reading at one time than today's subtitles or closed captioning require. (Historian James Steakley describes it as straining the medium to the breaking point.)[22] Hirschfeld pressed on anyway, repeating key aspects of his work in *The Transvestites*:

Nature is boundless in its creation. Between all opposites there are transitions, and that is true of the sexes. Therefore, apart from man and woman, there are also men with physical and psychological qualities of a women as well as women with all sorts of male characteristics.[23]

Hirschfeld goes on to compare the mistreatment of intermediaries to the persecution of heretics and witches (the literal witch hunts); he commands his viewers to rise up against prejudice. "May justice soon prevail over injustice . . . science conquer superstition, love achieve victory over hatred!" he exclaims, gesticulating for the silent camera. They were young rebels, and Weimar a new republic; the future was wide open to change, equal rights and justice tantalizingly close. But the film must also, Oswald was keen to remind him, have a plot—a story. For that, Hirschfeld chose the theme that had first moved him so many years previously: the suicide of innocents due to prejudice and blackmail.

The Wilhelmine era's bourgeois respectability had forced homosexuality underground, creating the perfect playground for extortionists. At the time Oscar Wilde was incarcerated, Hirschfeld estimated that at least 2,000 homosexuals fell prey to blackmailers each year in Berlin alone.[24] Harden's tactics with Moltke and Eulenburg likewise relied on threats and payoffs, and just before the outbreak of war, blackmail had even led to espionage. On May 25, 1913, an Austrian colonel named Alfred Redl committed suicide by bullet to the brain to avoid a trial for treason. Redl, chief of counterintelligence for Austria-Hungary, had leaked Austro-Hungarian and German war plans—specifically Plan III, the invasion of Serbia—to Russia.[25] Hirschfeld believed that Redl had "[fallen] victim to his homosexual love" for a Russian attaché who blackmailed him for state secrets.[26] Modern historians are less certain about Redl's motivations, but his treason and his homosexuality would be conflated for generations to come.

Hirschfeld's film intended to make it clear that extortion, and not homosexuality, was the ultimate crime. Remove Paragraph 175, and you remove the need for secrecy and the threat of blackmail.

The film would be titled *Anders als die Andern*, "different from the others."[27] To ensure the audience's sympathies, the protagonist, Paul Körner, would be played by film star Conrad Veidt. His haunted eyes, angular features, and hawklike nose would also appear in *The Cabinet of Dr. Caligari* (and later, *Casablanca*), and his grinning character in *The Man Who Laughs* would serve as inspiration for the Joker in the

Batman films. Veidt, easily the most recognizable film star in Germany, was joined by Fritz Schultz (as Karl), who had himself appeared in over one hundred films, and Anita Berber (as Else), a dancer and actress famous (and scandalous) for her androgyny and bisexuality.

The opening scene resonates with pathos. Körner, a successful violinist, opens the newspaper to read the obituaries and sees that three men of different ages and social standing have taken their own lives for "reasons unknown"—the phrase used most often in cases of homosexual suicide. Körner lapses into a daydream where he sees "an endless procession" of people "from all times and places" shackled to a single chain and walking beneath a suspended sword inscribed "§175." From the very first scene, the film foreshadows Körner's fate. It casts him as a relatable figure, a gifted musician, and a good son. He is also homosexual, and falls in love with his music student, Karl Sivers.

Through flashbacks and scenes with family members, we see Körner's struggles. Punished, chastised, and ridiculed throughout his life, he tries to find a cure through psychiatry and hypnosis, to no avail (Hirschfeld's little jab at those who didn't understand homosexuality as congenital). But Körner and Karl have an ally; Karl's sister Else, a seductive vamp, wants Körner for herself. He refuses her, explaining his nature. A reformed Else pledges her support of the couple—a reflection of the strong feminist influence on Hirschfeld and his SHC. The film gives viewers a moment of hope as the lovers dare to hold hands in the park, but a blackmailer from Körner's past intervenes. In flashback, we watch the extortionist trick the young Körner by leading him on, only to demand money; now he's back to ruin him completely.

In the grainy black and white of Hirschfeld's film, Körner's pale face flickers in dismay. He cannot afford to pay the blackmailer. With hesitation (and indignation), he decides to press charges. It's a risky move. Because of Paragraph 175, both Körner and his blackmailer may face criminal charges. As with the real-life trial of Oscar Wilde, it's the homosexual who is treated as a criminal. It's Körner who must go to prison. When he is finally released, he finds himself banned from performing as a violinist—but worse is coming. His own family disowns him cruelly, and Karl's parents break off all contact. Exposed and alone, Körner decides upon suicide. Shot in vignette with only his face in the light, Körner swallows a pill and dies. Karl rushes to his side intent on doing the same, but is prevented by Hirschfeld. "If you want to honor the memory of your friend, you must not take your life," he says, because "what matters now is to restore honor and justice to the many thousands before us, with us, after us. Through knowledge to justice!" The last scene closes on a copy of the law, as Hirschfeld strikes out Paragraph 175 with the firm stroke of a pen. Let their deaths not be futile; we must rise up and fight for acceptance.

THE FILM WAS BASED on the lived experience of many homosexuals. Its themes played out in the life of Dora Richter, too. She had tried to go home when the war began, but her father, ill-prepared to welcome an emancipated actress, demanded that Dora be Rudolf. So she traded Seifen for Leipzig, a city with half a million residents, ready work, and the safety of anonymity. By day, she bussed tables at an automat, a curiously popular restaurant of vending machine sandwiches. At night, at grand public soirées, she was the "beautiful little rose," well liked by the gentlemen.

One night as she walked home alone, a strange man began to dog her steps. A soldier, she thought, fired up with liquor. She walked fast and refused to speak to him. Angry, he took hold of her arms and pinned her against his body; he was trying to rape her. Dora's shouts attracted attention, and from the darkness came a young man. He chased off the soldier and offered to escort her home. Dora gladly agreed to take his arm. Before they reached the apartment, however, he had kissed her—once, twice, more. Dora's heart fluttered; she shouldn't, but he'd aroused her, so she invited him in. They never made it to her room. Once inside, he pressed himself to her, hiking her skirts. They had sex in the corridor, then he left. Dora didn't think more about it until a strange letter arrived; she opened the seal only to realize she'd been trapped. Her rescuer was a blackmailer who threatened to expose her as a man and as a homosexual—a horror to Dora, who considered herself neither.

For over a year, Dora divided her income between sending money home to her family and payments to her blackmailer, but his demands only increased. She could not buy clothes for herself; soon, she could not even buy food. When she faltered in payment, the letters contained threats to her life. Desperate, she begged the help of an older man she'd met at a masquerade, but his offer came with a catch. He lured her to his rooms, tied her up, and abused her. After four days, he put her on a train back to Saxony. Broken, emaciated, and frightened, Dora draped her meager frame in the male clothing she hated and returned once more to Seifen. She didn't admit to thinking of suicide, but this marked one of the lowest periods in her life, made worse because she still thought herself a lone sufferer. She would not see Hirschfeld's film, but many hundreds of other intermediaries would.

ANDERS ALS DIE ANDERN opened on May 24, 1919, at the Apollo Theater in Berlin. It was, without exaggeration, a box-office smash. Prints of the film made their way to Hanover, Cologne, Frankfurt; within a year, it showed in Austria and the Netherlands. In Berlin, it played to sold-out crowds for nearly a year. Letters poured in, some telling Hirschfeld that the film depicted their own lives, others saying that they understood homosexuality for the first time.[28] The SHC had the public's attention at last.

The film also sparked ferocious animosity. In the more conservative cities of Breslau (now in Poland), Bielefeld, Dresden, Leipzig, and Munich, protesters agitated for the return of censorship. Though Oswald threatened to sue anyone who called his work obscene, protests in the district of Friedenau shut down cinemas anyway. In Munich, an advisory board banned it before opening day and refused to let it be shown anywhere in Bavaria. As with the political divide, the hue and cry fell along geographic lines; "the film was being screened in Northern Germany over heated objections," writes Steakley, but "it was almost nowhere to be seen in the south." The turmoil would muddy the waters of bureaucracy, as the Weimar government was already struggling to gain ascendancy over municipal and state laws and regulations. The only way to quell the outrage was a national censorship law.

In 1920, the Greater Berlin Committee to Combat Smut (*Schmutz* in German) pushed for reform, and leading the charge was a man named Karl Brunner. His name should be familiar—and infamous. Brunner would one day join the Nazi SS and be responsible for the slaughter of Polish civilians. His animosity toward the film's "moral rot" was motivated partly by his rampant anti-Semitism. He disrupted one of the early screenings of *Anders als die Andern*, but Oswald shouted him down and kicked him out, humiliating him before a crowd. That, for Brunner, sealed it; he would have his revenge against Hirschfeld and his Jewish sex science.

In 1920, the government inaugurated a sweeping censorship code, the Lichtspielgesetz. So restrictive were its tenets that the Nazis didn't bother to revise it when they came to power thirteen years later. It required that all films be reviewed by a government committee, including *Anders als die Andern* even though it had already been released. In charge of the new censorship panel was Anna von Gierke, a close friend and ally of Karl Brunner, and she chose three long-standing rivals of Hirschfeld as reviewers: psychiatrists Emil Kraepelin and Siegfried Placzek and sexologist Albert Moll. The vote would be unanimous: Hirschfeld's film was banned, not because it was "ignoble" (so went the verdict) but because it was political. Moll at last had an opportunity to thwart Hirschfeld for what he considered unscientific bias; in angling for the repeal of Paragraph 175, Hirschfeld and Oswald were deemed to have "improper motives."[29]

The reasoning behind such a ruling is both genius and diabolical. The film did not show actual sex acts because, of course, it would have been banned as pornographic. But the ambiguity of content meant that "uneducated viewers" might assume that the law criminalized banalities such as the touching of hands or stroking of hair. The panel caught Hirschfeld in a double bind, first decreeing that the film was dishonest in its portrayal, yet also decreeing that it would "induce" homosexuality in its viewers.

There would be no winning against such pronouncements, but the final insult had far-reaching consequences: in the name of "public order," the law prohibited "any influence toward same-sex inclinations." How does one define influence? Or inclination? Power had seamlessly shifted toward aggressive intervention and regulatory control, and had done so with language that, Steakley writes, had "unmistakable parallels [to] Nazi rhetoric." The new republic, scarcely two years old, had already overturned one of its earliest promises; censorship under the Weimar government now exceeded censorship under Wilhelm II. Hirschfeld and Oswald would dutifully pursue an edited version of the film for later release, but suddenly, Hirschfeld had something else to distract him.

COMING HOME

The new censorship statute singled out homosexuality as a particularly immoral contagion, but there was still hope. Hirschfeld had acquired the palatial building at 10 In den Zelten. The president of the Berlin police, who was in charge of all charitable foundations, confirmed the status of the Hirschfeld Foundation—and now the building would house the world's first independent center for the scientific study of sexuality.

On the evening of July 1, 1919, a group of distinguished guests gathered for a dedication in song by Leo Gollanin, who would later become the cantor of Berlin's biggest synagogue. Hirschfeld stood before his peers to deliver the Institute's mission statements: first, "scientific research on all of human sexuality and love life, as well as the sexual life of all other creatures," and second, "to make use of this research for all."[30] He had lost several bids to overturn Paragraph 175. His film had been banned. Even so, Hirschfeld still believed the SHC had allies among the Social Democrats, and despite the censorship regime, print media remained largely free. Already, publications specifically for homosexuals—and, now, self-described transvestites too—were proliferating. Hirschfeld had reasons to be hopeful as he led his guests on a tour.

Entering through the front doors on Beethovenstrasse, they passed the room that would house the archive of slides, photographs, and other visual media. A lower floor housed an enormous and elegant dining room. There would be a reception area and rooms for consulting, as well as an apartment for Hirschfeld, while the rest of the building would be given over to myriad specialties: medicine, biology, endocrinology, psychiatry, anthropology, X-ray, continuing education, journal publication, film programs, public lectures, marriage counseling, and much more. The jewel would be the ever-growing library. Originally housed in a downstairs room and later relocated to a larger annex to the rear, it collected the resources of a burgeoning field: the science of sex.[31]

The Institute aimed to impress, but it still operated on the fine edge of a contradiction—a division that even Hirschfeld couldn't quite marry together. Laurie Marhoefer's critical work *Sex and the Weimar Republic* articulates the "fundamental dilemma" that had haunted the fight for rights all along: the struggle between "normal" and "abnormal" remained constant. Hirschfeld claimed repeatedly that homosexuality (and *Transvestiten*) represented natural diversification. The slides and photographs in his collection aimed to show how "sexual abnormals" differed physically (eugenically) from their hetero peers, right down to the measurements of hips and shoulders. Brand had objected to such things, even as he'd objected to seeing "homosexuality" as an immutable identity rather than a conscious choice. And he wasn't the only one.

Kurt Hiller, one of Hirschfeld's allies in the SHC, felt that the scientific literature was merely preaching to the choir. He wanted campaigns of public action—open homosexuals running for office, closeted homosexuals declaring themselves openly, even starting their own political party. Hirschfeld had seen this fail already. The way forward, he explained, was justice through science—rationality over religious morality. He wanted to do this through the existing governmental systems, not against them. Despite all the setbacks, he still considered the Social Democrats to be the heroes of the story and the Institute a "child of the revolution."[32] The conservatives might hate the Institute and everything it stood for—and they did, virulently—but Hirschfeld believed in public education and petitions to the state. In its very first year, the Institute played host to 4,000 people and 1,250 public lectures, plus private (and therefore legal) screenings of *Anders als die Andern*.[33] Would that be enough to bring about change?

It wouldn't if the audience was confined to the subset of people already considered "inverts"—but homosexuality wasn't the only sexuality about to undergo radical reshaping. We've seen already how the crisis of masculinity and the losses of war had a deep impact on expected roles for cis, heterosexual men and women. A year after the Institute's opening, scientific research would deliver its own moment of social crisis, giving new life to eugenic ideas about birth rates and breeding rights. It would shake up sexual terminology, too, even as it formed and contributed to something Marhoefer calls the "Weimar settlement" (that is, a new emphasis on three "abilities"—public/political ability, *dis*ability, and *respect*ability to determine who or what was permissible and what must be contained or eliminated).[34] Science would, just as Hirschfeld predicted, lead to more freedom and justice—for some. But it also created new insiders and outsiders, abnormals and normals, and it did so by returning (again) to that other impossible dilemma: what matters most, the body or the mind?

Hirschfeld's desk faced out through three windows onto his beloved Berlin. "For a long time," he wrote, those who studied the body's inner chemistry (endocrinology) and those who studied the mind (psychology) "passed each other by without regard."[35] The mind–body dualism of Descartes maintained an insistent hold, such that even in the 1920s, Hirschfeld described the division as "Here biology, there psychology—here body, there soul—here substance, there force, here *Steinach*, there *Freud*."[36] Freud had long established himself as a premier psychiatrist; Austrian physiologist Eugen Steinach had only just begun to make his mark. Steinach wasn't interested in sexual psychiatry, however. He was about to rock the world of endocrinology—and would, in fact, cement the future of the field. He'd discovered how to manipulate sex hormones and, by so doing, change sex itself.

6

THE ENDOCRINOLOGIST'S GAMBLE

SCIENTIFIC BREAKTHROUGHS RARELY FOLLOW A NEAT, LINEAR TIME-
line. We never have all the data, all at once, all in one place. Established,
well-worn science (like the principles of gravity) becomes so familiar
that it looks like unassailable truth, but science isn't answers. It's the
process of finding them: of observing, experimenting, and testing theories. Anyone who tells you otherwise is selling something. For this reason, sometimes even history must be told out of order, even back to front.

Eugen Steinach spent his best years in the animal house: Vienna's
Vivarium. The pseudo-Renaissance building had begun its existence
as a fanciful aquarium for the 1873 World's Fair.[1] A zoologist by the
name of Hans Prizbram, with botanists Wilhelm Figdor and Leopold
von Portheim, purchased the building in 1902 as a home for what they
called experimental biology. Universities, they complained, couldn't
keep pace with new discoveries, due to outdated technology. This was
not a problem for three like-minded and independently wealthy scientists, especially as they agreed upon one thing above all: rejecting "traditional descriptive and comparative" methods of research, they opted
for "invasive, innovative experimentation." Other naturalists and biologists called the Vivarium the Sorcerers' Institute.[2] It was, at least to our
twenty-first-century sensibilities, a bioethical nightmare. But for Steinach, this was the right sort of playground—and perhaps it's fitting that
the Institute for Experimental Biology could be found on the grounds of
the Prater, Vienna's amusement park.

Though a place of scientific research, the Vivarium looked—and
probably smelled—like a zoo. Inside, terrariums and cages housed

hundreds of animals from glowworms to kangaroos. A visiting zoologist, Charles Edwards, wrote about the lengths Prizbram and company went to in order to ensure environmental controls, including the use of a "carbonic-acid cooling machine" with circulating salt water and condenser (a sort of early air conditioning), heat lamps, light controls, micro gas burners, and drainage systems for the enclosures. The animals had to be kept and bred in a "natural environment," or as close to it as the facility could manage. The experiments depended upon it. This new kind of biological testing intended to deduce the "normal" character of animals by creating man-made abnormalities. In language that echoes lines from Mary Shelley's *Frankenstein*, Edwards praised the scientists for reproducing "monsters and variations."[3] By these means, science would strip away nature's mysteries and reveal the secrets of development, regeneration, adaptation, heredity, and—what most interested Steinach—sexual characteristics. Like Berthold with his roosters, Steinach sought to answer questions about internal secretions. What brought about sexual maturity? What decided an animal's sexual character? To put it plainly: which came first, the gland secretion or the nervous impulse, the body or the mind?

Hirschfeld's theory of congenital homosexuality privileged biological processes. His 1914 *Homosexuality of Men and Women* tried to connect theories of homosexual drives to secretions, even coining the terms "andrin" and "gynäcin" for the male and female types (though they never caught on).[4] He visited Steinach's lab to view "artificially feminized and masculinized" animals. Somehow, glands had been responsible, and the successful swapping of sex hormones suggested something momentous, "new and deep insights into the finer mechanisms of the body-soul [*Körperseele*]."[5] If an animal could be artificially turned masculine or feminine, then perhaps the origin of all sexes had been "hermaphroditic," by which he meant single-origin. This made sense of intermediary states of being; in fact, it seemed to prove Hirschfeld's boldest claim: that far from being anomalous or pathological, sexual intermediaries should be expected; they are natural, normal. He had claimed since 1903 that the idea of the "full man" and "full woman"—

creatures exclusively of a single sex—were abstractions, imaginary; they simply did not exist.[6] His conflicts with Brand and Friedländer, and even with Kurt Hiller, Hirschfeld's sometime advocate at the SHC, revolved endlessly around lack of proof. Steinach's work promised nothing less than confirmation for all intermediaries, a reconciliation of the parts to the whole, a return of edge to the center, and a complete exoneration of Karl Heinrich Ulrichs.

Hirschfeld also visited Sigmund Freud while in Vienna (Freud called Hirschfeld a "flabby, unappetizing fellow").[7] Had he been to the Vivarium, Hirschfeld asked? No, indeed; psychiatry and psychotherapy were interested in the mind, and sexology (still thought to be an outgrowth of psychiatry) ought to do likewise. He didn't know that sexology was on the cusp of realizing an endocrine dream.

The journey may have begun with Berthold's rooster testicles and Brown-Séquard's vitality serums, but getting from cocks and bollocks to a respectable field of study required repeatable experiments. It would cost the lives of many animals, kick off the first animal rights movements, challenge the Royal College of Physicians, and overturn the mind-over-matter debate. This is the story of an endocrinologist's gamble—and the scientific skepticism of an English physiologist.

THE PROBLEM OF A DOG'S GUT

Russian physiologist Ivan Petrovich Pavlov (who would win the Nobel Prize in 1904) conducted experiments on dogs. His aim: to sort out how the body's systems related to the external world. In his now-famous experiments, Pavlov played a sound, either of a metronome or a buzzer, before feeding a hungry dog. Originally the dog salivated because of the food, but due to this conditioning it began to salivate at the sound alone. "Why is it," Pavlov wrote, "that the glands produce and secrete in the digestive tract the very reagents needed" even in the absence of food?[8] How was information passed to the body about the object? His answer was twofold. First, he asserted that the nervous system sent messages to the body; second, something he vaguely called "body fluids" must be involved. He never bothered to explain the second bit, just privileged nerves and got on with things. For two of his young colleagues, however, the lacuna proved all too tempting to ignore.

Ernest Starling, with thick blond hair parted jauntily to one side and come-hither blue eyes, poses in photographs with all the aplomb of a would-be Oscar Wilde. He'd begun his medical studies at Guy's Hospital, London, at the age of sixteen, but it would be science that most intrigued him. After spending a year studying lymph nodes in Wilhelm Kühne's laboratory in Heidelberg, he rebranded himself a physiologist, like Pavlov. He also found a collaborator, the far less physically imposing (as well as timid and introverted) William Bayliss, soon to be Starling's brother-in-law. They'd begun with the heart, studied the immune system, and coined the term "peristalsis" for the contractions that move food through the digestive tract. Then came Pavlov's publications, and they found themselves in thrall to the mystery of secretions.[9]

In a way, the mind–body problem hadn't gone away so much as changed its address. The original division had been, like René Descartes's dualism, a matter of body and "soul" (or mind); now the divide rested between inner secretions and nerve fibers. Starling and Bayliss weren't willing to take it on faith that nerves acted as the information channel. So, they went looking for a stray dog.

The experiment took place in the middle of January 1902. Bayliss put the dog under anesthesia and opened the belly to get at nerves leading to the gut. If this sounds familiar, it's because—to a lesser degree—this was what Berthold had done with his cockerels: if you want to know whether nerves do the information delivery, an easy way to find out is by simply removing the channel. They severed the nerves, then fed the dog something acidic. Soon the digestive secretions were flowing from the pancreas, just as before. They had rediscovered what Berthold's experiments suggested: the messengers were chemicals, not nerves. To make doubly certain, they next excised a bit of the dog's intestine and injected it into a vein far away from the pancreas (a bit like putting a rooster's testes in its belly). Once again, without any input from nerves, the digestive system performed perfectly.

Starling and Bayliss worked to isolate the reaction-inducing chemical, originally calling it "secretin." Then they published a paper claiming to have debunked Pavlov's work, a move—as historian Randi Epstein writes—both daring and a bit foolhardy. Experts don't usually take kindly to the upending of long-held beliefs, especially their own. That, more than anything, drove the need for data-driven research. It would also land the scientists in court, but not by Pavlov's doing. They themselves were the accusers, in a defamation suit against some unlikely opponents. Like the Harden trials, what began with a case of libel was really about much, much more.

We may think of animal rights activism as a twentieth- and twenty-first-century concern, but anti-vivisection movements were in full sway at the turn of the last century. Feminists Lizzy Lind and Leisa Schartau founded the Anti-Vivisection Society of Sweden in 1900. Having heard of Bayliss's use of experimental animals, they posed as students at one of his lectures at University College, London. They were in for quite a show.

Excited about the Pavlov-disproving results, Bayliss performed the experiments again and again for his classes. That day, an assistant brought in a small brown terrier. This wasn't a new subject; the dog had already been experimented upon for a different demonstration on the pancreas (an important detail). For the day's lesson, Bayliss planned to focus on salivation. The details are not for the faint of heart; the dog was strapped down on its back and its throat cut open to reveal the salivary gland at the jawbone. Having exposed the lingual nerve connected to the gland, Bayliss attached an electrode. Electrical stimulation of the nerves should, so went Pavlov's theory, cause the gland to produce saliva. It didn't. No juices or secretions appeared. This offered proof, Bayliss lectured, that some other element did the work: a chemical messenger. Bayliss ordered the dog destroyed following the experiment, and it was killed right there, in the lecture hall, by a male student. This was just what the two women needed: they published their deeply troubling account of the event in a book called *Science in Shambles.*

Vivisection was not illegal. Reporting a procedure faithfully couldn't be considered libelous; it would just be journalism. The sticking point revolved around British legislation that prohibited the use of the same animal twice and required that all animals be fully anesthetized. Lind and Schartau claimed that Bayliss himself said that the dog had been previously experimented upon in class; they likewise reported that the terrier flinched in pain when cut open. Bayliss denied both accusations, sued for libel, and won.

The story became international news, not necessarily to the detriment of the researchers themselves. If anything, it unified the community of experimenters and scientists, just in time for Starling to face his peers at the Royal College of Physicians in London. The experimental data he and Bayliss had collected could be the future of endocrinology, but only if he could convince his colleagues of the importance—even the existence—of chemical messengers.

June 20, 1905, was sweltering, but, as usual, Starling exuded cool confidence as he approached the Royal College of Physicians. In this, the first of four lectures, he planned to explain chemical communication—but more than that, he wanted to excite his colleagues, to fire their imaginations. We know, he explained, that chemical processes may result from external stimuli, such as the development of antitoxin in response to the presence of bacteria. He could now prove that chemicals were also generated within the body without any input from the nervous system at all. Piece by piece, Starling explained the work. Neither the severing nor the stimulating of nerves had any effect on the production of saliva. Instead, he stated, the cells lining the stomach and small intestine release chemicals that tell the body to make digestive juices, whether the subject is consciously hungry or not. Secretin worked unconsciously; if a scientist could harness the chemical messages, Starling told them, why, he would have "absolute control over the workings of the human body"![10] A grand claim, it certainly got his colleagues' attention. Starling next proposed to give these amazing if obscure messengers a name all their own.

Starling (in conversation with biochemist and Chinese scholar Joseph Needham) chose the Greek word ὁρμάω—to excite or arouse. In English transliteration, ὁρμάω became "hormone."[11] The "recurring physiological needs" of the body ensured that hormones were continually produced and deployed into the bloodstream.[12] The hormones, not the central nervous system, acted as the arbiter of bodily change, and that meant that humans, in spite of their superior intellect, owed almost all biological activity to the same evolutionary process that guided all other living creatures. The tyranny of the nervous system (and of humans as the apex of the great chain of being) must give way. Welcome to the biological proletariat.

Starling's colleagues did not exactly relish the news. He knew they wouldn't. To soften the blow, he suggested that the nervous system offers more complex creatures (like humans) greater speed and flexibility. Humans and their big brains still had the upper hand. Even so, human development, desires, and needs resulted from unconscious responses to chemical messages. Given the assurance of backlash, Starling needed proof for his assertions and the courage of his convictions at the ready. That's where Bayliss and his dog experiments came in and why diges-tion, rather than sex characteristics, played the biggest role in his lec-tures. All the same, in undermining the hierarchy of bodily systems, Starling laid the groundwork for a brand-new understanding of male-ness and femaleness, on which Steinach (and a great number of frogs, rats, and guinea pigs) would build.

SEX, GONADS, AND THE MATING GAME

Eugen Steinach spent the early part of his career splitting time between research and teaching, which (as most academics will recognize) means more teaching than research. In 1907, he started his own laboratory in Prague, and then, in 1912, became the director of physiology at the Institute for Experimental Biology in Vienna—with its Vivarium. At last, aged fifty-one, he could dedicate himself to the study of sex.

Embedded in then-current sexism, Steinach took binary character-istics for granted; "everyone knows," he wrote, "that men are gener-ally hardier, more energetic, and more enterprising than women, and that women show a greater inclination for tenderness and devotion" and—conveniently—"a practical aptitude for domestic problems."[13] Steinach here elides sex-as-act, sex-as-characteristic, and sex-as-behavior, but the work of experimentation offered a possible means of disentanglement. The question at hand was: if sex drives us, what drives sex? What makes a man "manly"? What makes a woman "womanly"? Some degree of sexuality and sex characteristics must be present from birth (and determined by chromosomes)—but what is the extent of that inborn influence? Do hormones merely play along, or could these chemical messengers go against chromosomes by altering the physical, behavioral, and mental aspects of mating? True to the Vivarium's Frankenstein ethos, Steinach determined to discover the natural process by surgically creating unnatural ones. Far away from Bayliss and what was known as the Brown Dog Affair, Steinach set about making "monsters."[14]

The earliest trials involved mating frogs. At his operating station, Steinach selected several male frogs and transected their brain stems, cutting across them in a straight line. The frogs displayed the "clasp" reflex automatically, a grasping action of the front legs that they use to hang on to egg-laying females. To Steinach, this suggested that far from originating the sex drive, the central nervous system inhibited it; the brain, he reasoned, must "turn off" sex outside the mating season. Next, he experimented with testicular extracts; castrate a frog and it loses sex drive, but once injected with the extract, the drive returns. The brainless frog became a mating machine, while the castrati injected with testicle juice became amorous; not only had Steinach proven the chemical theory, he'd shown that the nervous center got in the way of things.

Time to up the stakes, and for Steinach, that meant mammals. He chose forty-four male rats and added extra transplanted testicle grafts. In the few that were successful (meaning that the extra testicles "took"), the animals became hypersexual; they force-mated with females who weren't even in heat. Next, he castrated rats and recorded that without testicles, they didn't try to mate, and young ones never reached mature sexual development. As he'd predicted, a rat without testes "withered" and one with implants "blossomed" in terms of vigor and sex drive— regardless of where in the body the testes had been implanted. (As

Randi Epstein puts it, "testicles work no matter where they dangle.")[15] Mostly, these early trials merely provided testable data for Steinach's already well-established assumption: hormones make a noticeable difference in the body. Perhaps, Steinach reasoned, the ovaries and testicles acted as "switches" turning puberty on and off. If so, you should be able to stimulate them (through grafts or injections), even to the point of manipulating sex itself. Back to the Vivarium he went, leaving both frogs and rats behind. It was time to swap some gonads—and for that, he wanted guinea pigs.

The operations weren't complicated. One by one, Steinach reversed the sexual organs of his subjects, putting ovaries in the males and testes in the females. He didn't have to wait long for results. The ovary-males grew larger nipples and softer hair, and developed a maternal instinct toward pups. Meanwhile, "the penis," Steinach wrote, "no longer deserves its name and appears to have been reduced to a clitoris." And the changes continued. The ovary-males soon grew breasts similar to pregnant guinea pigs, and some even produced milk and suckled young. Secondary sex characteristics, and also behaviors, had changed— and the same was happening to their counterparts. Testicle-females (as Steinach called them) grew rough coats and prominent, penis-like clitorises. They fought aggressively, chased and mounted females in heat, and in all other respects behaved like male guinea pigs.

Thrilled with his success, Steinach went on to develop intersex guinea pigs, which had some of both sexual characteristics and behaved masculine and feminine in turn—from which Steinach determined that the ovaries were cyclically active. But that wasn't all; though the greatest changes took place in prepubescent animals, castrating an adult male and transplanting ovaries into it still resulted in changes to body and behavior. In other words, despite going through a male puberty, reaching adulthood as a male, and mating as a male, surgically altered animals "changed" (as Steinach put it) to be like females—and the reverse. As Chandak Sengoopta writes in *The Most Secret Quintessence of Life*, these (s)experiments suggested that neither "somatic nor psycho-behavioral sexual characters were laid down permanently." By showing how easily sex polarities could be reversed, Steinach inadvertently "subverted the fundamental concept of sexual polarity" itself. The sex binary might not be so binary after all.

How many sexes are there, then? The World Health Organization defines sex (not gender) as "the different biological and physiological characteristics" such as "reproductive organs, chromosomes, hormones, etc." When chromosomes were first discovered in 1905 by Nettie Maria Stevens and her mealworms, it seemed they offered an easy and dualistic way of defining the sexes once and for all: you were XX or XY, female or male, woman or man. And yet, not everyone gets a standard XX or XY pair; there are other permutations, such as Klinefelter syndrome (XXY), Turner syndrome (X), and XY gonadal dysgenesis (Swyer syndrome), in which the structures are not fully formed. There may be XYY, and XXX, and in certain rare cases, a person is built of two different kinds of body cells (such as when twins merge in utero), ending up with both XX and XY cells at the same time.[16]

One in a hundred people are born with some kind of intersex makeup, and even those with the usual XX or XY display incredible variation in the way reproductive organs form (or don't). Rather than solidifying the division between male and female, some scientists now consider sex as bimodal rather than binary—as clusters of characteristics we can categorize as masculine or feminine, with some room between. Eric Vilain, director of the Center for Gender-Based Biology at UCLA, explains sex determination as a contest between two opposing networks of gene activity. Changes in the activity can sway an embryo toward or away from the sex "seemingly spelled out by the chromosomes."[17] John Achermann, who studies sex development and endocrinology at University College London, thinks there may be "much greater diversity within male or female," and "an area of overlap where some people can't easily define themselves within the binary structure." Meanwhile, developmental biologist Claire Ainsworth has written about new work in DNA sequencing suggesting that "almost everyone is, to varying degrees, a patchwork of genetically distinct cells, some with a sex that might not match that of the rest of their body."[18] Differences in Sex Development

(DSD) is a group of rare conditions involving genes, hormones, and reproductive organs, which result in genitals that look different from what is expected from a particular set of Xs and/or Ys. To put it another way, chromosomal sex might differ from anatomical sex.[19] Ainsworth is careful to explain that, for her, these complexities don't equate with new sexes, but rather create "a continuum of variation in anatomy/physiology" between the sexes.

That continuum matters.[20] Hirschfeld hadn't entirely dispensed with the gender binary either, but he embraced the idea of a third sex that included people who didn't fit into either camp while also exploding those categories into the vast spectrum of intermediaries. With his guinea pig experiments, Steinach muddied his own commitment to the binary sex/gender model; instead of clarifying it, he introduced a physiological foundation for intermediary forms.

If this fluidity seems like a revelation, now, consider Steinach's audience when he published the first paper on these experiments in 1912. The gonads, he wrote, "contain the essence of masculinity and femininity."[21] But neither the physical nor the psychological aspects of sex were governed by the chromosomes. That depended on the action of the sex hormones; without them, an animal would be sexless, even asexual.[22] As sometimes happens in science, Steinach overreached with this assertion; we are still teasing out the exactitudes of how genetic, hormonal, morphological, and environmental factors shape sexual differentiation. For Steinach, the either/or question mattered less than what came next: if a spectrum between absolute male and absolute female existed, hormones could be used to manipulate where on that continuum an individual sat. He'd already changed the sex character and behavior of his guinea pigs; now he wished to try it on human beings. Despite the experimental nature of the work, he would find plenty of ready volunteers.

Gender historian Katie Sutton describes the context of the hormone revolution in *Sex Between Body and Mind*. As the first large-scale technological conflict, the First World War deployed brutal weapons of destruction alongside some of the first really progressive medical interventions. From battlefields blasted by the shells and shrapnel of artillery, young men returned broken and torn—but they did return, and they lived. Injuries of the head, neck, and face were so common that the field of plastic surgery coalesced around their treatment. Equally horrendous were unexploded artillery shells that had buried themselves in the earth. A wrong step would trigger a blast, often between the legs of a soldier. Battlefield castration occurred so frequently that Austria funded the Biological Research Institute to explore glandular support for "demasculinizing" trauma. The First World War allowed Steinach to take experimentation out of the animal house and into the hospital, and his hormone research would take on new urgency in the fractured peace that followed.[23]

The gender crisis ongoing before the war grew more urgent as the population declined. Germany wanted babies, and wanted them so badly that non-reproductive sex came to be seen as selfish and immoral. This would have ramifications for birth control advocacy and the women's rights movement, but one of the most significant reasons for the drop in the birth rate had to do with the enormous death toll. There weren't enough young men left to marry and serve as fathers to children, and many of those who remained lacked glandular function. As Sutton describes, the situation further stoked nationalist and conservative fears about degeneration—physical and moral—which appeared in the media as attacks against homosexuals, "masculine" women, Jews, and "feminine" men, who were already under assault by Blüher's *Männerbund* ethos. The war and its aftermath created a boom for any therapy promising to reinvigorate faltering manhood and boost virility.

Robert Lichtenstern, who worked in Steinach's lab, performed a testicular transplant operation on a soldier to restore his libido after a traumatic wound and orchidectomy.* After the graft, the patient's sex life returned to its usual pitch, his face and body hair began to regrow, and he lost some fatty deposits that had appeared after the injury. Steinach was there to witness the surgery, and both men agreed that adding

---

* The removal of one or both testicles.

testicle grafts had "masculinizing" effects. If transplants restored castrated heterosexual men, then, Steinach reasoned, why not try it also on the homosexual?[24]

This requires some unpacking. The political vilification of homosexuals and the threat of Paragraph 175 lent urgency to the normative science of homosexual conversion. This was especially true in Steinach's Austria, where the statute criminalized lesbian homosexuality as well. The problem was that homosexual cures simply did not work. Psychosexual therapy and hypnosis, lampooned by Hirschfeld in *Anders als die Andern*, had failed. These were futile attempts to change the homosexual mind; with the discovery of sexual hormones, Steinach believed he could bring about the "cure" through manipulation of the body. Unlike Hirschfeld, he considered homosexuals aberrant and pathological; they were broken and they needed fixing. Endocrinology offered the means to control sexual identity, and by doing so, Steinach claimed, "the future of human nature" itself.[25] Steinach determined to try the experiment on a self-proclaimed homosexual man—and Lichtenstern had just the candidate.

The thirty-two-year-old patient suffered from tuberculosis; he was due for a double orchidectomy because the disease had painfully ulcerated both of his testicles. That would take care of the supposedly faulty hormones. Luckily, one of Lichtenstern's heterosexual patients needed an undescended but otherwise normal testicle removed; it would serve as the donor organ. Lichtenstern implanted the healthy testicle into the homosexual patient. Twelve days after surgery, the man reported erotic heterosexual feelings, and even had sex with a female prostitute. His voice deepened, he lost fatty tissue, and within a year he married a woman. In the patient's own words, "I am disgusted to think of the time when I felt the other passion."[26]

Steinach declared this an undeniable success, but he wasn't finished with the removed testicles yet. He took them back to the Vivarium and dissected them, along with those of preceding experiments—five supposedly homosexual gonads in total. In the microscope slides, Steinach located cells of an unusual size and shape. They weren't interstitial cells (the Leydig cells that produce androgen). They reminded him, instead, of the lutein cells he had seen in ovarian studies, which produce progesterone. He labeled them "F-cells" and claimed to have discovered, once and for all, the cause of homosexual tendencies. He immediately produced a series of papers sharing a scientific bombshell: he'd isolated sex hormones, he'd used them to "cure" homosexuality, and most importantly, he'd discovered (in F-cells) an intermediary cellular step, a physical difference that caused homosexuality and other intermediate forms in the first place. Scientists and clinicians, psychologists and psychoanalysts—even Hirschfeld himself—were utterly taken aback.

If what Steinach wrote were true, then it proved Hirschfeld's turn-of-the-century argument that homosexuality was a natural, inborn, biological phenomenon—and that sex and gender existed on a spectrum with intermediary forms. F-cells (if they really existed) offered visible, physical differences between the testes of the homosexual and heterosexual male, and presumably the percentage of such cells accounted for further variation.[27]

At Hirschfeld's Institute, all theoretical, empirical, and clinical work went on under the framework of intermediacy, and Hirschfeld was ready to use all scientific means—heredity, histology, physiology, and more—to popularize the concept.[28] He even created the "interstage wall," a presentation of photographs depicting intermediaries in 1913; it went with him to conferences and was then installed permanently at the Institute, a first stop on his grand tours. Hirschfeld's commitment to a testable means of demonstrating intermediate sexes led him first to patronize racial (and racist) anthropologists like Cesare Lombroso, using measurement of physique to claim that homosexuals demonstrated external variations. It next led him to publicize and popularize Steinach's work. Hirschfeld started his own lab study of testicular tissue in 1920, declaring that sexology, once "an appendage of the psychiatric clinic" and "lacking its own autonomy," had come into its own.[29]

It was akin to unveiling the first evolutionary theories about monkeys and men; if Hirschfeld's wall of intermediary photographs was the "March of Progress" illustration, then Steinach's findings provided the fossil record. But there were big problems, and for some of the same reasons. The March's tidy illustration of evolutionary progress from monkey to man was based on faulty assumptions and biased misreading of evidence; evolution is neither progressive nor linear. Hirschfeld's wall of photographs—and Steinach's F-cells—were likewise built upon presumptions and only reinforced the contradictions sexology had struggled with from the first.

Steinach's theory about congenital intermediary sexualities rebranded them abnormal and pathological—as disorders of the body, controllable and fixable. Instead of complex, mixed-trait selves on a sexuality spectrum, Steinach rendered human beings little more than hormone-driven machinery. Still, he wasn't without clients. Some of Hirschfeld's own patients would be willing volunteers, desperate to live a life without hiding and stigma.

ARBITRARY TRANSFORMATIONS

Dora bent over a letter, weeping silently.[30] It came from a young woman, the sister of a soldier Dora had fallen in love with during the war. One of the lucky ones, he survived. But he would never be hers—in fact, he never had been. I feel it is my duty, his sister explained, "to open [your] eyes." The soldier was engaged to be married, and the wedding day had come. All of his promises to Dora were a tissue of lies; he'd pretended affection in order to keep up the steady stream of money and gifts she sent to the front line. His sister's words were kindly meant; she thought Dora a good and honorable girl and hated to see the "cruel disappointment" her brother had visited upon her. Shaken and ashamed, Dora wrote a reply of thanks folded around the soldier's photograph—though she kissed it once more before sending it. She wanted to be angry; in place of anger she felt the hollow of despair.

For this false lover, Dora had quarreled with her parents. For him, she'd left her home region to live alone in a farm cottage, laboring on the land for money to send. Abandoned and estranged, mocked and used by everyone she cared about, Dora saw the future stretching out before her, "hopeless and tragic." Isolation gave her no joy. In desperation, she to wrote a woman friend from her youth; would she agree to a marriage of convenience? Dora would work hard, would do her best to appear the husband if only to end the loneliness. Her friend refused—she wanted to marry for love and have children, why would she make-believe a sham marriage? Dora could only agree and curse herself for asking; she had no right to expect that sort of sacrifice. So, she sat alone in her room, dressed in her favorite nightgown, and thought of home. Her youngest brother was about to be married. Everyone seemed to have someone. It wasn't fair. "I believe in God," she cried, "but cannot find true happiness"; would there never be a lover with the "heart to understand"? At last, homesick and weary to death of her solitude, Dora steeled herself for a terrible choice. To appease her family, she would try once more to live as Rudolf—and to advertise for a bride.

The war had taken many young men. Finding a marriage partner of their own age was increasingly difficult for the women left behind, and newspaper advertisements were common. In response to Dora's, letters poured in. One of them raised Dora's hopes: a clerk living in the Giant Mountains wrote with such a lovely style, perhaps they could at least be friends. Dora, having never been attracted to women, determined to try and change her nature. She sent a reply by post, promising to meet.

Dora dressed herself as Rudolf and took a train. The town was some distance away, so she planned to stay a few weeks. They might get to know each other by visiting theaters and taking walks. At first, all went well enough. She might not be comfortable in the trousers and shirts, but the girl was pleasant and good company. Unfortunately, she also had expectations. After a few dates, she desired to be kissed and held; she certainly kissed and caressed Dora, but Dora felt only repulsion. She tried to think of her soldier boy, his embrace, his face, his lips, anything to achieve some level of arousal. It just wasn't possible; she couldn't maintain an erection. Her would-be bride was bitterly disappointed, and Dora burned with a stomach-turning shame. How could she offer herself to any woman? Sickened by the experiment, she packed up and took the train back to her cottage on the farm.

It had all been a terrible failure; Dora could not change her inmost nature. Not for her family. Not for herself. Not for anyone.

THE ILLUSION OF CURE

We now return to Hirschfeld in 1920, gazing out those three lovely windows. He'd read Steinach's sixty-eight-page pamphlet "Rejuvenation Through the Experimental Revitalization of the Aging Puberty Gland." It must have been something of a shock, as Hirschfeld had once written that removing the seat of sexual instinct required removing the brain itself. Yes, he believed that homosexuality was natural, biological, and congenital, but he also considered sexuality a "psychical" identity—more than just psychological, "psychical" has to do with the inner self, the emotions, even the soul. He'd stated plainly "that castration has absolutely no influence on the orientation of the sex drive," and any attempts at changing the homosexual identity were therefore superfluous, painful, and fleeting.[31]

In the second edition of his *Homosexuality of Men and Women*, however, he added a preface that flew in the face of his original conceptions. Following Steinach's work, he wrote, "The decisive factor in contrary sexual feeling is not, as Ulrichs believed, in the mind or soul (*anima inclusa*), but in the glands."[32] He then set about collecting volunteers for Steinach. We have little in the way of reflection from Hirschfeld—did he have reservations? Was he perfectly convinced, in opposition to all he had previously claimed, that homosexuals could be "cured"? Did he wrestle with this about his own identity? We don't know, but Hirschfeld soon had reason to regret his support of the procedure.

A homosexual man in his forties volunteered for the surgical cure. He'd spent a lifetime trying to live as a heterosexual and had even married. His efforts failed; he remained attracted to other men and, suffering from a sense of inferiority, took to drugs and alcohol. He asked consent from his wife to undergo bilateral castration and have a "heterosexual" testicle implanted into his abdomen. She agreed, and the man went under the knife. More than a year after surgery, he would write a deeply unhappy letter to Hirschfeld. The new testicle had caused a brief period of body hair regrowth and other secondary masculinizing characteristics, but the man remained homosexual as before. He would confess only one real change to his nature: he'd lost all drive, all willpower, all sexual feeling. His zest for life had gone, leaving him less than before. "I am," he wrote, "destroyed as a man," and "I have examined the literature without finding a single case of lasting improvement after a transplant."[33] Would Hirschfeld publish that?

He would, and he did, in *Geschlechtskunde* (Sex Education, published in 1926), but Steinach had stopped treating or recommending the surgical cure by then. After his first ecstatic report, the procedure always failed, sometimes catastrophically. Knowing nothing about immunological rejection, the surgeons implanted tissue destined to decline. Sometimes the testicle simply failed and ceased to operate; in other cases, it caused a dangerous infection. By 1926, the cure had been thoroughly discredited, and so had F-cells. Surgeon Richard Mühsam performed two orchidectomy and transplant surgeries on patients referred by Hirschfeld; he didn't find any F-cells. Hirschfeld began examining excised tissue himself, but he never found them, either.[34] F-cells simply didn't exist. Not being a professional histologist, Steinach had mistaken some oddly shaped cells in testicles wracked by tuberculosis infection for evidence.*

Steinach's work now had doubters aplenty, but Hirschfeld remained a staunch supporter since—despite their differences—Steinach's experiments lent weight to the argument of natural sex and gender variations. Besides, Hirschfeld needed support; his enemies were many and his allies too few. In 1918, Emil Kraepelin, director of the German Research Institute for Psychiatry, attacked Hirschfeld and his Institute as though they were spreading a contagion, calling for a "containment" of homosexuality before it could infect the nation. Homosexual acts were worse than nonproductive in his eyes; not only could they not produce chil-

---

* In reality, the secretions and tissues of testicles look more or less the same, regardless of sexual identity.

dren, they "seduced" others into same-sex lifestyles.[35] His intent was to force Hirschfeld to cease his public campaigns touting the naturalness of homosexuality.

Hirschfeld published his reply in the same paper, the same year, using Steinach's imperiled but not yet questioned "cure" as a case study. It meant embracing the pathological theory, a deeply troubling capitulation. But we can understand his reasons. Steinach's work with hormones repudiated the psychological theory and the idea of homosexuality as contagious, a plague to be snuffed out. As Rainer Herrn writes, Hirschfeld saw the results of Steinach's flawed research to be "an indispensable prerequisite" for replacing the contagion theory of sexuality.[36] He was right to recognize its dangers; Hitler would, himself, refer to homosexuality as a plague. Better by far to espouse a biomedical explanation based in hormones, even if it meant embracing Steinach's theory of intermediaries over his own.

As for Steinach, in a culture bent on remasculinization, he next set his sights on turning heterosexuals into medical *Übermenschen*. Revered for its rejuvenation properties since at least the time of Brown-Séquard's elixir, male hormone (testosterone) had been elevated to something like a magic potion, even ushering in a craze for monkey glands. "Sex," as Steinach put it, "is the root of life."[37] One way to obtain more male virility (without transplant), he theorized, was to stimulate the gonads themselves into increased productivity. If the testicle made both sperm and hormone, then reducing one ought to increase the other—so went the reasoning. He started on rats, but quickly moved on to a middle-aged coachman. Supposedly, his human subject gained weight and strength, grew back "luxuriant" hair, lost his wrinkles and his stoop, and seemed at the height of his masculine sexual vitality. Ever the media darling, Steinach used the case to vault himself into the headlines once more. He called the procedure vasoligature; we know it today as an early type of vasectomy. Eventually, the procedure became synonymous with his name: everyone wanted to be Steinached—even Freud. It's little wonder that he held the public in thrall.

Hirschfeld consolidated his ideas (and modified versions of Steinach's) in later publications. The wall of photographs remained constant, and so did his theory of intermediate forms. Convinced that all human characteristics expressed themselves on a continuum of male to female, he busily measured genitals, stature, bone structure, pelvis, larynx, hair growth, and even breathing and perspiration.[38] About this, he would be wrong. However, he also believed that all people were mixed forms, a combination of male and female, with both types of hormones in operation to varying degrees. Here, he was closer to the mark.

Hormones offered another avenue of consideration, too. Leaving the "cure" behind, Hirschfeld realized that transplants and hormone preparations could be used in alignment with transgender desire.[39] "Practical experience shows," Hirschfeld wrote as early as 1918, "that the desire of transvestites goes . . . in the opposite direction," with men wanting ovarian tissue and women testicular tissue, because they felt that their bodies were inadequate—which Hirschfeld described as a mismatch between body and soul. One such patient wrote to Hirschfeld, having read about Steinach, but instead of "artificial rejuvenation," they asked to have their testicles removed and an ovary implanted. "[I am] more woman than man," the sender wrote; "perhaps I could serve as an important experiment."[40]

Steinach's popularity spread the news about intermediate forms, about hormones, even about gonad transplant surgery. Hirschfeld may not have agreed with his every tenet, but he would use Steinach to secure the foundation of sexual science. With the right patient, he could even take science in a brand-new direction, one that worked with the inclinations of intermediaries (including what today we refer to as transgender people) instead of against them.

7

THE LOVE AND THE SORROW

DORA WAITED IN A COLD CONFESSIONAL.[1] SHE WAS KNOWN HERE, AT the little Catholic church in Seifen; its records bore her birth and baptismal entry: April 16, 1892, Rudolf Richter. Now here she was again, full of trepidation—and about to say something unspeakable. The priest was seated, waiting, and it had to come out. "Father," she began, "I have committed adultery with a married man."

Life at the farm cottage had allowed Dora some freedom; she lived as she wished and dressed as she desired. But with only pet pigeons to keep her company, solitude had too little joy. She'd been celibate for a long time, easing her urges with physical exertion and weekly enemas, which gave her a sense of sensual relaxation. At night, she bathed and dressed in a women's nightgown before climbing between the sheets. She was a woman, alone in the dark, aching to be held. Dora craved sexual fulfillment, yes, but she also wished to be admired and adored; she wanted to belong to someone. And so, when the harvests were in and the masquerade balls in season, she once more donned a gown and went into town.

There were lights, laughter, dancing, and the opportunity to live in a moment of joy; it couldn't help but lift her spirits, and she left to walk along the river, singing as she went: "Do you hear the singing, do you understand the sound." Then, from across the water, came an answer, a man's voice, adding the next verse: "Thou shalt love me, sings the nightingale!" Dora peered across the water to see a young man; he crossed the bridge to join her, and they fell to talking as they walked. Had she seen him at the ball? No; he merely took night walks, he told her, to ease the pain of loss. He'd been married to a woman of "excellent character," he said, but she had died a young bride, and he lived alone and unhappy.

Dora wanted to comfort him; she told him that she too carried a "great heartache," and she meant it truly. They talked through the night and parted with a kiss, but without sharing addresses. He melted into the darkness and disappeared, but not from Dora's thoughts.

The season of masquerade ended, and without its distraction, Dora found herself thinking more and more about the sorrowful widower. How kindhearted and genuine he'd been! Truly, a fellow sufferer for love. Maybe she could find out more about him? It took some doing, but at last she managed to locate his address and sent him a note. Would he like to meet again? He would. And again, and again. They became fast friends, and then more than friends. Dora felt her reservations dropping away bit by bit; she had fallen in love with him, and he with her.

Then, the worst thing imaginable happened. He asked her to marry him.

For most women, this would be the greatest moment of joy, the fulfillment of promise, the resolution of a grand romance. For Dora, it brought on a storm of emotions—unhappiness, dread, and panic among them. It was one thing to fool a man in the hours they spent together. She'd become expert in playing the sexual part of a woman, too, even going so far as to insert a small bottle of Steinhäger, a type of schnapps in stoneware, into her rectum to stretch the sphincter. But a husband? He would discover her secret and feel betrayed. She'd been rejected and hurt too many times to face it again, so Dora fled. She packed her things and returned to the Ore Mountains. The widower wouldn't know what became of her, wouldn't know why she left—or with what heartache.

Every love became sorrow for Dora; she was a "pitiful" creature left "wandering from hope to hope without ever finding peace, much less attaining happiness." Of course, returning home didn't guarantee harmony, either, but Dora had learned that hiding her true self only caused more pain. She now referred to herself as a hermaphrodite. That, at least, would permit her the luxury of wearing women's clothes some of the time. It was a compromise, but she would try to live with it as it allowed her to increase her social circle. Dora visited her parents as Rudolf, but wore women's clothing at home in her rented apartment; she even attended a family party featuring a string band. Dora had a great fondness for music and played guitar, so she had agreed to don her male attire. But when the musicians took their places, she deeply regretted her choice. Among the players, as startling, striking, and talented as the protagonist of *Anders als die Andern*, was a young violinist. Delicate and nimble fingers danced on the strings, and Dora watched him in an ecstasy of delight. He had already "captured [her] whole heart"—but she'd met him as a man.

Dora hadn't seen Hirschfeld's film, possibly due to its poor reception in the south of Germany. By her own account, she didn't hear of him or the Institute for Sexual Science until 1923. But then, she didn't need to see *Anders als die Andern*; she lived it. Just as the lovestruck Kurt Sivers asks Körner for music lessons after hearing him in concert, Dora determined to be the violinist's pupil. The musician lived about an hour's walk from her apartment, and by happy chance, he walked past it every day. Dora determined to do a little acting of her own. Still dressed in men's clothes, as she had been at the party, she broke a string on her guitar. When the musician passed by, she flagged him down. Could he help her replace it? While he was kindly looking over the guitar, she uttered her wish: if only she could take lessons, she might truly improve herself. The violinist took the bait and agreed immediately. Her lessons would begin the very next evening. Dora could hardly contain herself; first of all, what should she make for supper? Because of course there would be supper, something warm on a festive table.

Dora had been something of a master flower gardener at the farm cottage; she knew exactly what she wanted, but roses were rare in the region, both hard to grow and expensive. No matter. She purchased the most beautiful red roses she could find. Next: what to wear? She had unfortunately trapped herself by beginning their association as Rudolf. She couldn't very well change that now, so on went the hateful trousers and coat (but with soft women's undergarments beneath). It was a little peculiar, falling in love with a man who did not yet know her as a woman.

The lessons carried on through the summer. The violinist had loved those first roses, his favorite flower. She determined he would never be without them. Dora's family lived just beyond the violinist's lodgings, so twice a week—on a pretense of visiting them—she left a bouquet of roses on his windowsill with an anonymous note: "star of my sleepless nights." And they were often sleepless. Dora waited to see his face as her daily gift, even when they didn't meet for lessons. This sometimes meant sitting at an upper-story window late into the night, just to watch his shape pass by in the darkness. That little flutter of feeling—of knowing the one she loved was safe and all was well—at last let her drift off to sleep. But her love was not reciprocated, and she knew it.

The musician was no fool. He knew Dora had feelings for him, and he took advantage of her charity. He first asked her to do a little errand for him, and she complied; then came more errands, little tasks, little gifts, but with no return. Dora spent money on lessons and also on good suppers and flowers and other pleasantries. In this real-world drama, the beloved musician did not fall in love with his pupil. Happy to be spoiled and doted upon, the violinist nevertheless kept Dora at a distance. It worried Dora to no end; did he think she was a homosexual man instead of a woman? How could she prove herself?

Dora had been an actress once, and she knew how to play the flirtatious debutante. A little subterfuge and a masked ball was all she needed, and the violinist gladly accepted her invitation. We'll bring the costumes to the ball, she told him; that way the reveal would be a surprise. Two gentlemen entered, but only the violinist emerged. When Dora stepped onto the dance floor, she was robed in a beautiful gown with false breasts and adorned wig. Now, she set out to seduce her teacher.

The violinist had been asking for Rudolf; had anyone seen him? When Rudolf didn't appear, he gave up and went to dance with the young ladies. Dashing and romantic, he had his pick of them, but he ignored Dora completely. She could not even raise his notice, much less engage him to dance. Dora felt her heart sink, and all the joy she usually took in dancing faded. She wandered into the more secluded and shadowed places, alone. Or, as it happened, not quite alone.

There, in the arms of a young girl, was her violinist. Half-clothed, rapturous; it was only too obvious what they were up to. "Self-control evaporated," Dora would recall; not only to be rejected, but then replaced so easily, so quickly, to know he had never been hers at all, was agony. Dora rushed back to the ball and found one of the violinist's friends. Could he please tell him his friend Rudolf was leaving? Let *him* interrupt the scene in the shadows; Dora wanted to be "alone with [her] great pain." Much to her surprise, however, the violinist returned after being apprised of the situation: Dora and Rudolf were one and the same. He was surprised by her appearance, but asked why she wanted to leave such a wonderful ball. He even introduced her to the man who had fetched him—who was impressed by her costume. Dora was in no mood for compliments, however, and wouldn't be swayed. "Am I the cause of your grief?" he asked. No, Dora lied. Then she went home alone, depressed and hopeless, feeling "as if [I] had been beaten all over [my] body." She took no joy in sleep, and shooed away her pigeon when it came to perch: "I have no more joy," she said, "not even in you!" What good was it to love when you weren't loved back? And then, despite everything, the violinist came knocking at her door as though nothing had happened—and he brought his friend with him.

Dora didn't bother trying to be Rudolf. She opened the door wearing her women's clothes and entertained as best she could, considering that she felt shattered inwardly. As twilight fell, the violinist took his leave. The friend, however, remained. He was older, married, talkative, and perhaps a little too friendly? He told her how shocked he'd been to learn that the nice girl he met at the ball was "really" a man. He wanted to sit close, intimate, but as his behavior grew more affectionate, Dora grew more uncomfortable. Was this a trap of some kind? Had the violinist sent his friend to try and discover her secrets?

She wanted the man to leave, but the weather had turned ugly, with heavy rain lashing the windowpanes. Would Dora give him quarters for the night, he asked? Dora did not want to. He coaxed, and she resisted. But as night fell, the storm went from bad to worse, and Dora's good nature won out over her suspicions. The apartment was small, but there were two beds. She left her guest so he could change for bed in privacy, slipping into her nightgown in the chilly confines of the kitchen. Now she just needed to cross the room and climb beneath her quilt—except, when she returned, her guest was not huddled beneath the blankets. Instead, he sat upright, bedclothes to one side, beckoning her to join him. "My wife and I are in discord," he told her, and had no relations. He wished to make love to Dora.

Dora stood in the cold room, unmoving. Whatever the man said about his wife, he was married. To do as he asked would be adultery. As a devout Catholic, Dora believed God forbade it. And yet, here was a man who must—despite knowing that she was both Dora and Rudolf—consider her a woman. Was it a trick? Was he moved by morbid curiosity about her supposed intersex qualities? Even Dora's most recent sexual partner had been more or less deceived. She determined that he was "looking for the woman in" her, and it pleased her. The man was attractive, likable; he spoke sweet things to her. She couldn't help but feel the stirring of desire; it had been so long since she'd had sexual satisfaction. The more he spoke, the more she wanted to give in. She climbed into bed with him, on the condition that he not reach for any part of her genitals. They had sex, but the act had scarcely ended before she regretted everything about it. He would surely tell the violinist. Worse, she'd violated her own ethics.

That is how she found herself in a confession booth in her hometown, at "odds with [herself] and the world." She'd tried to live as a man but could not—her spirit starved and shriveled. She'd tried to live as a woman, but her body always betrayed her. The priest listened with gentleness. "God forgives even the gravest of sins," he told her, because of her sincere repentance. But he said something more, too. We have only Dora's record of the encounter, but it seems he did not exhort her to live as a man. He didn't tell her to seek a doctor or psychotherapy. Instead, the priest told Dora that she wasn't alone. If the world had given her no peace, then perhaps she might try seeking entrance to a monastery.

There, he told her, she "would more easily meet people of a similar disposition to [hers] in the world." We can speculate on what he meant, but Dora took his message to heart.

Dora, like Karl Ulrichs, had long ago determined that her nature was not a sin. She could not help being born a woman burdened with the wrong body; God wouldn't punish her for that. Yet, it was her "lack of sexual satisfactoriness" that had led to adultery in a moment of weakness. If her nature brought her into conflict with everything, even her faith, then perhaps the priest was right; she could leave the world for a life of prayer and reflection. Still with plenty of misgivings, Dora wrote a letter to the local abbot about admission. Then, she told her parents.

Since well before the war, and now, two years after it, Dora had been sending her earnings home to the family, as was both common and expected for unmarried children. When she announced her plan to take orders, they pleaded with her to refrain. To please them, she withdrew her application to the monastery. Shortly after (and still to please them), she agreed to speak to her uncle, who, they explained, had a business proposition for her. In her intake interview Dora didn't explain their reasons, though it's hard not to suspect that they, too, took every advantage of her generosity and devotion.

Seventy years old, wealthy but stingy, judgmental and acrimonious, the elder Richter had never treated Dora with kindness, saying that her "feminine nature disgusted him." She couldn't imagine what he had to offer her, but Dora agreed to go and see him. As his home was too far away for a day trip, she expected to spend the night. True to the man's miserly ways, however, he didn't allow her the convenience of a spare room. Instead, a bed had been made up for her in a corner of his own sleeping quarters. The nature of the business proposal was equally lackluster. Over supper, the old man told her his plans—he was going to be married.

He'd wooed a wealthy innkeeper, widowed like himself. He knew that Rudolf had worked as a waiter and was a decent cook. He wanted her to come work at the inn, but Dora knew him better than that. Once there, she would become his servant, taken advantage of, given nothing but empty promises. This was no business opportunity; it would be as bad as slavery. Perhaps he planned to hang out an inheritance as bait, but Dora wasn't fooled by that, either. He had a living heir and was marrying again anyway; neither she nor her family would get a penny. Dora respectfully declined.

Her uncle was angry and disappointed, but his next question caught her off guard: Are you a hermaphrodite or not? Dora laughed at the question—possibly to make it seem ridiculous, possibly in realization that she did not owe him an answer, probably out of nerves. In any case, she left the table and retired immediately to bed. She would leave the next morning and get as far away from the man as possible. But her ordeal wasn't yet over.

In the darkness, Dora heard her uncle's footfalls as he entered the room. Closer and closer they came—and suddenly he grasped hold of the quilt and tried to wrest it away from Dora's body. He wanted to see this "anomaly" for himself; he wanted to see her genitals. As he yanked away the covers, Dora rolled quickly onto her stomach, clinging to the mattress so that he could not pry her up to expose her. But this assault was not enough. Her uncle, heavy and obese, climbed on top of her. She could not move him, and she could not climb out from beneath. Sick with horror, she was forced to endure while he performed *coitus interfemoris*—he did not penetrate her, but he climaxed between her thighs. I'm sure, he told her, you will "sleep very well following this gratification." Violated, betrayed, and feeling both angry and ashamed, Dora waited out the night in the same room as her rapist.

The date of this event is uncertain. From contextual clues, we might guess the year to be 1920—the same in which Steinach published his report on intermediaries and Hirschfeld began a public speaking tour to spread Steinach's science and popularize the concept of intermediate forms, which he saw as the basis for trans and homosexual rights. The year would not be kind to Hirschfeld either. By its end, he had nearly paid for his beliefs with his life. The intermediaries had enemies, enemies everywhere.

"WEEDS NEVER DIE"

Dr. Magnus Hirschfeld, the well-known expert on sexual science, died in Munich today of injuries inflicted upon him by an anti-Jewish mob.

—*NEW YORK TIMES*, OCTOBER 12, 1920

The October sun had set and darkness fell over Munich. Hirschfeld waited outside the Tonhalle on Briennerstrasse. He'd been promised a car, a safe escape after his lecture, but the car did not come. Voices in the distance told him not to tarry; he would walk to his hotel. At least, he would try. With each step came an echo. He was being followed. Suddenly, a stone went whizzing past his ear. Then another. He wouldn't see the third; it struck him on the back of the head, felling him instantly. A mob of attackers set upon his unconscious body and left him for dead in a gutter; so vicious were his wounds that newspapers reported him dead.[2] The *Brooklyn Daily Eagle* called his murder the first German pogrom—that is, an organized ethnic massacre of Jewish persons.

Hirschfeld wasn't ready to be a statistic, however. He suffered severe bleeding and concussion and was treated in the hospital, but was well enough to read his own obituaries. Then a letter came. A German Youth Nationalist expressed regret that his friends had failed to kill Hirschfeld; they would try again. The threats weren't only in the mailbox, however; they were in the news. In correcting their mistake about his death, a Dresden paper wrote: "We regret this shameless and horrible poisoner of our people has not found his well-deserved end," for it seems "weeds never die."[3]

Hatred was now a party platform. There were weeds all right, but they weren't growing at the Institute of Sexual Science.

Hirschfeld's troubles had begun at the start of the year, shortly after the banning of *Anders als die Andern* and, not coincidentally, the publication of Hans Blüher's third book. By now, Blüher had scaled up his anti-Semitic attacks, repeating the refrain that "feminine" Jews were emasculating Germany. Real men weren't homosexuals; real men were warriors like Greek soldiers of antiquity and, closer to home, the German Freikorps (volunteer militia).[4] As a *Männerbund* apologist, he'd picked the very worst "heroes."

The reason the Freikorps existed at all was that Germany had lost its large standing army. The Treaty of Versailles, signed after the First World War, restricted Germany's military capabilities to a small defense unit; but more than this, after demobilization, many soldiers simply melted into civilian life and didn't return to ranks. Even so, an army of some kind was needed, due to the perilous position of the ruling Social Democrats.

The Social Democratic Party, or SPD, traced its origin to an 1875 merger of the General German Workers' Union and the Social Democratic Workers' Party.[5] The first real test of this unity came when Austria-Hungary declared war on Serbia after the assassination of Archduke Ferdinand; many in the Social Democratic Workers' Party voted against declaring war in compliance with the treaty. History proved them right, but at the time they were labeled as weak pacifists. In response, Wilhelm Liebknecht, leader of the Social Democratic Workers' Party, and Polish-born revolutionary Rosa Luxemburg split away to form the communist Spartacus League. Because the Social Democrats had lost some of their members to the League, they held only the slimmest of majorities in the Reichstag. It seemed the Weimar Republic could be toppled at any moment, either by imperialists, who wanted a return of the monarchy, or by the Spartacus League. Without a sizable standing army, how would they have the force to remain in power?

Germany's first president, Friedrich Ebert, decided upon volunteer armed units. The Freikorpskämpfer, or "freebooters," joined up of their own accord, eating, traveling, and fighting together in bands that varied in size, age, and abilities—but a nationalist ideal they were not.[6] For one thing, most of them despised the new German republic (even though they were employed by it). But though they hated the Social Democrats, they hated the Spartacus League much, much more. The League had by this time rebranded itself the Communist Party of Germany, inspired by the new Soviet Union's support of women in the workforce and no-fault divorce, as well as the decriminalization of abortion and the elimination of anti-homosexuality laws. Many of the Freikorps men had grown up with the Wandervögel's masculinist ideals; they wanted nothing more than to stamp out the Communists and their liberal agenda. In December 1918, they got their first chance.

Communist Party leaders held a congress in Berlin from December 30, 1918, to January 1, 1919. They determined that the Social Democrats had no right to rule and staged an armed uprising of workers, threatening civil war even as the Weimar Republic drew its first breath.[7] In a moment of reckless optimism, Luxemburg and Liebknecht even declared President Ebert's government deposed. They were very, very wrong. The Freikorps hit the streets with artillery, flamethrowers, and armored cars. They mowed down Communists and their supporters, along with anyone who got in their way. "Civil wars are always brutal, but the zeal with which the Freikorps went about their business was out of all proportion," writes historian Robert M. Citino; they even "bragged about it in print." Luxemburg was abducted and clubbed to death, her body dumped in the river. Liebknecht's corpse would be stripped of valuables and left on the steps of a mortuary. The troops of Freikorps then dispersed to Bavaria, specifically to Munich, and to any other areas that might have pockets of potential Communist sympathizers (and more people to assault). They kept at it all winter and into spring, and no one—certainly not the Social Democrats—could rein them in. They might be volunteers, but they wouldn't go away.

There are several theories for the persistence of the Freikorps. First, most had no employment beyond their work as soldiers for hire. Many had no family ties, either. Blüher had been right about the bonds of warmongers; Freikorps men were divorced from the world of family and tied only to one another. Together, they participated in dangerous mythmaking. They would valorize the past as a time of *Übermenschen*; they considered the present state to be weak and feminized. But perhaps the greatest myth, and one they clung to like religion, was this: they did not believe Germany had lost the war. In rhetoric that will sound uncannily familiar to our ears, the Freikorps ardently believed that victory had been stolen from them. They blamed Social Democrats (and women, feminists, and Jews) for betraying the nation so that they might seize power. This gave them a scapegoat and absolved them of any failures; it also created the first inroad for fascism. Hermann Ehrhardt, leader of the Freikorps, called "for a powerful Germany united under a strong leader [Führer]," and a political system "stamped with . . . military virtues of authority and obedience." They embodied the natural evolution of Blüher's militant, misogynistic, nationalist ethos: wannabe heroes of belligerent masculinity.

In March 1920, President Ebert ordered the volunteers disbanded. They refused and attempted their own coup in Berlin, known to history as the Kapp Putsch. Ehrhardt gave orders to march on Berlin and "ruthlessly break" any resistance. With no military to resist them, they would have been victorious if not for the working class, who went on a strike 12 million strong. The coup ended six days later with the Weimar Republic intact, though Freikorps supporters had papered the city in flyers, listing those they targeted as enemies for extermination. Magnus Hirschfeld was among them. On his lecture tour, he would never be more visible—nor more vulnerable.

TWO SIDES TO EVERY THEORY

On his visit, years before, to Steinach's lab, Hirschfeld had enthusiastically encouraged Steinach's work on the "hermaphroditic" origins of all creatures. This concept appealed to Hirschfeld on several levels; first, it agreed with his concept of gender and sex spectrums, and second, it promised proof for single-origin theory, or monism.[8] Single-origin might not seem like an improvement on the binary model, and might even look like a contraction of the broader spectrum into a singular unity, but the theory of monism wasn't intended to reduce diversity. It aimed instead to explain it.

When Starling introduced the hormone to the Royal College of Physicians, he also introduced a democratizing idea: humans might not be so very far removed from the animals, all of us driven by chemical signals. Darwin's evolutionary theory had broken the age-old belief that humans were God's special creations. Evolution might answer some scientific questions, but it also allowed scientists to ask many more. What preceded humans? What preceded mammals? What preceded life itself? The great branching tree of life must start somewhere, and the race was on to discover that originary cell. Zoologist and evolutionary biologist Ernst Haeckel believed he'd located it: in the beginning was the egg.

If you compare the gestation of most vertebrates, you'll note surprising similarities; the study of this is called comparative embryology. In 1828, Ernst von Baer claimed that closely related species have similar embryonic development, and thought this could explain much bigger concepts. For instance, he linked the *ontogeny*, or the development of a single individual from ovum to maturity, to *phylogeny*, or the development of entire species as they differentiate from a common ancestor.[9] There's a reason the embryos of humans, pigs, and even whales go through similar stages; mammals share a common ancestor, a rodent-like creature that managed to outlast dinosaurs. Going back further, all vertebrates have a common ancestor, too: a very small water-dweller with a bristle spine. We know today that evolution is not interested in human advancement; traits evolve because they help a species thrive and are passed on by the top breeders. The process can go either way; some animals left the water, while other animals (such as whales) returned to it.

Theorists of the time, however, believed that evolution moved forever forward like an arrow from least to greatest. As a result, Haeckel linked evolutionary process to human concepts of progress, as though evolution had a semi-sentient goal to produce "higher" forms.[10] For Haeckel, each embryonic stage that an animal goes through in the womb enacted a chronological replay of past evolutionary forms. Consider the human fetus: it goes from a fertilized cell no bigger than the period at the end of this sentence, to an amphibious-seeming tadpole, to something scarcely distinguishable from a chimpanzee fetus, and then to a human in miniature. Haeckel believed that fetal development offered up evolution on fast-forward, and the developmental stages of each species represented the adult form of some distant evolutionary ancestor.[11] The idea wasn't just compelling; it almost approximated a religion.

Haeckel founded the German Monist Society to promote and share his findings. Both Hirschfeld and Helene Stöcker became eager members. Religion proper didn't appeal to either of them, as it was at odds with their progressive views and frequently their politics. Meanwhile, the monists' pantheistic approach promised unity in nature. Monism didn't erase difference; it demonstrated that differences had once mixed freely in one entity. This accorded beautifully with Hirschfeld's theory of gender unity, formulated in 1905; all humans existed on a continuum, "a long series between all male and all female forms, in which mixed characteristics are found in the greatest diversity."[12] If all of us evolved from a single deep-time egg, then of course the male would have a bit of female and the female a bit of male (with plenty in between). Hirschfeld manifested his appreciation for Haeckel in the most physical way possible. When he purchased the building next door to 10 In den Zelten (number 9a), he named it Haeckel Saal—the Haeckel Salon—with an inscription over the door: "Science not for its own sake, but for all humanity."

For Stöcker and other feminists, Haeckel's philosophy offered a way out of gender hierarchies by demonstrating that gendered social power structures were unscientific.[13] Why should sex difference determine "one's role in life more broadly," Stöcker asked, if everyone had a single origin? When she cofounded the League for the Protection of Mothers and Sexual Reform in 1905, she invoked Haeckel and Darwin's theory of natural selection as support.[14] These theories had repercussions for reproduction, too; if Germany was worried about the birth rate and better breeding, then women must have the right to choose or reject partners; left to their own devices, she claimed, women would "naturally" pick quality biological partners to "improve" the nation.

In *The Descent of Man*, Darwin argued that morality gave human beings a selective advantage. "In order that primeval men, or the ape-like progenitors of man, should have become social," he wrote, "they must have acquired the same instinctive feelings which impel other animals to live in a body." He lists the qualities that would arise from the arrangement: fidelity, courage, obedience, discipline, unselfishness, sympathy, faithfulness—the very qualities that inspired Darwin (within his cultural context). Accordingly, a tribe possessing these moral qualities would "spread and be victorious" over all other peoples.[15]

In the decades leading to the First World War, these ideas were increasingly turned toward explaining racial difference and defending existing inequalities. The ideas are monstrous, but many embraced them because social Darwinism provided some of the first real critiques against traditional structures—patriarchy, monarchy, the church—which stood in the way of equal opportunity.[16] Hirschfeld was attracted to monism and social Darwinism for their ability to bolster sexual freedom—but as Jewish and homosexual, he himself did not meet the criteria, which had been based on white heterosexuals of a certain class.

Here is where monism falls down; it might have helped to get rid of gender hierarchy, but it did not abolish the power structures that hierarchy established. Haeckel's philosophy didn't dismantle religion so much as become its own particular sect. It still held to power and privilege; where differences existed, monists saw hierarchies. When Stöcker suggested free choice for women in when, how, and with whom to procreate, she excluded those she considered inferior, suggesting that the disabled, those convicted of crimes, alcoholics, and "irresponsible" persons should be actively discouraged from breeding.[17]

Eugenics, or race hygiene, can never be divorced from the horrors it would cause or the racism and ableism it harbored. When these ideas first appeared, however, they had the veneer of scientific credibility. In the Weimar era, eugenics offered to empower people to make good choices—while simultaneously preventing those considered "incapable" from making bad ones.[18] The discovery of genes proved that certain traits were inherited (that is, carried in the genetic profile even if not apparent) and some were also congenital (genetic and present from birth); as a result, eugenics promised a future where only the "best" traits carried on, such that populations would evolve to become stronger.

It sounded good to most people, because they assumed they were on the side of the "capable." But who decides? By the turn of the century, most of Darwin's work had been married up to nineteenth-century fears of degeneration and notions of progress that (predictably) put white men at the apex. They, in turn, determined which were the "good" decisions and "best" traits.

In her critical work *The Hirschfeld Archives*, gender theorist Dr. Heike Bauer spends significant time unraveling the roles of race, politics, and eugenics in Hirschfeld's work. Though a victim of both anti-homosexual and anti-Semitic attacks, Hirschfeld wasn't immune to the cultural influence of social Darwinism—that is, the practice of race hygiene masquerading as science. He would have reason to change his mind (and his later work takes a very different look at racism), but in the 1920s, he believed that eugenics would "improve the health of the nation."[19] One of the largest departments of the Institute, Marriage Consultation, discussed both relational compatibility and breeding suitability with intended couples. At the Institute, eugenics sat right alongside social and sexual justice.[20] Leftist eugenics and marriage clinics did not generally consider race a determinant for or against reproduction, and the goal wasn't to prohibit but to educate.[21] Unfortunately, Haeckelian philosophy offered scientific grounding for right-wing, openly racist eugenicists, too.

Haeckel maintained that simpler creatures held inside them the "potential" for greatness if given the right set of circumstances, yet he still divided humans into twelve different species and even into genera, with his own race at the top.[22] Haeckel was Caucasian (white), and he supported the idea that Germans had Nordic roots—a tribe of people also referred to as Indo-European, Indo-Germanic, or (more recognizably) Aryan. He theorized that if natural selection allowed only the strong to survive, then those who survived in the harshest climates must have evolved to be the best. Since Nordic people lived in the harshest, coldest climates, they must have evolved to be better than all other humans.[23] Germans (Aryans) were thus on top, and on the bottom rungs, Haeckel put those from warmer regions: notably, African peoples and Jews.

Haeckel didn't invent anti-Semitism. Its roots go deep, but this particular branch of racist theory emerged, in part, from a series of essays published in the mid-1850s: Joseph Arthur, Comte de Gobineau's *Essay on the Inequality of the Human Races*, which contributed to the myth of Nordic superiority as well as degeneration through racial mixing. German anthropologists embraced the idea, mixed it with Darwinism, and combined it with the race-hatred of Theodor Fritsch, a German writer and publisher often called the godfather of anti-Semitism. Yet it would be Darwin that Hitler referenced in *Mein Kampf*, and Haeckel's theories that Hitler later endorsed (and enforced),[24] as they justified his anti-Semitism and supported his burgeoning political aims. Survival of the fittest increasingly meant survival of the white German; the rest should be eliminated from the gene pool. It was called racial extermination, and it had already been practiced—in America.

Journalist and painter Rudolf Cronau used social Darwinism to support the extermination of indigenous tribes across the United States. A four-volume work on ethnology by Friedrich Hellwald quotes Cronau's claim that "the current inequality of the races is an indubitable fact. . . . [Indigenous Americans] naturally succumb in the struggle, its race vanished and civilization strides over their corpses [sic]."[25] Racial cleansing in the United States did not restrict itself to race alone, however. The father of the American eugenics movement was a Harvard-trained zoologist named Charles Davenport. Like Steinach, he had his own experimental lab, but Davenport wasn't working with rats and guinea pigs. He used people. His protégé Bleecker Van Wagenen, president of the American Breeders' Association, described their work at an international conference on eugenics in 1912; even then, they were long past the theoretical stage. Confinement centers like the Virginia State Colony for Epileptics and Feebleminded would house the "genetically unfit" and remove "defective strains" from the population via forced sterilization. Little more than prisons, such places performed cruel surgeries and confinements based upon racist, classist, and ableist justifications; in the category of unfit were included "epileptics, criminals, deaf-mutes, the feebleminded, those with eye defects, bone deformities, dwarfism, schizophrenia, manic depression, or insanity."[26] Eight American states already authorized forced sterilization. Hitler admired Davenport's eugenics work as much as Haeckel's theories, and would introduce his own eugenic measures for eliminating *minderwertig* (inferior) people.[27] As he would later remark, "Only the born weakling can view this as cruel."[28]

ON FEBRUARY 24, 1920, Adolf Hitler ascended the podium to deliver the platform of the newly formed National Socialist German Workers' Party (NAZI for short). It had been the German Workers' Party, but with Hitler as spokesman, its aims had changed. The NAZI planned to strengthen German citizenship by excluding and controlling Jewish and other "non-German" people.[29] Using fiery oration and catchphrases like "Germany, awake!," Hitler leaned into earlier concepts of dominant masculinity to claim that Jews were eating away at Germany's core the way bacteria eat healthy tissue. The weak were usurping the strong and must be stopped.

The argument appealed immediately to one group in particular: the recently disbanded Freikorps. Hitler made the most of the *Dolch-stosslegende* myth; it means "stab in the back" and blamed Jews and women for Germany's loss of the First World War. Right-wing papers ran caricatures of Jews with knives standing over troops, or masculinized women with monocles and tuxedos, and insisted that both groups represented degeneration and moral decay. They attacked the Social Democrats, too, convinced that leftists were conspiring to feminize Germany. Hitler used it all to his advantage. The separate threads of misogyny, anti-Semitism, homophobia, and conservative nationalism had been there all along; they just needed a charismatic champion to pull them together.

Hitler—fan of Davenport and social Darwinism—chose to unite his party under the auspices of evolutionary and eugenic "science." He even had a textbook for the occasion. Erwin Baur, Eugen Fischer, and Fritz Lenz had just finished writing *Human Heredity Teaching and*

Racial Hygiene. It would be Hitler's basis for eugenic sterilization—and much worse to come. Eugenics would be a tool of evil. It would sweep monism along with it.

Not long after Hitler's debut, Hirschfeld received an invitation from Wilhelm Ostwald, then president of Haeckel's Monist Society, to speak in Hamburg about Steinach's work and its support of the single-origin theory. Hirschfeld gladly obliged but was prevented from speaking moments before approaching the lectern. A warning had come by anonymous tip: the podium had been compromised with firebombs set to go off during the speech. The police arrived to remove them safely, but before Hirschfeld could resume, protesters launched live fireworks into the crowd. Chaos ensued, and Hirschfeld left horrified and "trembling with indignation."[30]

The German Nationalist Protection and Defense Federation took official credit for the disruption; they counted Freikorps men among their members and were avid supporters of Hitler. As the largest and most active anti-Semitic group in Germany, they openly rejected the Weimar Republic and accused Jews, and especially Hirschfeld, of introducing homosexuality and other "foreign" notions.[31] They missed their target in Hamburg, so they followed Hirschfeld to Munich—Hitler's base of operations. That's how he found himself outside the town hall, waiting on a car that never came, at the mercy of a mob bent on ending his life.

Hirschfeld made lighthearted pronouncements about the effect of reading his premature obituaries, but the incident would haunt him and the threat would continue to dog his steps. He was a marked man.

Hitler received news of Hirschfeld's recovery while dining at a favorite beer hall. It was a bitter disappointment. He blamed the Weimar Republic for allowing "Jewish swine" to poison the German people, calling Hirschfeld "the most dangerous Jew in Germany."[32] Why had he conceived such a hatred for the Berlin sexologist? In part, because it was expedient. Hitler drew upon associations between Jews and sexual rights—along with the myth of Jews as sexual pariahs—to advance a conservative agenda, playing on existing fears and exciting new ones. He put Hirschfeld's image on Nazi campaign posters, one of ten "un-Aryan" opponents Hitler intended to crush.[33] Using Hirschfeld, he could unite prejudice against the feminine with xenophobia and homophobia, simultaneously accusing Jews of undermining German strength and homosexuals of preying upon young men and boys. The strategy worked only too well.

It had been just over a year since the hopeful opening night of *Anders als die Andern*, but it didn't seem like the same Germany. Rifts had opened even among those Hirschfeld had once considered allies—from Brand and Blüher to Albert Moll to members of the Social Democratic Party (who still had not fulfilled their promise of homosexual rights). In cruelest irony, those who disrupted the Monist Society meeting and attacked Hirschfeld in Munich were probably followers of the same Haeckelian beliefs that Hirschfeld professed. Monism, Darwinism, Steinachism: Hirschfeld promoted these theories because he wanted science to lead to justice. Unfortunately, science cannot speak for itself and may be as easily misused. At its best, science offers a means of asking questions and testing hypotheses. Distorted by bias and prejudice, it can be used for evil as easily as for good.

The year was coming to a close, and Hirschfeld continued his recovery at home. Christmas was almost upon them, a holiday he cherished. Despite being born Jewish, he considered himself non-practicing. He did not agree with the revival of the Hebrew language, which he thought promoted isolation, and likewise distanced himself from the idea of Jewish racial purity. Considering himself a "dissident," he celebrated the Christian holidays not as a convert so much as a cultural participant.[34]

Yet Hitler and his Nazi party had, violently and suddenly, forced Hirschfeld's Jewishness upon him. He could see the humiliation, the degradation, and now the danger that Jews faced as a minority in Germany, even those who had been born and raised there. "The question: where do you belong—what are you really? Tortures me," he wrote; he was not a German or a Jew but both, and a "world citizen," too.[35] Hirschfeld had never been open about his homosexuality, fearing (among other things) that it would cost him the authority to speak on homosexuals' behalf. He did not generally speak of his Jewishness, either. Now, both aspects of his identity were public ammunition. But, in his sickbed on the second floor of 10 In den Zelten, he was at least no longer alone. There was Karl.

Karl Giese and Magnus Hirschfeld had met after one of Hirschfeld's lectures, shortly before or during the ill-fated *Anders* project. Tall and angular, with deep-set eyes and hair swept back from the temples, Giese arrived in "dirty work clothes," stammering that he was "like that, too." From a working-class family, he lacked formal education, but was bright and willing to learn. Hirschfeld trained him in archival work and as a personal secretary, but he became much, much more; he was "the absolute link between Magnus Hirschfeld and the environment."[36] Now, at Christmas, the young man bustled about, looking after Hirschfeld. There is nothing warmer in a cold room than company; Giese liked needlework and fashion and put himself in charge of Hirschfeld's wardrobe (the man was appallingly negligent, he claimed). By all accounts, Giese was "the woman of the house," and the house, at last, was full.[37]

Hirschfeld wasn't giving up. His collaborators weren't giving up, either. Eugen Steinach was in the midst of making his own film, which would popularize the concept of intermediate sexuality. It would be viewed so widely that, in 1923, Dora Richter would see it. One day soon afterward, she would approach the Institute for Sexual Science, read the inscription above its front door, and walk inside. It did not read "From science to justice," though that had always been the SHC motto. Instead, it read *"Amori et dolori sacrum,"* sacred to love and sorrow.[38] Nothing for the intermediary had ever been easy, but there could be celebration even through grief.

8

THE DOCTOR WILL SEE YOU NOW

A TWENTY-FIVE-YEAR-OLD FORMER MILITARY OFFICER LAY UPON THE operating table in Dresden. It was March, 1921. He'd been prepped for surgery in the clinic of one Dr. Richard Mühsam and now awaited the doctor—and the knife.* He wasn't ill, not in the way of disease or wounds you could see, but he'd been suffering since boyhood from a sense of imbalance, anxiety, and depression. Most of all, he felt trapped in the wrong body. Mühsam had a reputation for performing Steinach's homosexual "cure"; he believed that surgery could succeed where psychological intervention failed and was prepared to take experimental risks. First, he removed the patient's testicles and implanted an ovary. Now, he was preparing to give him a vagina.

The officer, whose patient identity was protected by record and whom I will refer to as M, had spent the previous year under the attentive care of Arthur Kronfeld at Hirschfeld's Institute for Sexual Science. Kronfeld wrote that the returning veteran was "psychologically completely broken and completely adrift." M had many of the hallmarks of *Transvestiten*, as Hirschfeld conceptualized them; since his earliest childhood, he'd felt like a woman, and even military life had not suppressed his feminine nature. He still found himself attracted to women and not to men (thus, he was not, in the terms of the day, a homosexual), but had never performed a sexual act with another person. Considering himself

---

* The patient chose to retain masculine pronouns, thus the use of he/him.

addicted to masturbation, he begged Kronfeld give him an immediate double castration.[1]

Kronfeld refused. He had been a soldier himself. After suffering a war injury, he had helped found a *Nervenstation*, or mental hospital, at the military reserve in Freiburg, for soldiers suffering what we would call PTSD today. After the Weimar Revolution, Kronfeld served as spokesperson for the Freiburg Soldiers' Council before taking work at the Herzberge municipal mental hospital in Berlin. He understood very well the trauma war could inflict upon the mind.[2]

After speaking to the "highly nervous" patient, Kronfeld rejected the idea of anything so rash as immediate surgery. The man first needed counseling and care and psychotherapy. In response, M said that he had a revolver and a vial of morphine. Should he be refused an operation, he told Kronfeld, he had ample means of ending his own life.[3] Kronfeld wrote the referral. The resulting changes to M's body are recorded in the case history by both Kronfeld and Mühsam; M lost body hair and developed fatty deposits that allowed him to pass more easily as a woman. But this surgery, often cited as one of the first attempts at surgical body modification, is not the earliest case on record. It's not even the earliest case published by Mühsam.

We must ask, what counts as the earliest surgical intervention that could be considered transgender? Historian Rainer Herrn cites a report of bodily manipulation for the purpose of feminization around 1905, when a Dutch father of four castrated himself and subsequently attempted to enlarge his "breasts" by injecting air beneath the skin.[4] Does that make it the earliest modern example? Some of the difficulty in unearthing this history comes from the variant evolution of the language we use to describe it. In *Before We Were Trans*, Kit Heyam points to these problems of expression: the "literary canon" (by which we mean classic works, books you learn about in school) doesn't provide space for "messy" identities, because the fringe, aberrant, and non-normative are frequently weeded out.[5] That doesn't mean such stories don't exist, even if we must pry them from history's grip. Medical texts—especially those of Richard von Krafft-Ebing—offer us the earliest glimpses in the time before Hirschfeld or Havelock Ellis. By publishing letters and autobiographical accounts of his own "invert" (transgender) patients, Krafft-Ebing "enabled voices to be heard that were usually silenced."[6] Therein lies the power of representation.

Written reports of what we think of today as gender dysphoria don't appear much before the turn of the century, but this doesn't mean the condition didn't exist. It was frequently treated as a mental disorder, a psychological problem, some form of hysteria, or the result of being seduced by bad actors of the same sex. Krafft-Ebing described "inversion" as a "contrary sexual feeling"—it joined "uranism" and "homosexuality" as medical terms to replace the punitive "sodomite" and "pederast"—but he originally saw deviant sexuality as an aspect of more fundamental mental problems. In this view, mental illness caused a person to feel they were in the wrong body, rather than the experience of being in the wrong body causing mental illness.*

Krafft-Ebing would shift his thinking in later works, suggesting that "inverts" might be biologically determined, and that sexuality was a salient feature of identity and culture.[7] This was "gender" in its infancy, and despite the misalignment of cause and effect, its arrival coincided with (almost grew out of) the recognition of gender dysphoria. It's a crucial development, because as medical treatises provided the terminology (or, at the very least, the experiential examples), they gave others a framework to articulate their identity. Especially when employed by a popularizer like Magnus Hirschfeld.

Hirschfeld coined the word "transvestite" in 1912, and not by coincidence, Mühsam saw his first female-to-male patient in 1912. The term would eventually replace "inversion" as the best descriptor for those who felt they had the wrong sex characteristics, though it doesn't exactly equate with our modern conception of transgender. For one

---

* It's not the first time in history cause and effect have been confused by medicine; epilepsy, which may be preceded by sensory auras of certain sounds, lights, or smells, was thought to be caused by them.

thing, it focused (as the name suggests) on clothing; for another, the terms were used in somewhat the reverse of today's terminology. Mühsam's patient, a thirty-five-year-old assigned female at birth, dressed in men's clothes and experienced back pain and feelings of "foreign bodies" inside them. They wished to have breasts and uterus removed because, as they said, "the organs did not belong to [me]." Today, they would identify as a trans man; Mühsam identifies them as a female transvestite, saying (with the pronouns of the time) that "she thought she was a man in disguise."[8] Mühsam at last agreed to perform surgery, taking away the secondary sex characteristics. At the time, medicine could not produce a phallus.

Or at least, not literally. Five years earlier, a curious little book appeared on Berlin shelves titled *Aus eines Mannes Mädchenjahren*— published in English as *Memoirs of a Man's Maiden Years*. The pseudonym playfully read as N. O. Body but told the story of Karl M. Baer. Named Martha at birth, the German-Jewish Karl had a genetic condition known as hypospadias. This not uncommon condition causes a malformation in the opening of the male urethra. Instead of appearing at the end of the penis, a ventral opening develops along the penis itself. This results in a grooved or "butterflied" glans—or occasionally, a urethral hole midway along the scrotum. In infancy, Karl's unusually shaped genitals confused physicians, and they declared him a girl. Today, intersex and DSD (differences of sex development) activists castigate attempts at quickly resolving ambiguous gender—particularly the once-common practice in which doctors, sometimes even without the parents' consent, would choose a single set of sex characteristics for intersex babies. Hirschfeld argued something similar. He felt that those with ambiguous genitals should be allowed to choose their sex (and so also gender) when they reached the age of responsibility—and for good reason.[9]

Growing up, Baer felt different from the other girls, but wasn't sure why. Then (much like Dora Richter), he happened to glimpse the genitals of a playmate. Both were supposed to be girls, but "down there," he wrote, they "were certainly very different! And a nameless fright took hold of me."[10] Puberty made things worse; instead of developing breasts, he sprouted chest and facial hair. He developed sexual feelings for girls instead of boys, and at the age of twenty-one fell in love with a married woman. Baer at last sought the advice of medical experts about his condition and they, in turn, referred him to Hirschfeld.

Hirschfeld writes about his examination of Baer in the first volume of *The Transvestites*: having a large frame, Karl-as-Martha had tightly waist-trained with a corset to emulate other women's body shape. The patient even modulated the way he breathed. Hirschfeld did not consider him a transvestite; instead, he diagnosed Baer's condition as *hypospadia peniscrotalis* and pronounced him a "pseudo-hermaphrodite," biologically male, and thus—despite what his genitals looked like—permitted to legally change name and gender. Today, the condition can be adjusted with surgery to create a more usual-looking penis. Karl Baer, however, chose to remasculinize himself in a different way. In addition to choosing male clothes and mode of address, he formalized his gender through narrative. A journalist named Presber encouraged him to pen an autobiography, saying, "on the path of this first task that you perform as a *man*, you may find your way," and the "rusty fetter" that once oppressed will fall away.[11]

Even without surgical intervention, it was possible at the time (if difficult) to change one's gender legally, and Baer isn't the only patient Hirschfeld helped to do so. Since at least 1909, Hirschfeld, together with Iwan Bloch and psychoanalyst Karl Abraham, had negotiated "transvestite certificates," or licenses to cross-dress. Instead of being harassed by police or arrested on spurious charges such as "causing public nuisance" or "disturbing public order," those with the certificate could move about freely.[12] On its own, the license did not confer a legal change of identity—only permission.

Hirschfeld attempted to obtain a legal change of gender for a patient named Katharina T., by means of an expert opinion. He explained all of his medical and psychological reasons, but authorities refused on account of "her completely normal sex organs."[13] It may have been a setback, but it also taught Hirschfeld to amend his tactics. First, he altered his definition of the term "hermaphrodite" to correspond with his new understanding of intermediary sexuality (and monism). Just because dual gender didn't appear in the genitals didn't mean it was absent, he argued; hermaphrodism could be a psychic condition. In 1912, he tried this new tactic on behalf of Louise S., asserting "a case of hermaphroditism, not in a purely external sense, but rather in a deeper sense," and "gender transitions occurring in all conceivable nuances." Though, as in the previous case, the external genitalia still looked female, Hirschfeld was stating that there were hidden depths to sexuality. The surface cannot be the only indicator, he argued, nor should it determine sex "to a greater degree than the overall sexual personality."[14] This time, officials agreed to change the civil register: Louise, previously regarded as a lesbian and a transvestite, was now Louis and permitted to marry their longtime girlfriend.[15] In neither Baer's nor Louis's case was a phallus artificially created, but neither was it required for the patient to become "male." In the epilogue to *Memoirs of a Man's Maiden Years*, Hirschfeld writes that a person's sex originates "more in the brain than in the genitals"—all of Steinach's theories aside.[16]

Let us return to 1920. Back in Dresden, Mühsam performed a complex second surgery on the young, castrated officer. He made an incision and cut from the scrotum to the perineum (the thin layer of skin between the scrotum and anus), tucked the man's penis into the wound, and sewed it up, hiding the penis from sight. He fashioned the remaining scrotal skin into something like labia. Mühsam published the case as "Surgical Interventions for Sex Life Abnormalities," proclaiming the first surgically created "vagina-like structure" and declaring the surgery a success.[17]

The patient, however, did not agree. Eight weeks later, he returned to the Dresden clinic to demand a reversal. He no longer wanted to dress or live as a woman, he said; he'd acquired a girlfriend and wished to have his penis restored so that he might have sex with her. Mühsam complied on August 23: the scrotal labia were removed, the perineum reopened, and the penis fished out. Apparently, all went as smoothly as a one-of-a-kind surgery can be expected to go, and the man went merrily on having erections and sexual relations. (He also finished medical school and become a pathologist.) All of the officer's surgeries took place in the span of only fourteen months,[18] and no reason was ever given for the sudden change, whether psychological, social, economic, or practical (pathology would have been a difficult career to enter as a woman in 1921). The patient evidently considered himself wrong to have wanted—or received—surgery, but haste hadn't allowed for healing and reflection, nor had any counseling or psychological examination been provided (that we know of). Kronfeld, following Institute protocols, had been keen to avoid just such a mistake.

As a result of its reversal, the Dresden case is not usually considered the first successful gender affirmation or transition surgery. What it demonstrated, instead, was a problem of too heartily privileging only one type of therapy—Steinach's transplants, Mühsam's surgeries, or Starling's hormones—or even one type of sex characteristic as pointing the way to definitive sex and gender identity. The case also allows us to differentiate between the ethos of the Institute and other practitioners; Hirschfeld's goal was to provide supportive care, healthful confirmation, and a sense of belonging. The intermediaries might display any number of sexual characteristics, but they were individuals and must be treated as persons, not pathologies or anomalies.

Before 1792, those considered hermaphrodites didn't have to choose a "true" gender under Prussian law; that is, they weren't seen as a defective version of one of two immutable sexes. The sex binary wouldn't be codified until 1899, when the Civil Code of the German Reich claimed that "there are neither sexless nor both sexes united in themselves, that every so-called hermaphrodite is either a sexually malformed man or a sexually malformed woman."[19] The idea of strict binary sex might be recent, but once systematically rooted in medicine and law, it proved very hard to shake. Even Hirschfeld struggled to be free of it in his first expert report about an intersex patient, in 1904. Friederike Schmidt had lived her life as a woman, but in addition to labia and a vagina, she had a microphallus and mini testicles.* Hirschfeld's notes show that he advocated for a legal change of gender to male, which would provide social and economic advantages, but to his astonishment Schmidt refused; she "was shy of the attention this would attract and feared that she would lose her position, which she found comfortable"—most likely meaning her occupation or her living arrangements.[20]

Twenty years of experience taught Hirschfeld better. In 1924, German law required that Anna, an intersex patient with ambiguous genitalia but functioning internal testicles, be declared a man. Hirschfeld's testimony took the patient's side; since Anna "feels like a woman, looks like a woman, and loves a man whom she wishes to marry," then medicine had no right to disagree. "We have no right to say to a man who wants to be a woman: *You are a man*," he wrote, "or to command someone who wants to be a man: *Stay a woman*."[21]

If the body's glandular systems, its hormone-producing tissues, produce physical as well as psychological characteristics to varying degrees in various individuals—something that Starling's work and Steinach's tended to agree upon—then we should not be surprised to find varieties of gender. In addition to intermediate physical conditions, there would be intermediate psychological conditions. "I am of the opinion," Hirschfeld wrote of Friederike Schmidt, "that in such cases only mental behavior can be decisive for determining sex."[22] This he referred to as "psychological hermaphroditism," a mixture of different sexual "characters."

He went on to further differentiate four types: 1) *hermaphroditism genitalis*, those with intersex characteristics; 2) *hermaphroditismus somaticus*, those with an androgynous or "mixed" body type; 3) *hermaphroditism psychosexualis*, those with "mixed" sexual characteristics, by which he meant homosexuals; and 4) *hermaphroditism psychicus*, those with mixed psychic characters, something Hirschfeld

---

* Her photographs would later appear in the Institute's Wall of Transvestites, both a highly revealing photo where Hirschfeld pulls the labia away to reveal the microphallus (with Friederike's helping hand), and a triptych showing her in men's attire, semi-nude, and in women's attire.

sometimes calls "soul" and is related to how the person feels about their identity—the *Transvestiten* or transgender persons.[23] This expanded view is what allowed Hirschfeld and the staff of the Institute to declare "transvestite" patients "hermaphrodites" even in the absence of intersex genital formations.

We can see how terminology expanded to create space for complex and varied identities long before words like "transsexual" (coined in 1923 by Hirschfeld) or "transgender" (coined in the 1960s) came into popular usage. Most patients at the time would have called themselves transvestites, but being labeled a hermaphrodite—officially, by Hirschfeld—meant they could legally change their name. This has understandably introduced a lot of confusion for latter-day historians. The famous Lili Elbe, for instance, is sometimes described as intersex— she wasn't, but formal name registration required the "hermaphrodite" seal of medical approval.[24]

According to Haeckelian monism, all things begin in unity and branch out in diversity. Hirschfeld's unity is plurality. Already hidden in the germ—in the originary cell, rather—are all the ingredients for every variability. Even those who aligned with cultural expectations could be placed somewhere on the spectrum he created, not on a scale of normal-to-abnormal as in good-to-bad, but as evidence of brilliant natural diversity—even if the spectrum was still, in some ways, tethered to the man/woman binary.

ENTER DAS WUNDERLAND

A couple wait in the counseling room. They want a divorce on grounds of sexual incompatibility. The man complains that his wife won't have relations with him; she complains that he's impotent. Hirschfeld listens, makes suggestions, and advises them to give it another try before calling it quits. Down the hall, a woman has come for advice about contraception (still tightly controlled, even during the Weimar Republic), and a man is examined before referral for a Steinach rejuvenation procedure. Physicians meet with patients suffering from venereal disease, psychiatrists see those with troubled mental health, a homosexual man is treated by X-ray for removal of his beard, and "a considerable number" of *Transvestiten* come to Hirschfeld "just for advice."[25] Of the 3,500 patients who visited the Institute in its first year, Hirschfeld reported that at least 30 percent of them were intermediaries, among them homosexuals, intersex, and transgender people ("hermaphrodites" and "transvestites").[26] For them, the Institute of Sexual Science offered much more than mere medical treatment.

The Institute operated as a center—a hub. Artists, writers, thinkers, leftists, feminists, and activists toured the grounds, regaled by Karl Giese's descriptions of the sex toys in the museum and the books in the extensive archive. The erotica collection certainly turned heads, displaying whips, lingerie, high-heeled thigh boots, and masturbation devices (one powered by tricycle pedals). Self-described transvestites took tea on the grounds, staff dined below stairs, and the public turned up a few nights a week for Question Evenings—open discourse about sexual and medical matters. Then there were the private rooms for tête-à-têtes; Christopher Isherwood, novelist, playwright, and seemingly endless diarist, would pop round to Giese's sitting room with poet W. H. Auden and British archaeologist Francis Turville-Petre. It was just the place for coffee and gossip, especially on dark winter afternoons, a "cozy little nest lined with photographs and souvenirs" and Giese, "giggling [and] touching the back of his head with his fingertips, as if patting bobbed curls."[27] There were costume balls and Christmas parties, places to laugh and to play. The Institute had life in it and, increasingly, a significant piece of that life dressed, lived, and identified across expected gender lines.

Counseling for homosexuals and transvestites fell to one of three staff members: Hirschfeld, Arthur Kronfeld, or Felix Abraham. Most psychotherapy practiced at the time focused on the elimination of the same-sex drive. Hirschfeld instead developed something he called adaptation therapy, later referred to as psychic milieu therapy. In the case of *Transvestiten*, this meant allowing them to wear the clothing in which they felt most reassured and comfortable. The basis of treatment worked much the same for homosexuals; in the first place, Hirschfeld and his team would reassure the "homosexual personality" by explaining that "it has to do with an inborn orientation of the drive for which no one is to blame, which is not a misfortune in itself, but rather made so by the unjust prejudice" of others.[28] In the second place, Hirschfeld made sure to emphasize that a happy and fulfilled life was possible—the very thing Dora most longed for. Therein lies the joy and laughter of the Institute, the reason for balls and music and dinners and dancing. It's also the reason, today, for community networks and for making the right sort of friends.

Hans Grafe came to the Institute as a teenager.[29] He'd been sent there by his father, a medical doctor familiar with Hirschfeld's work. Hans would board at the Institute for a month for adaptation treatment, which, Hirschfeld explained, meant to steel him against such dangers as blackmail and threats, give him an awareness of himself and of proper comportment, and above all, prevent thoughts of suicide.[30] The point wasn't to cure him of his homosexuality but to help him live with it in a society where—despite all the SHC's efforts—homosexuality continued to be illegal and considered immoral.

The day often began with therapy, a session with Hirschfeld or another therapist (at least four a week). Then came induction into the network of intermediaries. Hans met Englishmen, other Germans, travelers visiting from abroad. He frequented the medical museum and the photographic material devoted to Hirschfeld's theory of intermediaries—enormous cabinets of filed folders with measurements and types intending to demonstrate 40 million variations on a theme. Then would come teatime and the importance of social mixing. Hans joined the staff, the patients, outside friends, visiting doctors and scholars, and of course several transvestites in colorful outfits. All of this, Hirschfeld explained, aimed at "bringing the patient into an environment which corresponds to what he is." For that reason, the day's therapy often ended with a trip to a gay bar, from which there were many to choose.[31]

We might be surprised at this sort of training, but supervised interactions at these establishments offered a safe way for young homosexuals to meet others. The elders could help them steer clear of bad influences and coach them on proper etiquette, not unlike a debutante's coming-out. The teenage Hans made his debut at the Bei Elli, in Skalitzerstrasse— relatively safe environs. There were more famous (and infamous) locales, like the Mikado or the Eldorado, which were also frequented by tourists. John Henry Mackay's novel *The Hustler* (1924) makes frequent reference to the Adonis Lounge, based on the Marienkasino, or Marie's Casino, which was full of "respectable" gay couples and also homosexual and transgender sex workers.

Hirschfeld makes plain that prostitution is as much a part of intermediary as of heteronormative culture, driven similarly by "a miserable livelihood, unemployment, lack of accommodation and probably greatest of all problems, hunger."[32] Did Hirschfeld intend that his teenage charge meet such characters while on nightly trips to Bei Elli? Yes he did, along with transvestites and blue-collar homosexuals, as Skalitzerstrasse bisected a working-class district.[33] (Isherwood and Turville-Petre preferred the Cosy Corner on Zossenerstrasse; also working-class, it suited Turville-Petre's eagerness to bargain for cheap sex workers.)[34] To sample the other side of the social spectrum, Hans would attend a grand ball at the Institute, just like the one in *Anders als die Andern*. Prominent, uncloseted intermediaries gathered to show their finery, sometimes with famous guests. On one occasion, Conrad Veidt himself made an appearance to drink champagne beneath the glittering chandeliers.[35] Adaptation therapy attempted to teach homosexual patients to accept and to enjoy themselves while remaining medically, physically, and legally safe.

For the *Transvestiten*, adaptation therapy took a similar course. Felix Abraham adopted Hirschfeld's approach, though in addition to counseling, he served as a medical advocate and cofounded the transvestite organization Vereinigung D'Eon (after Chevalier d'Eon, an eighteenth-century transgender French diplomat).[36] By the mid-1920s, even the word "transvestite" had undergone a radical shift; following Hirschfeld's own broadening of the terminology, transgender people increasingly used the word to refer to themselves. No longer a diagnosis, it had become an identity. As gender historian Katie Sutton writes, self-identified transvestites "constituted an increasingly vocal presence in German cultural life from the mid-1920s, not only organizing into associations with links to the contemporary homosexual rights movement, but also producing newspapers and magazines aimed at entertaining, encouraging, and furthering the political rights of 'like-minded' individuals."[37] The transvestites at the Institute were encouraged to meet others with their inclination—to make friends, to meet for tea, to wear their favorite clothes and discuss fashion, and above all, to be themselves.

BUT WHERE ARE THE WOMEN?

Nearly all of Hirschfeld's transvestite patients were assigned male at birth and wished to wear the clothing of women. In general, women and those assigned female at birth are pushed to the margins. The stories of Louis and Katharina T. are among the few female-to-male cases mentioned by Hirschfeld. That doesn't mean that there weren't far more cases, only that Hirschfeld's interest in women was somewhat peripheral; he rarely speaks about lesbians, either, despite the fact that women were increasingly involved in the SHC and its work. Hirschfeld joined forces with them for good reasons; Stöcker and other sexologists and feminists like Henriette Fürth, Grete Meisel-Hess, Adele Schreiber, and Mathilde Vaerting were veritable powerhouses of activism.[38] So where were the lesbians and female-to-male transvestites? With little attention paid to them by either science or the law, they largely spoke for themselves.

Three different lesbian magazines circulated in the Weimar years, sometimes including serialized novels and poems as well as essays. They boasted female staffers and editors, and one of them—*Girlfriend*—had 7,000 subscribers. In 1928, Ruth Roellig published *Berlin's Lesbian Women* as a guidebook, including clubs for lesbians and also for female-to-male transvestites; soon short novels appeared, along with plays and even a film, *Mädchen in Uniform*. Lesbians were visible enough in the

Weimar era to raise complaints from conservatives who regarded them as proof of moral decline. Social clubs celebrated "girlfriends" with dances and cruises, evening parties and "transvestite balls." Historian Laurie Marhoefer writes that "the fact that social clubs enjoyed a lot of success while more explicitly political groups did not" misleads some into thinking that lesbians were apolitical; they weren't. Women, some of whom were uncloseted lesbians, had been members of the SHC for years, and they joined other rights groups as well, even though Paragraph 175 didn't apply to them. The social clubs themselves had political significance, including social welfare and social reform; for lesbians and gender nonconformists, the social and the political were intertwined.[39]

Lesbian leader Ruth Roellig wrote that her club's mission was "to offer the same-sex-loving woman a kind of home" and a shield to protect "differently oriented" women.[40] The lesbian subculture also provided space for transvestite culture; two magazines especially for male-to-female transvestites appeared as inserts inside *Girlfriend* and a related publication, *Garçonne*. Transvestites had their own societies, too, such as the League of Human Rights' Coalition of Transvestites and the German Friendship Association's Vereinigung D'Eon.[41] The ability to share through media and meetings meant that people could discuss and debate how, exactly, they interpreted their chosen identities. Were you a transvestite only if you wished to dress in the clothes of the opposite sex? Or did it refer to those whose "true" sex wasn't their birth sex— people like Dora, who wanted to transition from one to the other? How did that relate to sexual orientation? They weren't the only ones asking; Hirschfeld had been trying to codify and differentiate between identities for years.

Most of his patients who were assigned male at birth and transitioning to female still sought relationships with women. Today, we would consider them to be lesbians, but Hirschfeld considered them heterosexual, as it was then the practice to assign sexual desire to the original sex identity. As a result, he deduced that a primary feature of transvestism must be heterosexuality. Yet even then, he could not claim this was universal. Significant differences between heterosexual and homosexual male-to-female transvestites existed, and caused serious rifts about what terminology should be used by each group. It was, to say the least, confusing; it could also be divisive. So-called heterosexual (attracted to women) male-to-female transvestites refused to associate with so-called homosexual ones, and so-called homosexual transvestites remained suspicious of the so-called heterosexuals, mistrusting their desire to live as women.[42] In trying to defuse the constant conflicts that erupted around masculinity, Hirschfeld separated male-to-female transvestites, with their performative femininity, from homosexuals who might, like Brand, eschew all things feminine—while remaining circumspect about most female-to-male cases.

This only drove the wedge further. Masculinists distanced themselves from the "feminine" transvestites; so-called heterosexual transvestites rejected the concept of homosexuality and even tried to claim a moral high ground—what Sutton calls the "respectability imperative." Marie Weis, leader of the Vereinigung D'Eon, claimed that "genuine" transvestites conformed to the binary ideal of the modest woman—meaning that she disdained those who were of lower socioeconomic standing as well as those who could not "pass." Those attitudes, Sutton argues, necessarily led to peer policing, division, and insiders vs. outsiders—the very tensions that had once split the SHC.[43]

The neat theoretical categories Hirschfeld designed, and the moral standards called for by upper-class (frequently self-identifying heterosexual) transvestite groups, simply didn't hold; they sidelined homosexual male-to-female transvestites (i.e., those who desired men) and very nearly erased female transvestites. Those who didn't fit into orderly categories were, writes Sutton, "excluded from the terms of 1920s transvestite citizenship." What started as a union between male-to-female transvestites and lesbians never extended to homosexuals in general; heterosexual transvestites who engaged in feminine dress nevertheless described themselves as "normal" and "manly." Masculinity still managed to define a subculture "whose one shared point of identification was its challenge to gender normativity."[44] Part of that normativity meant accepting the genitals you were born with; "respectable" hetero transvestites were still men, and they used that position of power to critique homosexual transvestites for having too much femininity. How dare they want to change their bodies?

It had become clear that the terminology needed shifting; the word "transvestite," at least, didn't cover all the divergences. Hirschfeld compromised by describing people who wanted a surgical realignment as "total" or "extreme" transvestites. He also described his hesitancy about such procedures; he considered them "both very dangerous and unnecessary."[45] That would change in 1923, not because of new discoveries in endocrinology, or the political goals of the SHC, or the machinations of their enemies. Transgender people advocated for the change themselves. The world's first gender affirmation surgeries would take place with Hirschfeld's blessing and the Institute's support due to the earnest wishes of patients—patients like Dora, the blue-eyed girl from Saxony.

Once again, everything, everywhere, was about to change.

9

1923 IN FOUR ACTS

WE LIKE OUR STORIES TO HAVE BEGINNINGS, MIDDLES, ENDS. HIS-
tory gives us none of these. It provides instead repetition, variations on a
theme, and something we might call entanglement.

The Weimar government stood on shifting sand. Divisions had widened between factions, and unrest grew as Germany struggled to meet
the reparations demanded by the Treaty of Versailles. Tensions ran high,
the economy threatened to collapse, and Germany seemed on the edge
of civil war—again. In the midst of the chaos, the SHC would band
together with their sometime opponents, the masculinists, in an attempt
to finally sway the teetering Reichstag. And in the south, an Austrian
orator with a Charlie Chaplin mustache would go from "unimportant
agitator" to rising politician. The year is 1923, and four stories are about
to find their point of convergence.

ACT 1: TROUBLE IN THE RUHR

In accordance with the Treaty of Versailles, Germany owed reparations
in cash and in kind (coal, timber, chemicals, dyes, pharmaceuticals) for
the damages wrought by the war.[1] Germany asked for a moratorium
on payments; exhausted by the war and the seemingly never-ending
postwar crises, it didn't have the resources. Meanwhile, the value of
the Deutschmark sank precipitously, meaning that more of them were
required to meet the minimum payment.[2] Taxes could only be raised so
much—and the German people already resented the treaty's exacting
conditions (especially since Austria and Hungary, now separate nations,
were not held to the same punitive standards). Negotiations broke down,

and the Inter-Allied Reparations Commission found Germany guilty of default. France had the excuse it had been waiting for, and 45,000 French and Belgian troops marched into the Ruhr Valley in January 1923.

On the doorstep of Belgium and the Netherlands, the Ruhr Valley was declared a demilitarized zone by the Treaty of Versailles. German troops could not enter either to police or to protect it. This valley, fifty kilometers across, was modest in size, but it was among the most valuable land in all of Germany. Black seams of coal ribboned the ground beneath, and industrial smokestacks clouded the sky above; home of refineries, steel mills, and armaments manufacture, the Ruhr drove the German economy. It had lifted the Krupp family to its place of power; it had provided the raw materials for mortar shells in the Franco-Prussian War; it had weaponized Germany in the First World War.[3] To the rest of the world, the Ruhr represented both economic and military might. So, when Germany defaulted on reparation payments, France and Belgium seized their moment—and the cities of Düsseldorf and Duisburg.

This had no doubt been the plan all along; relations between France and Germany—never rosy—had degraded to simmering hatred. The last thing Allied neighbors wanted was a robust German nation; crippling the economy and cutting Berlin off from natural resources meant forestalling a "war of revenge."[4] At the same time, adding the Ruhr's coal riches to its own iron ore meant that France could claim a position of power in Europe while simultaneously breaking the back of its enemy.

With the protection of the Allied demilitarized zone, it seemed that victory was in sight for the occupiers—but they hadn't counted on the unions. Mining operators, civil servants, transport workers, and others simply refused to obey the occupiers' orders. Trade unions led with passive resistance and withdrawal of labor; railwaymen left their posts and sabotaged tracks, engines, and signals as they went. French troops tried to seize the means of transport, arrested and court-martialed various actors, but even when able to run trains found that the general public boycotted them.

In an attempt to control communications, the French banned German newspapers in the Ruhr. That didn't help either; volunteers took on the dangerous role of distributing news leaflets under cover. When French troops seized the mines, workers siphoned off benzole through sewers into unoccupied territory, while others covered coke reserves with mud and hid ammonia underground. Outmaneuvered, France responded by sending more troops, and then by seizing property. Coal would be shoveled into trucks, a skeleton rail service would be reinstated, homes and schools seized, and machinery and goods requisitioned. The invasion of the Krupp factories was the first blood spilled in the occupation.

On March 31, 1923, Easter Saturday, shots rang out in the Altendorferstrasse garage of the Krupp Works in Essen. Troops had come to seize automobiles stored there, and a fight ensued. In the midst of the skirmish, a French lieutenant gave orders to open fire. Thirteen people were killed, eleven of them where they stood, with two others dying in hospital shortly after. The funeral attracted hundreds, with long processions of mourners in black following the plumed coffins. But it wasn't over. French officials laid the blame upon chairman of the board Gustav Krupp. He would be ambushed and abducted, put on trial, and sentenced to ten to twenty years in prison. With Krupp and others publicly convicted, the Ruhr's willingness to resist faltered. The French enforced new regulations to bolster weakened German laws and prevented anyone from leaving occupied territory, by force if necessary. They changed the currency to the franc, made resistance of any kind illegal, ended free speech, and enforced a five-year prison sentence for refusing—or even doubting—orders by French authorities. The local economy crumbled. German citizens had no food, and the already beleaguered Reich was forced to send supplies to stave off starvation. They sent money too, hidden in luggage with false walls, inside shoes, and even in a fire engine. Unfortunately, there wasn't enough to go around.

Wilhelm Cuno, acting chancellor of Germany, hoped that strikes in the Ruhr would damage the French economy and compel France to withdraw. However, both France and Belgium had Allied support. When coal didn't come from the Ruhr, they imported it from Britain. In the end, even Germany was forced to do the same. The strikes did have a powerful effect on the economy, but the most damage was done within Germany. Industry in the Ruhr, the beating heart of Germany's wealth, collapsed and unemployment soared. The government printed banknotes—even the cities of the Ruhr printed banknotes—but they weren't backed by anything tangible and soon were worth less than the paper and ink. Food riots broke out across the nation as people shopped desperately against the falling Deutschmark. Germans resorted to looting and theft in cities, while armed bands raided farms in the countryside.[5]

Inflation had destroyed the mark (or rather, the *papiermark*, as it was no longer backed by gold). In one anecdote, a student at Freiburg University went to a café for a cup of coffee priced at 5,000 marks, then decided on a second; when the bill came, it amounted to 14,000 marks. If you want to save money, he was told, order both cups at once. In another, a workman described the turmoil of payday: "At 11 in the morning a siren sounded, and everybody gathered in the factory forecourt, where a five-ton lorry was drawn up loaded brimful with paper money. The chief cashier and his assistants climbed up on top. They read out names and just threw out bundles of notes. As soon as you had caught one you made a dash for the nearest shop and bought just anything that was going"—before the prices went up again, and again.[6]

Germany, driven to its knees and hemorrhaging money, was ripe for another revolution. The British ambassador to Berlin reported to London that "almost everybody was in favour of a restoration of the monarchy" or, indeed, "any man who appears to know what he wants and issues commands in a loud bold voice."[7] Cuno resigned in August; the new chancellor, Gustav Stresemann, ended passive resistance in the Ruhr. To halt the runaway devaluation, he introduced a new currency: the *Rentenmark*, equal to an astonishing one trillion papiermarks and backed not by gold but by real estate (land used for agriculture and business). It would be his only win in what was now a four-way war against "the invaders, against inflation and hunger, against Communists, and against separatists."[8] The once united front against France and Belgium in the Ruhr had crumbled.

France was now pushing for a "Rhenish republic"* free of

---

* The river Ruhr is a tributary of the Rhine. The suggested "Rhenish republic" would have encompassed the whole of the Rhineland, including the Ruhr Valley.

Germany—and in the rest of the nation, fury at the Weimar government's capitulation to foreign demands caused both the Communists and the right-wing German Nationalist Party to denounce the republic.[9] Stresemann responded by declaring martial law—but the regions of Bavaria, Saxony, and Thuringia flatly refused to obey. In October, a paramilitary group called the Black Reichswehr attempted a coup in the eastern state of Brandenburg. That putsch failed, but there would be more. One month later, Adolf Hitler stepped to the podium in a Munich beer hall intent on overthrowing the Weimar.

ACT 2: THE BEER HALL PUTSCH

Bavaria, the largest state in Germany, representing approximately one-fifth of the country's overall area, remained deeply conservative. It had resisted the Weimar government and continued to operate very much on its own. When Chancellor Stresemann abandoned the Ruhrkampf defensive on September 26, 1923, Ritter Gustav von Kahr, leader of Bavaria's League of Patriotic Societies, determined to sever those ties more thoroughly. Kahr had served as Bavaria's prime minister; now he took over as General State Commissioner, a role with dictatorial power.[10] Bavaria, he claimed, would once more be an independent monarchy—an act of treason against the Reich.[11] Berlin didn't have the financial means or manpower to stand firm against this rebellion; it looked to be the final crisis of the Weimar Republic, and Stresemann's government began to fall to pieces. But Kahr never completed secession. He didn't have the chance.

On November 8, 1923, a crowd gathered outside the Bürgerbräukeller, or "citizen brew cellar," one of the largest beer halls in Germany.[12] Inside, Kahr planned to give an address articulating the confused political situation and the aims of his regime. The Bürgerbräukeller grand hall could seat 3,000 people under chandeliers hanging from the steel-supported ceiling; it filled to capacity. Those turned away huddled near the entrance and blocked the streets, but Kahr rejected the idea of having the only remaining military, the Reichswehr—a small group of defenders, limited by treaty to under 100,000 men—serve as guards. It might look weak, or as though he feared his own people. As a result, a police detachment of about 150 remained outside.

Inside the hall, a mixed assortment of Bavarian civilians gathered along with businessmen, bankers, manufacturers, and press—and some of the most politically important men in the region. The sun had long set and introductory speeches came to an end; Kahr took the podium.

At a little past eight in the evening, Adolf Hitler arrived at the beer hall. The crowds and the police presence didn't suit his evening plans, however. He approached one of the officers and made a "helpful" suggestion: such a rowdy group, most of them well into their beer tankards, might incite panic—why not have the waiting police clear the streets? The officer agreed. Off went the police to disperse the crowd, leaving the streets in shadow-cloaked darkness. Then, exactly on cue, the trucks began to arrive. Hitler went inside to hear the speech as 55,000 of his own followers and 4,000 *Sturmabteilung* (shortened to SA or Storm Troops in English) surrounded the hall.[13] Any remaining police were stunned into inaction by men in steel helmets carrying army rifles. Everyone inside the Bürgerbräukeller was now a prisoner; they just didn't know it yet.

Kahr droned on, rehashing earlier talking points with an additional denunciation of Marxism. Hitler waited in the antechamber with a glass of beer, like any other guest, until Ulrich Graf arrived to give him the all-clear. It was time for theatrics. Hitler smashed the glass to the floor and pulled out his Browning pistol. Together with his bodyguards, he pushed his way through the throng to the podium—arriving just as a battery of additional Storm Troopers blocked the entrance with a machine gun. He marshaled Kahr and his associates into the next room, where he encouraged them to support his coup by promise and by threat. "There are five rounds" in the pistol, he told Kahr, smiling, "four for traitors, and, if it fails, one for me."

Small-scale negotiations had never been Hitler's strong suit, however; when Kahr proved recalcitrant, Hitler returned to the anxious, captive crowd. They threatened to bolt in confusion, so Hitler fired a shot into the plaster ceiling as a warning: there would be order! An eyewitness account recorded by historian Karl-Alexander von Müller described the strange scene as it unfolded.

Hitler spoke softly. Perhaps this ensured the room's silence, as people strained to hear. He had nothing against Kahr, he told them, and Kahr would of course remain regent in Bavaria. But a new German government must be formed. As he spoke, the emotion in the room began to shift. What had been a dangerous energy diffused and realigned. "Hitler turned them inside out, as one turns a glove inside out," wrote the eyewitness; "it had something of hocus-pocus, or magic about it." After mere minutes, applause roared forth, and with it Hitler raised his voice: "Outside are Kahr, Lossow, and Seisser. They are struggling to reach a decision. May I say to them that you will stand behind them?" Yes! Yes! came the answer. Now, full of emotion, Hitler shouted over the crowd: "In a free Germany, there is also room for an autonomous Bavaria! I can say this to you: either the German revolution begins tonight or we will all be dead by dawn!"

Having won the crowd, he also won Kahr—who had no choice. Once loyalty had been pledged, Hitler returned to the crowd. "I am going to fulfill the vow I made to myself five years ago," he thundered, "to know neither rest nor peace until the November criminals had been overthrown, until on the ruins of the wretched Germany of today there should have arisen once more a Germany of power and greatness, of freedom and splendor." Then, however, he made an error: he left the hall to oversee difficulties at the army barracks, where the Storm Troopers had been unable to shift the German soldiers. Hitler's commanding charisma faded in his absence; the crowd dispersed and Kahr escaped. The next day, Kahr sided with the Weimar government against Hitler.

The putsch was over as quickly as it had begun. It resulted in the death of sixteen Nazis and three police officers; Hitler himself suffered a dislocated shoulder (and was saved from worse by his bodyguard). He would be arrested two nights later, on the 11th, and taken to Landsberg, another city in Bavaria, for trial. The coup had not been well planned; the surprise was not its failure but that it occurred at all. To many, Hitler's popularity seemed to come out of nowhere.

In 1920, the German National Socialistic Workmen's Party, as it was officially known, had been "making itself rather conspicuous" to the British consul in Munich, who noted that the group had a violent turn and seemed virulently anti-Semitic—but its leader was "little known" and little cause for concern. Even in 1922, Hitler was dismissed as a "chauvinistic but rather unimportant agitator," almost "comic" and beneath real notice.[14] Hitler didn't have the family connections or political clout of Kahr; he hadn't even finished his education. After trying and failing to get into art school, he lived a precarious, bohemian life by scraping together funds painting postcards and advertisements. He was even rejected by the military during the First World War because he lacked "physical vigor," but he successfully petitioned to join the 16th Bavarian Reserve Infantry Regiment later in the conflict. Gassed at the Second Battle of Ypres, he ended the war in hospital, but not before earning two Iron Crosses for "bravery in action."[15]

These were his first real accolades; little wonder that he adopted the *Männerbund* belief that war would make boys into men. Hitler admired the discipline and camaraderie of the military and had found ready friends in Munich, where disbanded and dissatisfied Freikorps had gathered. British diplomats still thought of him as "unbalanced"—even a "clown."[16] Yet, in less than a year, he'd become the face of a dispirited population. British consul general William Seeds warned that the middle classes "look upon him as their Mussolini"—the man who had just led a successful coup in Italy and introduced fascism.[17] Now, the Bavarians had their own demagogue. They wanted a powerful leader, a Führer who would retake the nation from the liberal-minded Social Democrats—by any means necessary. Seeds predicted that Hitler would never bow to Kahr and sent probably the most prescient warning ever delivered: "The governing parties in Bavaria," he wrote, "are faced by a Frankenstein monster, originally of their own creation, with which they may well prove powerless to deal."[18]

With Hitler's arrest, many assumed the battle was at an end. They couldn't have been more wrong. A public trial was coming, and Hitler knew how to work the public. On the day of his arrest a message circulated among his followers, supposedly from his hand: "Germans, be united and faithful. Do not desert the Fatherland!—Hitler." On November 11, 1923, a new order was given, this time by Walter Buch, a Storm Troops official under Hitler. It read as follows:

> The first period of the national revolution is over. It has brought the desired clearing [of the air]. Our highly revered leader, Adolf Hitler, has again bled for the German people. The most shameful treachery that the world has ever seen has victimized him and the German people. Through Hitler's blood and the steel directed against our comrades in Munich by the hands of traitors the patriotic combat units are welded together for better or for worse. The second phase of the national revolution begins [now].

The second phase would involve placards, newspapers with false fronts to disguise Nazi communication, speeches in the streets, and leaflets "handed to passers-by, thrown into barracks, dropped from airplanes." Before Hitler had spent a full night in prison, the Nazi propaganda machine was fully operational.[19]

ACT 3: THE ACTION COMMITTEE

When tensions began to rise over reparations and the conflict in the Ruhr, Social Democrats lost a considerable number of seats in the Reichstag and no longer held a majority. A coalition government followed, with far more conservative ministers of justice. Luckily, from Magnus Hirschfeld's point of view, the new chancellor, Joseph Wirth, remained well left of center; he was an enemy of the growing nationalist parties and committed to democracy and the republic. But would he risk his tenuous hold for the sake of homosexual emancipation? It seemed unlikely.

Hirschfeld had become the face of homosexual emancipation. But he had also become the old man of the movement, and the SHC itself a conservative elder. If Paragraph 175 was ever to be rescinded, fast action was needed—and the old guard needed new blood. That meant courting younger, more assertive homosexual societies. At the SHC's general meeting in 1920, Kurt Hiller—a younger and more radical member of the SHC—stated the case in no uncertain terms: all pro-homosexual associations must unite as an Action Committee, including the German Friendship Society and Adolf Brand's self-owners, the Gemeinschaft der Eigenen.[20]

The German Friendship Society was everything the SHC was not: fresh, heavily populated by youth, open about its sexuality, and broad in its support base. It had formed from the merger of numerous "friendship leagues" in Berlin, Dresden, Düsseldorf, Frankfurt, Stuttgart, Hamburg, and Hanover. They had no wish to merge with the SHC, which was made up almost entirely of professionals and scientists, many of them closeted; they preferred mass public involvement.[21] The Gemeinschaft der Eigenen didn't hold much affinity for the SHC either—more like a quietly simmering disdain—but the Action Committee needed them even more than the Friendship Society. If they planned to reach politically conservative homosexuals and overcome the problem of homosexual feminization introduced by Hirschfeld and supported by Steinach's endocrinology, they needed to make amends—again. It might seem a very unlikely union.

The German penal code had been redrafted, and the draft was published in 1921 before being debated in the Reichstag. It not only upheld Paragraph 175, it also dealt a serious blow to the science of sexology by claiming that homosexual acts were both "reprehensible" and "worthy of punishment" whether or not homosexuality was an inborn disposition.[22] In the eyes of the law, same-sex love remained pathological—and illegal. Frustrated and furious, Brand conceded to join the fight with the SHC, as did the Friendship Society. Meetings of the Action Committee would still be held at the Institute for Sexual Science, as the first of many soon-to-be established sexual clinics and as the clear leader in public health campaigns with government approval (stopping the spread of sexually transmitted diseases, eugenic counseling, and the care of mothers and infants had unilateral support).[23]

The first order of business was to create their own propaganda. There would be press statements, counterstatements, lectures, and pamphlet drops. The Action Committee would also rewrite the penal code and submit it to the Reichstag commission as a counteroffensive. Meanwhile, it seemed that the best strategy would be to begin abroad—gain international status, such that national support must follow. In a clever move, the First International Conference for Sexual Reform on a Sexual-Scientific Basis was held from September 15 to 20, 1921. This wasn't just the first such meeting to take place in Germany; it was the first international meeting of any kind since the beginning of the First World War. Representatives arrived from Holland, Sweden, Switzerland, Austria, Czechoslovakia, Russia, Italy, and even Japan, and the arrangement of topics made Paragraph 175 a principal focus.[24] By design, the conference made Germany look good, once more a significant player on the world stage of scientific endeavor; meanwhile, the content of its panels made legislation against homosexuality look bad. Therein lies the genius of it: officials wanted to fête the convention as a credit to the nation but could hardly do so without acknowledging that its focus criticized the redrafted law.

The mind—and might—behind the Action campaign was not Hirschfeld's. Ostensibly the SHC remained the parent group, but this "new phase of political action" fell once more to Kurt Hiller.[25] Hiller, who was younger, rather dashing, and steeped in legal and political matters as a jurist and journalist, took his contribution even further. He compared anti-Semitism (directed at Jewish minorities) to anti-homosexuality (directed at sexual minorities), and called Paragraph 175 the "anti-Semitism of its century."[26] A gauntlet had been thrown down. The Action Committee would aspire to be the antithesis of the Nazis; they planned to fight for homosexual and Jewish rights and, by their next conference, for women's rights as well.

Hiller, himself also Jewish and homosexual, did not align entirely with Hirschfeld's theories. Like Brand, he disagreed with the strategy of relying on the biological argument as the basis of homosexual rights. That reliance had—partly due to Steinach—reshackled homosexuality to pathology, even as it freed it from the panic of gay contagion. More than this, it had not been effective; under the proposed new law, whether you were born with a particular orientation didn't matter. The law aimed to get rid of the orientation altogether, either through "cure" or eugenic breeding selection. Hiller preferred the Nietzschean concept of sovereign individuals living "free from the collective moral restraints" of both the public and the state.[27] He struck a balance between the members, with masculinist individualism on one side and Hirschfeldian science on the other. When the conference ended, Hiller circulated the findings—which demanded the elimination of penalty for sexual offenses—to justices, ministers of the German states, and various Reichstag parties.[28] Then, the Action Committee invited Reichstag members to the Institute itself, not only to hear Hirschfeld but to hear from his intermediaries.

On November 11, 1921, the Institute's presentation hall hosted representatives of government—those who would rule on the legality not just of actions but of identities. Before them, a small group of men and women awaited their turn at the podium; they had volunteered to share intimate details and feelings, to be publicly vulnerable. The first was a homosexual man who gave listeners "an image of his emotional/inner life." Next came a man already accused under Paragraph 175; two days hence, he might no longer be a free man. One by one they told stories of suffering and persecution, about families that rejected them or tried to have them forcibly cured. Then, at the end, two couples emerged—a pair of women and a pair of men. They explained their love to the crowd, their happy hours, the joy of being together as succor against a hard world. When they finished their moving testimonies, the Action Committee put forward their petition against the new law, and asked—if the listeners had any heart to be moved—if they would sign it. Many did. One of them was Gustav Radbruch, the Reich Minister of Justice.[29]

Radbruch styled himself a legal philosopher and served on the faculties of several universities. Influenced by neo-Kantian principles, he believed that law was defined by constantly changing moral values.[30] Concepts like "right" and "just" weren't absolute, but relative to time and place. Heather Leawoods, of the University of Washington School of Law, summarizes his outlook this way: "only by allowing the individual, in truly extraordinary times, to take the moral stand that a legal system has gone too far will citizens truly protect themselves from the intolerable perversions" of their leaders.[31] Radbruch saw, in the Action Committee and in the personal stories of homosexuals, individuals taking just such a moral stand. As the year ended, he invited Hirschfeld to a private meeting. There, he encouraged him not to worry about the draft penal code; it was a "private work." The "government draft" would be different, but it wouldn't be ready until autumn 1922.[32] It may seem a brush-off, but then Radbruch did something truly surprising. He promised to involve Hirschfeld in the final discussion over Paragraph 175. Would Hirschfeld agree to speak before the Reichstag in March to inform other party leaders?

He most certainly would, and with him came Heinrich Kopp, the Berlin Criminal Commissioner and detective superintendent, another signatory of the petition. Hirschfeld's speech gave the scientific basis for eliminating Paragraph 175; Kopp lectured on the law's untenability from the standpoint of a practicing criminologist. By the summer of 1922, the Institute had become the "premier lobbying institute on the subject of homosexuality," hosting police detectives from all of Germany's larger cities and providing lectures to the public.[33] The Action Committee had finally moved the needle; in October, Radbruch delivered a more liberal draft of the law, and for the first time, non-prostitution homosexual acts between consenting adult men would not be punished. He planned to introduce it for debate in the Reichstag. The one thing all factions agreed upon—the overturning of Paragraph 175—might finally be realized, and for a time, positivity papered over the schisms within the Action Committee itself.

Well, almost. The Friendship Society had begun to fracture from within. Many members broke away to form the League for Human Rights, which quickly outgrew its origin group. For the League, the fight was not primarily about sexuality; it was a fight for the rights of "legal individuals."[34] Some of this agreed with Hiller's stance; the League wanted mass organization, true politicization, and active attempts at liberation. Unlike Hiller, however, the League dismissed the scientific outlook as useless to their cause. Neither did they care to align with the "aesthetics" of masculine friend-love. Leaders of the League for Human Rights renounced the chief publication of the Friendship Society as "insufficiently political" and founded their own publication on three principal goals: 1) to produce and distribute "propaganda" on homosexuality (something which the SHC approved of); 2) to explain the legal dimensions to other homosexuals; and, most importantly, 3) to organize the masses in favor of political rights for "respectable" homosexuals.[35]

Respectable. The word returns, as it did in the divide between heterosexual and homosexual transvestite culture, as it did in the words of Helene Stöcker and the feminists. The new League for Human Rights didn't want rights for all humans. They believed the law should protect "law-abiding" homosexual citizens, as opposed to the "socially disruptive" subculture of prostitutes, their clientele, and *Tunte*—that is, effeminate homosexuals. Hirschfeld—who was known to familiars at the Institute as Tante (Aunt) Magnesia—fell into that last camp. So, too, did Dora Richter. The rift that tore apart the SHC years earlier had come full circle. No one could keep the components of the Action Committee from rocketing apart at the first strain—and a strain of magnitude was about to rock the entire nation.

AS THE YEAR 1923 approached, the proposed new penal code still had not come up for debate. We return to the winter stalemate over the Ruhr: Germany had defaulted on reparations, France threatened retribution, and French and Belgian forces occupied cities in the valley. Chancellor Wirth had run his campaign on fulfillment of the Treaty of Versailles; this now seemed both impossible and deeply unpopular. His own party leaders doubted him; he probably doubted himself. Unable to find a solution to Germany's debts, Wirth resigned, and the coalition government that had allowed the Social Democrats to retain some semblance of power collapsed.[36] Wilhelm Cuno took over, restructured the government, and replaced minister of justice Gustav Radbruch with the far more conservative Rudolf Heinze. There would be no debate. The penal code passed to the executive branch, where it stalled indefinitely. Christmas came and Christmas went, and nine days into January, troops rolled into the Ruhr and the Deutschmark began its precipitous decline. Germany had entered into crisis, and so had the Action Committee. All their work had been for naught, and Adolf Brand once again broke ranks with the SHC.

The League for Human Rights reported Brand's resignation in their journal; he "had come to the impossible and alienating view," they wrote, that the "grave distress" of the Fatherland must take precedence over any fight for homosexual rights.[37] In other words, the masculinists sided with nationalists against the left-leaning liberal politics of the other groups. This presaged dangerous allegiances to come. *Der Eigene* had fostered, published, and supported anti-Semitic views, just as Hans Blüher had done; the masculinist–nationalist did not depart overmuch from sentiments at home in the Nazi party. Brand's beliefs were influenced by Ewald Tscheck, a young man who "flirted" with the fledgling Nazis and likely joined Hitler's Storm Troops in 1924. Tscheck had been introduced to Hitlerism by Karl-Günther Heimsoth, the lover of Ernst Röhm, Hitler's right-hand man.[38] These seemingly loose connections would have consequences for the Institute as yet undreamt of—but for now, the loss of Brand was trouble enough. Without him, the center would not hold; a last gasp of cooperative energy went into the Action Committee's April conference, where the SHC and the League for Human Rights attempted to sort out separate spheres. They couldn't overcome the new terrain of limited funds and political instability. In the end, all three groups would compete rather than collaborate.

Hirschfeld returned to his little kingdom at the Institute. The SHC had been on the cusp of a victory three decades in the making; now, they waited to see if the Institute itself could remain afloat. In 1918, the exchange rate had been 4.2 marks to the dollar; on January 9,

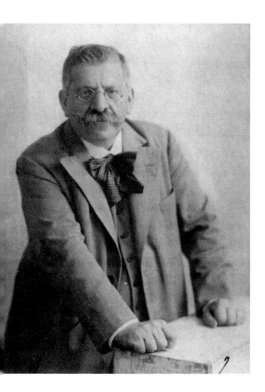

Dr. Magnus Hirschfeld, circa 1927.
COURTESY OF MAGNUS-HIRSCHFELD-
GESELLSCHAFT E.V., BERLIN.

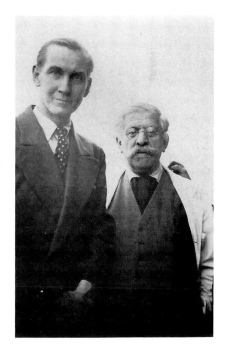

Karl Giese and Magnus Hirschfeld. COURTESY OF
MAGNUS-HIRSCHFELD-GESELLSCHAFT E.V., BERLIN.

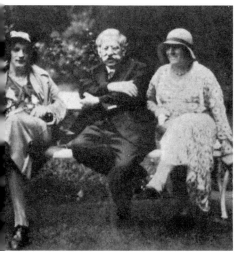

Magnus Hirschfeld and two *Transvestiten* outside
the Institute for Sexual Science. On the right is
Dora Richter. VOILÀ / GALLIMARD, PUBLIC DOMAIN.
COURTESY OF MAGNUS-HIRSCHFELD-GESELLSCHAFT
E.V., BERLIN.

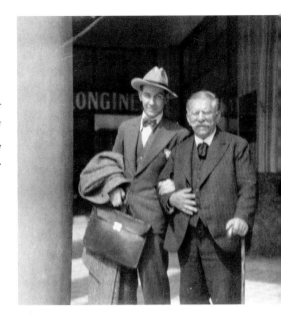

Magnus Hirschfeld with his partner Karl Giese, 1934. COURTESY OF MAGNUS-HIRSCHFELD-GESELLSCHAFT E.V., BERLIN.

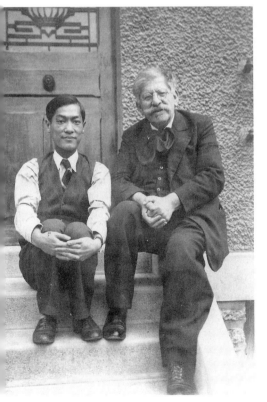

Magnus Hirschfeld and Tao Li in Nice, 1935. COURTESY OF MAGNUS-HIRSCHFELD-GESELLSCHAFT E.V., BERLIN.

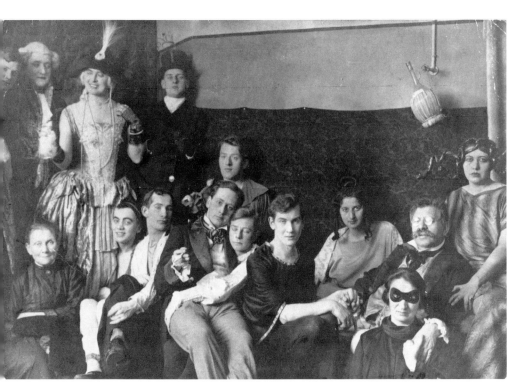

...stume party at the Institute for Sexual Science in Berlin, date unknown. Magnus Hirschfeld (in ...asses) holds hands with his partner, Karl Giese (center). COURTESY OF MAGNUS-HIRSCHFELD-...ESELLSCHAFT E.V., BERLIN.

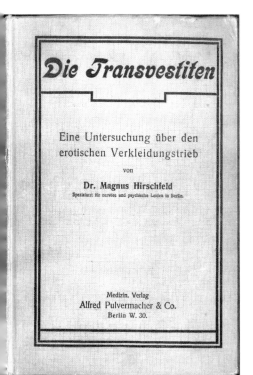

Die Transvestiten by Magnus Hirschfeld, 1910. COURTESY OF MAGNUS-HIRSCHFELD-GESELLSCHAFT E.V., BERLIN.

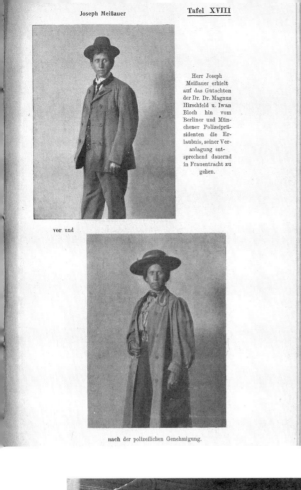

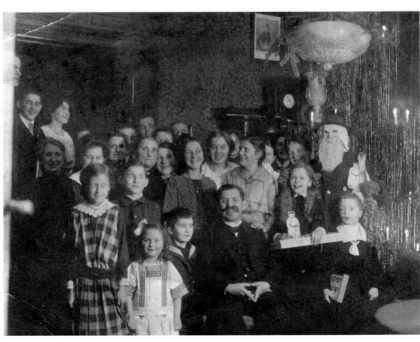

Dr. Magnus Hirschfeld with children of the domestic personnel at the Institute,
Christmas, 1917. COURTESY OF MAGNUS-HIRSCHFELD-GESELLSCHAFT E.V., BERLIN.

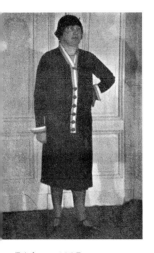

ra Richter, 1927.

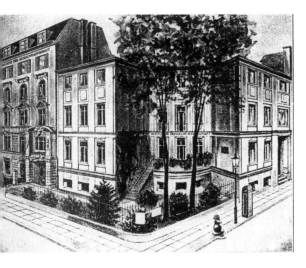

Dora Richter in dance costume
in Dr. Kankeleit's pamphlet,
December 1927.

The Institute for Sexual Science,
c. 1921. COURTESY OF MAGNUS-
HIRSCHFELD-GESELLSCHAFT E.V.,
BERLIN.

The wall of sexual interme-
diaries, 1928. COURTESY OF
MAGNUS-HIRSCHFELD-
GESELLSCHAFT E.V., BERLIN.

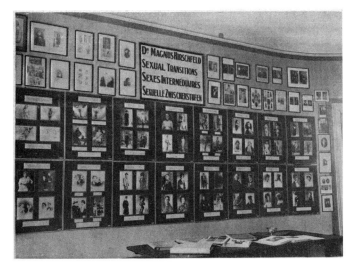

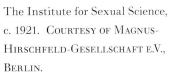

Magnus Hirschfeld's fourth, seventh, and sixth patients, c. 1910. Originally published In *Die Transvetiten*.

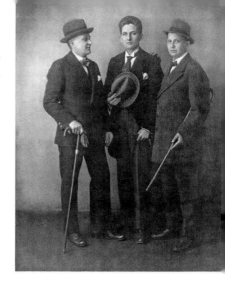

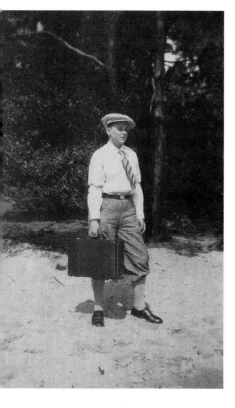

Gerd Katter (born Eva Katter), one of Magnus Hirschfeld's transgender patients at the Institute for Sexual Science, c. 1929.
COURTESY OF MAGNUS-HIRSCHFELD-GESELLSCHAFT E.V., BERLIN.

Hirschfeld's medical assessment of Gerd Katter under his birthname, Eva, enabling him to get a transvestite certificate.
COURTESY OF MAGNUS-HIRSCHFELD-GESELLSCHAFT E.V., BERLIN.

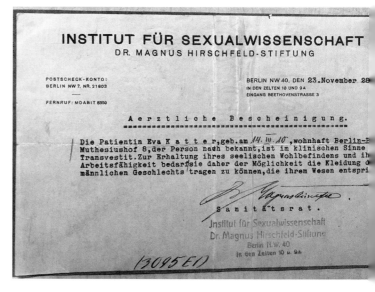

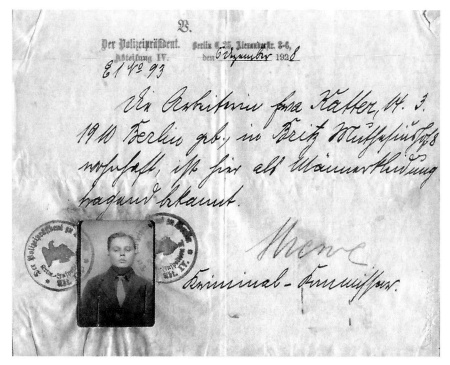

Katter's transvestite certificate, issued by the Berlin police department. COURTESY OF MAGNUS-HIRSCHFELD-GESELLSCHAFT E.V., BERLIN.

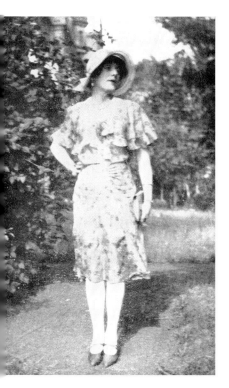

Lili Elbe, one of Hirschfeld's patients, from her book *Man into Woman*. COURTESY OF THE WELLCOME COLLECTION.

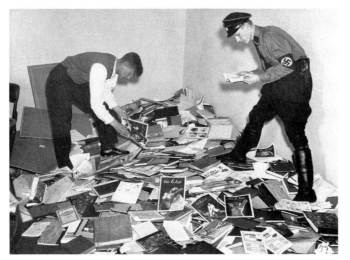

German students and Nazi Stor
Troops plunder the library of
Dr. Magnus Hirschfeld,
1933. COLLECTION OF THE
UNITED STATES HOLOCAUST
MEMORIAL MUSEUM.

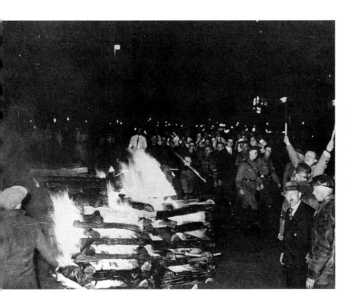

Inspired by a speech by Minister
Propaganda Joseph Goebbels, students gather around a huge bonfir
to throw "un-German" books into
the flames on the evening of
May 10, 1933, in Berlin.

On November 22, 1943,
the Institute building and
grounds suffered exten-
sive damage during an
air raid. COURTESY OF
MAGNUS-HIRSCHFELD-
GESELLSCHAFT E.V., BERLIN.

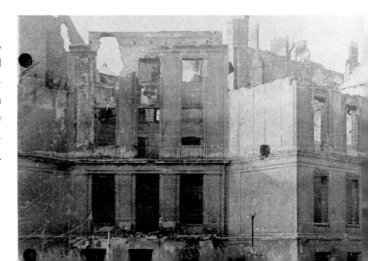

1923, a dollar was worth 10,000 marks, and by the end of the month, 49,000 marks.[39] The storm of hyperinflation that followed can scarcely be exaggerated. As explained by historian George J. W. Goodman, "When the 1,000-billion Mark note came out, few bothered to collect the change when they spent it. By November 1923, with one dollar equal to one trillion Marks, the breakdown was complete." Currency had lost all meaning.

The Institute's capital, which had been invested in the Reichsbank for security, should have earned around 8,000 marks in interest every year. Now, the bulk sum had been reduced to a pittance, with no income at all. The *Yearbook for Sexual Intermediaries*, so long the SHC's greatest publication and weapon against prejudice, closed for lack of funds. Hirschfeld had always intended to make the Institute building part of his foundation, and it was time to safeguard what he had built. On February 2, 1924, he solemnly handed over the Institute for Sexual Science to its state-sanctioned nonprofit foundation, with the hope that it would become a state institution.[40]

This seemed the only way to secure the future, though it also meant renting out the property next door for cash. Rooms would be let to paying guests including writer Christopher Isherwood, and in 1926, Hirschfeld would rebrand a hormone preparation of his own devising, with the alluring name of Titus Pearls, for public sale. Nothing should stand in the way, he announced, of the foundation's "self-preservation and self-administration" until such time as the state could run the Institute in the "spirit of its founder."[41] There were fiscal casualties, however. Funds for scientific research had entirely dried up. In place of research, the Institute would add an inpatient department to its therapeutic protocol. One patient, in particular, was already on her way.

ACT 4: ARRIVING AT THE BEGINNING

Dora put on her party clothes.[42] It had been some time since she'd had a reason to do so; the previous year was a difficult one. Still pining for the violinist, she fell ill with pleurisy, likely the result of pneumonia, and spent the better part of a month hospitalized. She needed a change of scenery; it was time for a new start, new surroundings, and new acquaintances. She'd taken a job in a liquor factory some distance from home and rented rooms at a nearby inn. The distance, she thought, would help free her from her angst-ridden and pointless passion. Besides, the inn had charms of its own. During the day, at the liquor factory, Dora had to be Rudolf and wear men's clothes; at night, she donned women's clothing, helped to serve guests, and even gave performances. For those in the audience, it offered pleasant entertainment. For Dora, it meant freedom.

On this night in February 1923, however, Dora headed off to a masked ball, determined to enjoy herself. Perhaps she might even fall in love again. After all, as she said, "life, without love, is a flower without fragrance."

Masked balls had long been a mainstay of the transvestite community; several were held at Hirschfeld's Institute, and many more at establishments in Berlin. For the normative world, wearing a costume offered a chance to be someone else; for Dora, it meant being her truest self. She caught the eye of a dashing young man; they danced and made conversation. He liked her a great deal, and asked Dora to write him a letter when she returned home so they might plan a second rendezvous. Dora sent a note agreeing to meet him; it seemed the perfect arrangement. He lived in the next town; she could travel there regularly. Their friendship passed into intimacy, but Dora took all the necessary precautions so that he would not guess her secret. All precautions except one—in writing to him, she'd given her address. It simply hadn't occurred to her that this new paramour might seek her out at home.

He meant to surprise her. Having business in the town, the young lover paid her a visit at the inn, but he didn't know her room. He inquired at the desk, saying he was there to see his girlfriend, Miss Richter. There was no Miss Richter—only a mister. Assuming a mix-up, the innkeeper fetched Rudolf and said a gentleman was there to meet him but didn't give his name. Dora had no warning. She stepped into the inn's public room without her wig, false breasts, or dress. Despite these subtractions, the young man recognized her immediately.* Dora flushed with embarrassment and began to apologize desperately, much as she had done when her first sexual partner saw the truth—but she had better words now. She told him she was a hermaphrodite; she must work in men's clothing in her professional life but was otherwise a woman. Like Hirschfeld, Dora adapted language to help identify herself; she wasn't apologizing for who she was, only for failing to disclose it. And to his credit, her lover accepted this explanation. More than this, he comforted her for the "suffering" she must experience at so cruel a fate. He had developed "great affection" for her and was happy to call her his "girlfriend."

Such acceptance astonished Dora; it should not astonish us. By 1923, sexology had meaningfully changed the public discourse: hormones and the body, with its frequent sexual ambiguities—rather than the mind or morals—had become a determinant of gender, and surgery a means of changing it. Dora never provided the young man's name, but they continued to see each other—and, on his insistence, she would watch a most unusual film. He'd seen it himself, he told her excitedly, and believed it could solve her problems.

Der Steinachfilm had premiered in January 1923 at the Ufa-Palast am Zoo in Berlin, the flagship cinema of the German studio UFA.[43] Seventy-five minutes in length, the film packed the 2,100-seat cinema for weeks before being released nationwide. Unlike Hirschfeld's film, this one had no plotline. The silent film featured Steinach himself, and alternating footage of animals and people with "animated diagrams" and explanations of glandular function—*all* the glandular functions. Steinach described the thyroid and pituitary as well as the suprarenal glands, providing visuals for how "disturbances" in each result in "deviance" from the bodily norm. Then come the sex organs—the testes and ovaries—and, of course, the rats. In graphic laboratory footage, rats are castrated and implanted, and the viewer observes their change from masculine to feminine body type and vice versa. Steinach sets the stage long before

---

* It says something about his attention to Dora that he did so; the violinist failed to see Dora and Rudolf as the same person until she made herself known.

introducing human sexuality, but in the last two segments of the film, he introduces the term first used by Hirschfeld: sexual intermediaries.

Film historian Maria Makela provides a breakdown of the fourth section. First, Steinach presents a "true hermaphrodite," an individual who has both male and female genitalia. He then provides "variations" on the theme. Two women appear on the screen, one with full breasts and large nipples, the other with slight breasts and small nipples. The first he describes (in titles) as normal, and the other as masculinized. The pageant continues: clinicians compare the hip and shoulder width of two men, one with wide shoulders and narrow hips (normal) and one with narrow shoulders and wide hips (feminized). The "inner secretions," the film explains, are out of balance: a masculinized woman doesn't make enough ovarian hormones and a feminized man lacks enough of the masculine hormone made by the testicles. He even claims that imbalanced hormones cause men to seek out women's jobs and the reverse—tapping into an already rampant fear about reversals of the "natural" (patriarchal) order. Steinach suggests that, for men, this is easily fixed; the film presents surgical footage of a homosexual man receiving a "heterosexual testicle." The fifth and sixth parts of the film concern rejuvenation, something Steinach's vasoligature surgery (with its supposed boost in masculine virility) promised—and which would outlive his homosexual "cure."

Steinach's film succeeded where Hirschfeld's had failed—at times, in spite of Steinach's own wishes. Film had not been especially kind to scientists (or sexologists), and Steinach resisted the idea of a film at first, hoping to preserve his reputation. Convincing him took the intervention of state, namely the Federal President of the German–Austrian Peoples' State and Highest Official Agencies. It also required a promise from UFA to fiscally support his experiments.[44] Thus, the scientific version of the film debuted in 1922—but that wasn't the film Dora and her boyfriend would see. Without Steinach's consent, and very likely without his knowledge, UFA reworked the film for public release. Only then did the film run afoul of censorship, but not for the same reasons Hirschfeld's had; the censorship board rejected it for release because the medical interventions it suggested (including testicle transplant) weren't proven safe or effective.

The decision would be overruled, and Steinach's work entered popular culture. Hormones, sex surgery, and sexual intermediacy were now in the public forum—and late-coming physicians began publishing their own papers on the glands.[45] Unfortunately for Steinach, these new sexologists explored the topic on their own rather than privileging his work. As Rainer Herrn and his coauthors explain in *Not Straight from Germany*, Steinach's approach to explaining diversity of forms through a single focal point, or monocausal theory, had already been outpaced by the scientific thought of the time.[46] Apart from the great number of new vasoligatures that followed (filmmakers even provided the names and addresses of doctors performing them in the closing credits), the popularization of Hirschfeld's Institute might be the film's most lasting legacy.

With its wall of intermediaries and archive of "deviant" types, the Institute served as the premier research stop for those interested in homosexuality, sadism and fetishism, transvestites, and sexual ethnography.[47] Dora learned of its existence at the cinema. She bought a train ticket and headed for Berlin in May 1923.[48]

DORA CHOSE A PALE blue dress to match her eyes, low-cut to expose her neck. It was simple, close-fitting, but not ostentatious; she didn't want to draw too much attention to herself. She'd always been modest and even a bit timid, but of course modesty would be impossible under the circumstances. Soon she would be entirely naked: vulnerable, bare, exposed. And it seemed likely she'd have to repeat this process, this time in front of a photographer.

Neat, economical, discreet Dora would never have considered such a thing on her own, but this was a consulting room in the Institute for Sexual Science. A young doctor and his stenographer recorded her intake interview and measured her every feature—from the shape of her chin to the centimeters between the iliac spines of her pelvic bone. Into his notebook she went, with all her bits and bobs, and so too her most inti-

mate secrets. For this she'd left her home in the Bohemian Ore mountains: she wanted to be made whole—and to live free.

Can you tell me, asked Werner Holz, the physician, why you have
come? For once, Dora knew exactly what to say. She fixed him with her
gray-blue eyes and gave voice to her greatest desire: free me from the
genitals I hate, she told him, so that I will "no longer be a man." "I had
to torture my entire brain with thoughts of [those] who never understood me," she told Holz; why couldn't she "simply be and live as [she]
wished to be and live?"

Holz copied everything into a notebook, and would eventually submit these details as part of his doctoral thesis, "The Case of Rudolf R."
He calls Dora "a man in good nutritional condition," measuring 150
centimeters (4 feet 11 inches), and misgenders her throughout. She had
"good blood flow to the skin," and "somewhat greater accumulation of
fat around both nipples is noticeable, as a slight suggestion of gyneco-
mastia." Both Steinach's film and Hirschfeld's photography suggested
that homosexuals and transvestites could be recognized, that their bodies in some sense betrayed their mixed natures. Holz expected Dora
(whom he considered a homosexual man) to have wider hips, more fat,
and soft shoulders. "The facial expression is quite feminine," Holz continued, "facial features are very soft," the blue-gray eyes have a "dreamy
expression," and the Adam's apple "protrudes only slightly." To these
observations are added a table of measurements—hips, shoulders, upper
and lower body height. It would go into the files with the other intermediaries, along with photographs.

Rainer Herrn and Alex Bakker write at length about how these
photographs served as visual evidence for Hirschfeld's argument that
transvestites were a "natural" third category of sex. Hirschfeld had
even played a kind of game in the publication of *Geschlechts-Übergänge*
(Sexual Transitions), asking readers to guess whether a photo is "man
or woman." By the time Dora was examined, Hirschfeldian sexology
located sex/gender "in" or at least "on" the body itself. Measurement
and illustration do more than reinforce ideas; they offer up their own
kind of argument.[49]

Holz dutifully describes Dora's testicles (of "medium size" and "firm consistency") and her penis (medium in size, covered with foreskin), then notes that she has come with "the urgent desire to be surgically freed" from them.[50] What Holz does not say—but which Hirschfeld would later record—is that Dora claimed she would "lay hands on herself" if the doctors didn't give in to her desires. This calls to mind Mühsam's patient—an "emergency operation" to "save the patient from worse."[51]

Dora's intake interview ends with Holz's assessment of her condition. "Liked by everyone," says the intake form, "mood is steady," "shy and docile," "soft" and "good-natured." She qualified as an "extreme" case—considered a homosexual transvestite (for her love of men), and seeking dangerous surgical intervention. But Dora was not homosexual. Her understanding aligns more naturally with how we perceive transgender sexuality today: She "could not understand how two men could take a liking to each other," writes Holz in her intake interview; "the patient perceived [her]self so much as a woman that it does not even occur to [her] that [she] is homosexual."

To Holz, the physical assessment lined up nicely with this pronouncement; "a deviation from the heterosexual norm can be observed . . . that the lower body height as expressed as percentage of the upper body length is greater than 100, in that it amounts to 105 here, while in the average of heterosexual men it is less than 100." The numbers are, we now know, wholly arbitrary—but Holz used them to support his final assessment: "Since our patient has been dominated since [her] earliest youth by the thought of being freed from [her] genitals, and has come to Berlin solely for this purpose, and thus it is to be feared that [she] would fall into a deep depression if [she] had to travel back without having [her] wish fulfilled, without further ado I consider the indication for castration to be present in this case." The "only thing" left, Holz continued, "is the extent to which the intervention is to be performed, and which precautionary or preventive measures have to be taken."[52]

Thus, Dora entered the sanctuary that was Hirschfeld's Institute—and she would remain there for the next ten years. The journey to become herself had begun.

10

LIVES IN TRANSITION

BLOOD SOAKED THE DRESSINGS, SWELLING UP THROUGH GASHES carved in flesh. Only sixteen years old, the patient had already lost far too much blood, and Dr. Ludwig Levy-Lenz shouted for an immediate transfusion. He knew the patient well—they had come to him a few days before asking for surgical breast removal and he'd turned them away because of their youth: "we considered that, at the age of sixteen . . . mental development was not complete."[1] Assigned female at birth, the girl, as Levy-Lenz called them, had responded by attempting self-amputation with a razor blade. Now, the surgeon worked both to amputate the lacerated breasts and to save a life.

It wasn't the first time Levy-Lenz had encountered a transgender patient. That had happened at his private gynecology clinic nearly a decade earlier. Levy-Lenz opened his practice in 1918; he was then twenty-eight (the same age Hirschfeld was when he began his career in sexology). In those early years, a "very elegant woman" appeared in his surgery; she sauntered across the room, the scent of her perfume kissing the air, and perched herself upon Levy-Lenz's desk. "It is scarcely necessary to say that my profession had hardened me against feminine charms," he wrote, "but to prove the rule there must be exceptions." He found himself flustered by her sex appeal, "just the kind . . . that I liked," and couldn't help noticing the flash of shapely legs as she crossed them over the edge of the credenza. In charming embarrassment, she told him she'd been "led into committing an infidelity" and worried she might have caught an infection from her partner. Levy-Lenz invited her to sit in the examination chair—the sort that provided stirrups for performing a gynecological exam. "Oh, that won't be necessary," the lady replied; it would be just as easy to examine her standing up—and with that, she raised her skirt to present a penis and testicles.[2]

Levy-Lenz was shocked to the core. He couldn't know then that he would one day be the principal surgeon at the Institute for Sexual Science, where he would be responsible for surgical remediations from castration and penectomy to the creation of an artificial vagina.

Surviving photographs of Levy-Lenz show him in later middle age, bald and bespectacled. But with wit, good humor, and a movie-star cleft chin, he'd been something of a charmer in his youth. He loved to tell stories from medical school which, he admitted, preserved more "inventive power" than truth.* Reading his memoirs, it's easy to think of him as a jocose, fun-loving wiseass. But Levy-Lenz could also be quick to judge and to assert his own moral superiority; in later reflection, he wrote that he had spent his youth "wallowing in a morass of superstition and ignorance . . . gossip, backbiting, and stupidity."[3] In the case of Magnus Hirschfeld, awakening to the plight of intermediaries had come as early as discovering his own homosexuality. For Levy-Lenz, it required the loss of a friend.

Levy-Lenz earned his degree in Heidelberg, a beautiful town on the river Neckar. Home to famed sociologist Max Weber, it blossomed with the liberal, open-minded spirit thinkers like Weber had fostered, but prejudice is hard to stamp out. As a student, Levy-Lenz belonged to a circle of four friends who coalesced around a mutual interest in investigating (and debunking) spiritualism and quackery. Among them was a youth named Fredy. He had what the others described as "delicate sensibilities"; he never took part in their search for female partners and rebuked them for being promiscuous. Over a period of weeks, Levy-Lenz noticed that Fredy had been "cut dead" by another member of the group.[4] When he demanded an explanation, the student explained that his fraternity forbade him to socialize with Fredy because he was homosexual.

Levy-Lenz first responded with confusion, then with "a kind of savage

---

* Such as the woman who believed a mouse lived in her stomach, and the crafty doctor who performed a fake operation and produced a live mouse in a cage as evidence (it backfired; the woman later became convinced the mouse had given birth before its removal).

rage." How dare Fredy pretend to be like them, he thought. No wonder "it was so easy for him to pretend to be morally superior" regarding the women! He seethed with (utterly unearned) moral indignation and confronted Fredy with brutal words, calculated to hurt him. Fredy made no reply. He just sank to the floor in a flood of tears and heaving, desperate sobs. This took the rage out of Levy-Lenz but replaced it with confusion. He stood by, helpless. When the tears subsided, Fredy told him a story the young doctor would go on to hear hundreds of times: he could not help who he was.

Levy-Lenz went home feeling disgusted at Fredy, but also at himself. He couldn't sleep. He needed answers. The next morning, he hunted in the university library for what science had to say on the subject of homosexuality—and found the work of Magnus Hirschfeld. "I devoured his books and all other works on the subject," Levy-Lenz wrote. "How infernally blind and stupid I was." For the first time, he understood that homosexuality was not a moral sin and that it did not lead to pedophilia, as he'd been led to believe by the use of the word "pederast." The suggestion that homosexuals were a danger to children worked during the Liebenberg scandal; it had permeated even the liberal culture of Heidelberg University; it's still an arrow in the quiver of some conservatives today. Upset and full of regret, Levy-Lenz set out for Fredy's rooms. They were vacant, swept bare. Fredy had left the university.

Distraught, Levy-Lenz wrote to Fredy's father. The reply was short and final: friendless and humiliated, Fredy had gone to America. His absence so haunted Levy-Lenz that, forty years later, he published a plea in the American edition of his memoirs: "My dear Fredy, if you ever read these lines in some far country I want you to know how deeply I regret the injustice I did you. . . . Forgive me. I am ashamed at my conduct in insulting you without reason and in presuming to set myself up as judge in matters I did not understand." He knew, and admitted, that there was no excuse, no taking it back, no balm for the wounds inflicted, "but I have tried to make good the wrong which I and your other friends did you by becoming a disciple of enlightenment."

After leaving university, Levy-Lenz declared himself a sexologist. He joined the Institute for Sexual Science in 1925 and would go on to perform numerous gender transition surgeries, mostly on male-to-female patients. "Female transvestites," he wrote, meaning female-to-male, had the greater quandary; years before the invention of phalloplasty, they could not easily change the nature of their sex organs. But the "strength of their desire," he wrote, "is powerful to a degree which a layman cannot possibly imagine."[5] The self-mutilated child on his operating table proved it. The surgeon had supposed a teenager too young to know their own mind; he was very wrong. Levy-Lenz completed what the patient had begun and sewed up the wounds.

The patient survived, went on to pursue legal recognition under a new name, became a carpenter, lived through the Second World War, and died in 1995. Levy-Lenz doesn't tell us this; rather, some sixty years later, an elderly trans man named Gerd Katter reached out to the Magnus Hirschfeld Society in Berlin. Describing himself as a carpenter, artist, and amateur sexologist, Katter claimed that Levy-Lenz's anonymized case was his own. Born Eva Katter, he had sought aid and refuge at the Institute in the mid-1920s, considered Hirschfeld like a father, and described the years spent at the Institute as "among the most interesting of my life." Like Dora, Katter realized that he wasn't "like the others" at an early age. Unlike Dora, Katter's parents supported him; his mother even accompanied him to the Institute. He would spend the next year attaining a transvestite license through Hirschfeld's expert diagnosis, and then attempted to change his name; the "patient," wrote Hirschfeld, suffered "difficulties in [his] professional life" because the name Eva contradicted his masculine qualities and appearance. Sometime after this, Gerd requested breast removal and was denied, before taking the task upon himself.[6]

Was Katter the sixteen-year-old Levy-Lenz describes? Discrepancies exist between his account and that of Levy-Lenz. Additional details in Hans Abraham's dissertation on Katter and eleven other female-to-male patients at the Institute don't match up either.* Either way, the

---

* For this reason, I have used "they/them" to describe Levy-Lenz's patient and "he/him" to describe Gerd Katter.

stories indicate that a much larger number of female-to-male patients transitioned at the Institute than was recorded by Hirschfeld. Possibly, this is because female-to-male did not fit his tidy definition of "transvestite"; possibly it's because science and medicine, even when "enlightened," still valued male experience (as it was seen at the time) over female experience.* Then again, none of the earliest transition surgeries, despite their groundbreaking nature, left behind more than a trace.

We know of four surgeons who performed gender transition surgery: Heinrich Stabel, who performed Steinach's rejuvenation surgery on Hirschfeld's patients; Erwin Gohrbandt, chief consultant at the surgical department of the Urban-Krankenhaus in Berlin; Kurt Warnekros, a Dresden gynecologist and former head of the University of Berlin Women's Hospital; and Ludwig Levy-Lenz, the only one to write about the experience. As for scientific publications, we have a single report in 1931 by the Institute's Felix Abraham, referencing both Levy-Lenz and Gohrbandt, but if it weren't for the relative fame of Lili Elbe's autobiography (in which she outs her surgeons) Warnekros's involvement might never have been known. Rainer Herrn suggests that the reluctance to publish likely stemmed from the explosive nature of the subject matter and fear of professional backlash.[7] If any further articles or news reports existed, they have since been lost or destroyed, such that the words of Levy-Lenz, "Institute surgeon," provide the only professional perspective on patient transitions, and on the great changes taking place at the Institute itself. It's partly from this work that we learn the extent to which hormones became part of transition.

THE HORMONE DEBATES

The science of hormones had come a long way since their discovery in 1905. Important milestones included Steinach's work on intermediate

---

* Once again, the binary makes talking about these cases endlessly difficult. Hirschfeld's contemporaries tended to regard female-to-male as female transvestite and male-to-female as male transvestite in their categorization.

forms, but physiologists and biochemists were undermining his "beautifully clear scheme" of gonads operating in isolation as independent organs. Instead, it would be seen that they function in conjunction with the entire the endocrine system—including thyroid, pituitary, adrenals, and other glands.[8]

In the United States, from 1914 to 1920, Chicago embryologist Frank Rattray Lillie studied freemartins to determine that hormones and genes worked together to determine sex. In 1925, endocrinologist Carl Moore effectively demonstrated that an ovary implanted into an uncastrated male guinea pig did not feminize the animal. Viennese gynecologist Otfried Otto Fellner, working in the early 1920s, was among the first to extract hormones from testicles, ovaries, and placenta for comparison. They were "identical in color, solubility, and odor" and even in action—when introduced into a female animal's reproductive tract, all three brought about "pregnancy-like" changes. Male and female gonads, he determined, must be "hermaphroditic in a secretory sense"—something that would hardly have been a surprise to Hirschfeld but may have shocked other endocrinologists. Then, in 1927, researchers at the Dutch school of Ernst Laqueur found female hormones in healthy heterosexual men (as we now know, all people generally produce both testosterone and estrogen). The discovery made testicle replacement surgeries obsolete but drove new interest in the hormones themselves; once isolated, could they be injected? Animal models again led the way.[9]

In 1930, gynecologist Bernard Zondek published a letter in *Nature* that turned the hormone debate on its head.[10] His subject: horse piss. He'd discovered that the urine of pregnant mares provides an excellent reservoir for extracting ovarian hormone (by then called *strogenic* hormone or *s. œstrin*)*—500 to 3,000 times more than a sexually mature woman. This was useful but not groundbreaking news. The real shock came

---

* Horses are a source of estrogen even today. Public outcry about the treatment of the animals has led to a greater reliance on artificial hormone, but Premarin (pregnant mare urine) continues to be used in the United States.

when Zondek examined the urine of stallions—that is, non-castrated, sexually mature male horses. Dr. E. P. Häussler (in the scientific laboratory of Hoffmann–La Roche in Basel) had been the first to suggest that stallions also excrete estrogen, but Zondek wanted to quantify it. He collected the urine of four stallions, added mineral acid, boiled for five minutes, and then extracted the hormone with benzol. The resulting numbers were astounding. Not only did the stallions make estrogen, they made more of it than female horses! His conclusion: "the testis of the horse is the richest tissue known containing estrogenic hormone" at 500 times the hormone content of both ovaries in an (unpregnant) mare. How could this be possible?

Zondek posited that testosterone and estrogen begin as basically the same chemical compound, and even that one could be converted to the other; he considered the sexes to be "at the hormonal level" essentially interchangeable. Testicles contain something called cytochrome P450 aromatase; it's capable of converting androgens into estrogens.[11] We know now that estrogen (and estradiol in particular) is necessary for healthy male fertility, and that it's produced not only in the testes but also in the male brain.

The findings confused early endocrinologists; they struggled to see how estrogen aided or influenced the male of the species. And the analysis worked in both directions. According to Nelly Oudshoorn's study of medical indices, the first report of male sex hormones in female urine appeared in 1931, by the German gynecologist Harald Siebke.[12] The findings shook the then firm conviction that the "essence of femininity" and "seat of masculinity" were located in the gonads—but things took a hard right into eugenics first.

In 1934, German scientists led by Adolf Butenandt and Ulrich Westphal isolated progesterone, a steroid hormone produced by the adrenal cortex as well as by the ovaries and testes.*[13] That same year, Lennox Broster asserted that the female fetus went through a "male phase,"

---

* Estradiol and testosterone are steroid hormones too.

directed by the adrenal glands, between the eleventh and the fourteenth week; hormones from the pituitary gland at week fourteen returned the fetus to the "female phase." Broster (no feminist) thus considered women to be physiologically unstable. As a result, he claimed, stress could cause the adrenal glands to reassert their influence later in a woman's life, making her more masculine. The "social consequences," he warned, would be dire; masculinized "intersex type" women threatened all of humanity, and the women's emancipation movement proved that the downfall had begun.[14] For Broster, selective breeding was the only solution (though he never worked out how this was to be achieved). Plenty of eugenicists agreed—but endocrinology would at last pull free from its influence.

Hormone science had worked several minor miracles by the 1930s. The discovery and isolation of thyroid hormone and insulin offered the first real treatments for hyperthyroidism and diabetes, and the isolation of estrogen, testosterone, and progesterone earned several Nobel Prizes. Steinach, however, was not among the winners. He claimed that his Progynon extract was the "very essence of Eve," powerful enough to restore sex function and menstruation and, of course, offer further rejuvenation to the patient.[15] Unfortunately (and ironically, given his Vivarium past), it only worked in rats. The first truly effective ovarian extract was produced by American anatomist Edgar Allen and biochemist Edward Doisy in 1923 to treat menstrual and fertility problems in women. Allen and Doisy won the Nobel, but even so, hormone treatment didn't catch on in the gynecology clinic.

Testosterone did better; Butenandt and colleagues synthesized it in 1935, and these androgens finally achieved what Brown-Séquard's crushed dog testicles could not: improved muscle mass, lifted mood, greater strength, sexual appetite, hair growth, and so on.[16] Not surprisingly, some sexologists immediately attempted to cure homosexuality with testosterone, just as Steinach had tried with testicle transplant. The idea that having more of the masculine hormone made you more male remained potent, though erroneous. Alternatively, some theorized that homosexual men had too much estrogen. Hirschfeld even used the

Allen–Doisy test for measuring estrogenic activity to analyze the urine of homosexual patients at the Institute; he assumed that homosexuals must make elevated levels of estrogen compared to heterosexual men.[17] They didn't—as Zondek's stallion studies proved.

Despite all this work, hormone extracts and hormone replacement therapy did not come easy. It would be decades before they became therapeutically useful to both male and female reproductive anatomies, but that doesn't mean experiments weren't ongoing. Long before the Nobel Prizes were awarded, Iwan Bloch developed Testogan and Thelygan, which were said to contain "extracts of the male and female gonads" respectively.[18] Hirschfeld developed his own hormone extract, collaborating with Bernard Schapiro; they called it Testifortan (later rebranding it as Titus Pearls). A treatment for impotence, Testifortan boasted an 80 percent success rate. Critics felt this was due to the power of suggestion, but that didn't stop Hirschfeld and Schapiro from advertising in brochures, ads, and journals. A great number of patients came from the upper and middle classes, which helped to prop up the Institute financially.[19]

The first concoction included West African aphrodisiacs as well as testicular hormone; the second contained ovarian extracts to treat the "sexual coldness" of women.[20] But the preparations weren't only for cisgender heterosexuals. At the "urgent request of transvestites," Hirschfeld injected "female organ preparations" into male-to-female patients.[21] Results included the development of small breasts and a decrease in beard growth (also treated by electrolysis and X-ray depilation). Sadly, his male hormone extracts did not have the same salutary effects on female-to-male patients; that would come later. In 1946, for instance, the English Michael Dillon (born Laura Maud Dillon) took testosterone and had breasts removed—followed by the first phalloplasty, conducted by Sir Harold Gillies. "Where the mind cannot be made to fit the body," Dillon wrote in his autobiography, "the body should be made to fit the mind."[22]

History demonstrates that "transvestites"—that is, transgender people—were the first to decide upon surgical change, and the first to (as Hirschfeld puts it) "urgently request" hormone replacement therapy.[23] They turned to doctors for help, but surgical and hormonal transition occurred at the intersection, with patients and doctors working together. Hirschfeld played an extraordinary role, partly in providing a place for these transitions to take shape, partly in connecting patients with surgeons, partly in fighting for the rights of those patients to exist at all. The protagonists of this story, however—heroes who dared question sex and gender binaries and who exhibited the courage to risk everything for their truth—have always been the transgender patients: Dora Richter and those who came after her, embarking on journeys of *Genitalumwandlung*, or genital transformation.

DEFINING A SCATTERED HISTORY

From 1923 to 1933, the Institute treated numerous transgender patients for whom we have no record, and only a few for whom we do. To tell the story of surgical and hormonal transition at the Institute requires piecing together a scattered history—and sometimes conflicting documents. The most detailed description of Dora's surgery comes from the work of Felix Abraham, yet in what is probably a typographic error, he puts the year at 1922 (before Dora first heard of the Institute). Werner Holz's intake interview shows that Dora arrived in 1923, and in May was under evaluation and awaiting Hirschfeld's decision.

For Hirschfeld, Dora represented an anomaly: a transvestite whose life history and desires ran counter to his theories. He'd initially assumed that transvestites assigned male at birth were heterosexual, in the formulation of the day—in other words, that they were sexually attracted to women. Some, like the original patient treated by Mühsam, had asked to be castrated, but Hirschfeld considered surgical intervention dangerous and the impulse for it rare. Now, in his consulting room, Dora told him that if he did not authorize surgery, she would take matters into her own hands. Why, Holz had asked, would she want to do something so drastic? Dora answered with emphasis born of lifelong yearning: "Then at least I will no longer be a man!"[24]

Hirschfeld at last referred her to surgery for castration. Levy-Lenz had not yet taken his post at the Institute, so Heinrich Stabel performed Dora's first surgery, and did his best to convince her not to pursue penectomy.[25] He assured her that her desire for such a drastic course would fade with time. It wouldn't.

"It was not easy for us to decide on the described procedures," Felix Abraham wrote in the *Journal of Sexology and Sex Politics*, "but the patients were not to be dismissed" because of their "mental state that made it probable that self-mutilation, with life-endangering complications, could be possible." He went on to describe the results for Dora: castration caused "the body [to become] rounder/fuller, the beard growth to decrease, breast initiation to be noticeable." Endocrine discoveries would reveal why; since the male body makes both testosterone and estrogen, the effects of Dora's estrogen production became noticeable once the testes were removed. We don't know if Dora took estrogen preparations as well, but even without them, Abraham wrote, the surgery caused "the fatty tissue of the buttocks and in the rest of the body to take on a more feminine form."[26]

Dora would wait eight years before taking the next surgical step, and by then, Hirschfeld had radically altered his opinion on how rare such cases really were. In 1926, around two years after Dora's surgery, Hirschfeld published one of his most influential works: *Geschlechtskunde* (roughly, *Sex Education*). Hirschfeld had begun by dividing sex and gender into four subgroups, from which any number of combinations might be made. But as his understanding of *Transvestiten* grew, he further extrapolated. Soon, there were ten intermediary subgroups. The first he called total or "full" transvestites, who have the desire to change clothes and behaviors completely. The second were extreme transvestites, "who have changed not only their artificial dress, but also their natural dress," meaning the body itself. The male-to-female accomplished this by depilation (removal of the beard and other hair by electrolysis or X-ray), castration, penectomy, and finally the creation of a pseudo-vagina; the female-to-male transvestites had ovaries and breasts removed, and in at least one case a testicle added. The remaining subdivisions include various permutations of changing dress or mannerisms, and the final two demarcate the "bisexual" and "homosexual" transvestites (i.e., those attracted to the sex assigned to them at birth). Regarding those interested in surgical transition, he admitted his earlier error: "These cases," he wrote, "are much more frequent than was previously even remotely suspected."[27]

It was for this reason that Felix Abraham wrote about Dora's surgery and those of another patient, Toni Ebel—not just castration but penectomies and vaginoplasties. Surgeons themselves had yet to describe the practice, but Hirschfeld felt sure that "patients with the same inclinations exist, who desire similar procedures, but do not know of any means and ways to achieve [them]."[28] Dora's story led the way.

THERE IS A PHOTOGRAPH: on a bench in the sun sits Magnus Hirschfeld. His hair has lightened, his mustache appears white above a broad grin. He holds his elbows as if just recovering from a laugh, one pinstriped leg tucked playfully beneath the other. Next to him, so close that their elbows touch, is a round-cheeked woman in a floral dress and sunhat. She's looking at Hirschfeld, a soft smile on her face. He called her Dorchen: little Dora.

We know Hirschfeld would have counseled her, though we have no record of the conversation—only a statement taken years later: "When [Dora] came to us at the age of twenty-five," Hirschfeld wrote, she told him she was ready to put an end to a frustrated and lonely life.[29] The suicide of desperate homosexuals had first brought Hirschfeld to sexology; there were few other subjects that could so move him as the snuffing-out of young lives full of promise. Dora, wrote Holz, "is well liked everywhere because of [her] friendly and genuinely feminine nature." He would have cause to know her very well as he took her on as a housemaid at the Institute, doing "all the feminine work" with "exemplary faithfulness" and "untiring diligence."[30] She had been accepted as a patient and also as staff. She became the Institute's first transgender maid; she would ultimately serve as the elder in a small group of five. Levy-Lenz talks about the first time he went into the kitchen one evening after work to find the "fair ones" sitting "peacefully around the grate, sewing, embroidering, polishing silver, and singing old German folk songs." There in the firelight, Dora would be at her lace-making pillow, the perfect "picture of domesticity."[31]

A DECADE OF TRANSGENDER SURGERY

Body modifications are made all the time: breast implants and reductions, penile enlargement, injections to increase the size of the buttocks, Botox, hair removal, and hair regrowth are only a few of the more popular types. We may think of these as very modern, but because of Sir Harold Gillies's groundbreaking work on facial reconstruction during and after the First World War, body augmentation was within reach in the 1920s and 1930s. Today, gender affirmation may include facial surgery (adjustments to masculinize or feminize features), top surgery (for breast removal or augmentation), and bottom surgery (genital reconstruction). When Dora began her own surgical odyssey, all of these were available except the artificial creation of a phallus. At the time, any surgeon might express an interest in "plastic" or cosmetic surgery, and every procedure was also an experiment.

Castration was a straightforward procedure; it had been practiced well before Steinach's testicle transplants in various cultures throughout history. Ovaries and breasts had been removed, too, in cases of disease or tumors. As a result, these operations were not usually recorded in detail, except in cases where patients had attempted to remove their own.

In 1927, a German doctor by the name of Kankeleit published an article with case studies and illustrations he procured from Karl Giese at the Institute, titled "Self-Harm and Self-Mutilation of the Sexual Organs."[32] He detailed six assigned-male-at-birth and two assigned-female-at-birth patients at the Institute who swore to "lay hands upon themselves" in an attempt to remove their genitals, and began with Dora Richter.

Two images stand side by side in the text. One presents her as a naked patient against a white wall, knees together, hands down, eyes and most of the upper face covered by a blindfold. Dora appears vulnerable, help-less. The photo was taken, most probably, to demonstrate the results of castration; she has slight breast swellings and rounded thighs. The blindfold may represent a desire for anonymity—but Kankeleit paired the photo with her name and a second photo in which she looks at the camera, coy and smiling. She poses in a costume something like that of a belly-dancer: a bejeweled camisole that exposes her middle, a matching beaded and tasseled skirt, and low heels, with a veil held up behind her head. We can imagine her attending one of the Institute's grand balls, but the caption reads merely "after castration." Her inclusion in Kanke-leit's article seems to hinge upon her early experiment with a length of yarn—but also on the ideation of self-harm.

Kankeleit, an ardent eugenicist, considered transgender people to be "sexual perverts" "under delusion." In his introduction, he sees the drive for castration as a means for "deviants" and "primitives" (by which he means non-white people) to remove themselves from the gene pool, sav-ing Germany from "inferior offspring." For him, the "desire for elimina-tion or damage of the sexual organs" was "a hint of nature to eradicate the degenerate." People like Dora were not always in sympathetic hands, and some who successfully treated transvestites would later counte-nance Nazi genocide and the repression of sexual intermediaries (if not their extermination); the complexity of seeking life-affirming care from a conservative medical establishment continues today. Kankeleit does not respect the identity of his transvestite subjects in the way Hirschfeld does, but it's through his article that we learn of those who would join Dora as the first of the Institute's trans patients. His single contribution is to name these transgender pioneers.

Ossy (born Oskar S.) came to the Institute at the age of thirty. Ossy said she felt like a girl of thirteen; she was "servile" and "submissive." She had regular intercourse with men but felt that both her sex drive and her genitals were at odds with her wish to be a "pure young girl." If denied surgery, she planned to try castration on herself; Hirschfeld agreed to refer her, and she was castrated in 1926 or 1927 (based on the date of Kankeleit's publication). Gertrude (born Paul H.) received a transvestite certificate that permitted her to present her female persona in public. Like Dora, she had managed to conceal male sex characteristics from her lovers. Kankeleit includes her picture; with traditionally feminine features, she poses with her boyfriend, though Kankeleit never says whether she went through with castration. Next comes Willy (for whom we are not given the chosen name): homosexual (i.e., assigned male at birth and attracted to men) but consenting to intercourse with women by imagining herself a woman, too—more successfully, apparently, than Dora had done. She loathed that arousal caused her to have erections and underwent castration at the age of forty in hopes of relief.

Heterosexual transvestites also appear in Kankeleit's report. Detlef S., thirty-nine, was married with children; she felt "completely female" and desired full physical feminization. He also mentions Christabel (born Erich S.), a civil servant, married with children, but living entirely as a woman. The final two transvestites mentioned were assigned female at birth and had come to the Institute seeking mastectomy: a second Dora (whose chosen name was omitted) and Alex K. (born Lotte). Alex began to live as male at age fourteen "by permission"—probably with a transvestite certificate. He went on to earn an engineering diploma and to work as an aviator. While a patient at the Institute, he underwent mastectomy and the only reported testicle implant—sadly, it failed.

Together with Levy-Lenz's patient, who may or may not be Gerd Katter, these are the only female-to-male patients for whom we have identifying records. There were surely others, but the cases here may be representative. In all the literature that remains, male-to-female transvestites are the principal focus; for them, surgery could go much further. The amputation of the penis, creation of a vagina, and cosmetic changes to the face offered new vistas for experimental procedures—and Levy-Lenz was an eager learner.

"The difficult problem of outward appearance," Levy-Lenz wrote, required complex and multifaceted treatment. He suggested that male-to-female patients begin with the elimination of facial hair. In the early years, the Institute's X-ray lab had been fitted out for this purpose, but Levy-Lenz objected; X-ray depilation worked but often caused severe burns. He recommended electrolysis instead, and because "treatment with a needle takes a long time" patients should begin while awaiting orchidectomy (testicle removal). "After that," he continued, "the penis was amputated . . . and then an artificial vagina" created; in some cases, patients would also ask to have their faces reshaped.[33] Levy-Lenz performed facial surgery on both genders, making some more "masculine" and others more "feminine" as the need required. Every patient incurred risk; they were guinea pigs for brand-new techniques, some of them in the most tender and vulnerable of places. "I had, of course, read books on the subject," Levy-Lenz wrote of his foray into the field, "but in plastic surgery theory counts for very little, and practice is everything."[34]

His first successful artificial vagina and vulva, he claimed, was covered by the international press. Letters came from all over the globe and "lots of people came to see us to have the same . . . performed on themselves"; in short, Levy-Lenz soon had "a great deal of material on which to experiment."[35] These reports have been lost to history. We know with certainty of only three complete surgeries performed at the time—that is, castration, penectomy, and vaginoplasty—though no doubt there were more of them. The first was Dora's; the second, Toni Ebel's; the last, Lili Elbe's. We know, too, that American dancer Charlotte Charlaque was a patient at the Institute; her male-to-female transition seems to have occurred around the same time, but no written records remain.[36] She appeared in a film, *Mysterium des Geschlechts*, along with male-to-female footage of Dora and Toni. In the years that followed, Charlotte and Toni would become lovers, living together until Nazi forces tore them apart.

Dora's castration took place in 1923; the amputation of her penis occurred in 1930.[37] The dates of Toni's surgeries are less precise; Rainer Herrn speculates that they began in 1929 and finished in 1931. The two would live and work together at the Institute as maids, two of the five Levy-Lenz saw clustered about the domestic kitchen fire. Toni, born Arno, made a living as a painter. Though homosexual, Toni married a woman and she bore a son, but the match was never a happy one. Toni's inclinations grew stronger as she matured, but her wife refused to allow her to wear women's clothing. Soon, Toni felt she could not paint while wearing the hateful clothes of men; it filled her with nervous distress, making her "worthless" (as Felix Abraham put it). When her wife died, Toni decided to live entirely as a woman; at fifty-two, she had waited a long time, which might explain the speed at which she went through the stages of surgery–recovery–surgery. Levy-Lenz performed both castration and penectomy on Toni (only the penectomy on Dora), but despite his work on creating artificial vaginas, a budding plastic surgeon completed both of these vaginoplasties: Dr. Erwin Gohrbandt, director of the surgical clinic at the Urban Hospital of Berlin.[38]

The penectomies took place at the Institute. Levy-Lenz first removed hair from the area and cleaned it carefully; "the most scrupulous hygiene is a prerequisite."[39] Today, total penectomies performed for gender affirmation remove the entire penis, including the root that goes into the pelvis. At that point, the urethra, or the tube through which urine flows, must then be rerouted to a spot in the perineum (between scrotum and anus).[40] Current surgical methods even allow for the glans (the tip of the penis) to be removed and reused as a clitoris, while penis and scrotal material are fashioned into vulva, labia, and vagina.* Levy-Lenz lacked the ability to fully relocate the urethra (or, at least, to do so without complications), so he removed the penis but left a "penile stump" behind, through which urine could flow. He then reattached scrotal skin to the area just beneath, allowing it to heal over; in future, he would use this tissue to fashion the labia (much as is done today). Dora remained at the Institute to recuperate. Then, in 1930, she arrived at Gohrbandt's clinic, ready for the last act of a lifelong drama.

After another scrub-up and additional hair removal, Gohrbandt inserted a catheter into the stump of Dora's remaining penile tissue.

---

* The current version of this procedure is known as peritoneal pull-through (PPT). It has been used in the reconstruction of cisgender women's vaginal canals and is also used in trans women.

With the patient fully anesthetized, he used a scalpel to make the first vertical cut into the muscles of her perineum. Slowly, he deepened the opening, stopping once he reached the peritoneum, or the membrane that supports the abdominal organs. The neo-vagina had a depth of about four and a half inches. Left to itself, the cut would close, blood vessels and muscle reknitting together. The surgery's next phase was designed to prevent that possibility. Gohrbandt used a speculum to stretch the new vagina open, and inserted a rubber sponge fitted with a wooden rod into the cavity. Lining the entire outer surface of the sponge were thin, nearly transparent slivers of flesh: skin taken from Dora's thigh. This allowed a healing layer to form inside the newly opened vagina.*

The sponge remained in place for three weeks, absorbing any "secretions" from the wound. When the time came to remove it, Gohrbandt first took out the wooden dowel, then gently removed the pliant sponge from fresh tissue. In recovery, Dora continued dilation techniques to stretch the vaginal walls and applied ointments to protect new skin. Abraham ends his report by saying that "one could raise an objection to this type of surgery [as . . .] some kind of luxury . . . with a frivolous character," but "to perform this surgery was in these cases (and probably it will be the same in many other cases) a kind of emergency . . . to save patients."[41]

The Institute and its affiliated physicians had performed the first complete male-to-female surgical transition, and they did it nearly a century ago. Dora was first. She wouldn't be the last.

IN 1931, LILI ELBE published her autobiography in Denmark; it was followed a year later by a German translation and, still later, an English one. The German title was *Ein Mensch wechselt sein Geschlecht*, lit-

---

* This technique, known as the Thiersch method, was introduced by Munich surgeon Karl Thiersch in the late nineteenth century to shorten the duration of postoperative skin repair.

erally "a person changes their sex." The English title would be *Man into Woman*.

Born Ejnar Wegener, Elbe worked as an artist with her wife, Grete. Grete supported her in her transition, standing up for her when a doctor called her a hysteric.[42] Like Dora, Lili Elbe came to the Institute and met with Magnus Hirschfeld, but she did not like what she saw there. The good doctor would have diagnosed her as an "extreme transvestite," but Elbe refused the term; such persons "disgusted" her.

In her autobiography, Elbe described herself as two complete persons; her male self and Lili. The male self, it seemed, had been slowly dying away, while Lili was ascendant; she wanted to have the rest of the male cut out so she could be Lili entirely. Like Dora before her, she considered herself a hermaphrodite, and Hirschfeld's assessment (to her) confirmed this. There is little hard evidence that she was intersex; as we know from other histories, Hirschfeld made a practice of providing the diagnosis of hermaphrodism so that patients could legally change their names. Elbe checked into the Dresden Women's Hospital for removal of the testicles and penis (performed by Gohrbandt, though in her book she changed the name to Gebhard).[43] Kurt Warnekros performed the vaginoplasty. He didn't use the skin graft as Gohrbandt had on Dora but instead the Schubert operation, named for a surgeon who transplanted a piece of the rectum* a few centimeters long into the newly formed vaginal opening.[44] Elbe returned to the surgeon in 1931 for a third surgery; she wanted a uterine implant and an opening into the vaginal canal that would permit her to become pregnant and to give birth. Sadly, the procedure did not go as planned. "I cannot write about my last operation," Lili explained in an entry of August 15; "it was an abyss of suffering." At the beginning of September she wrote a final letter to her sister, telling her that she'd dreamt of their mother, who called her by her chosen name: Lili.[45] She would die shortly after, possibly due to necrosis; the

---

* The technique was developed for cases of vaginal hypoplasia (when the vagina forms incompletely); other methods used a small section of bowel.

other procedures had used her own tissue, but transplanted organs cannot survive without immunosuppressive drugs.

Lili Elbe's autobiography would be published after her premature death—and yet she has a name we know, a gravestone we can visit. She has a legacy. Glamorous, a painter with money, education, opportunity, and support, Elbe offered up an ideal. The media covered her case and portrayed her as a pioneer and an icon—not only because of the surgery but because she "die[d] as a woman."[46] Dora's story, meanwhile, has mostly been forgotten; we have none of her words after the intake interview, and only Levy-Lenz's description of the happy maid plying her craft by the kitchen grate. Then again, this might not have displeased Dora. Modest and retiring, Dora lived in the uncelebrated hallways of domestic servitude and the voiceless anonymity of the laboring class. She was a woman of her time, that is, in every sense.

11

ALL THE DEVILS ARE HERE

LATE WINTER SNOW FELL ACROSS BAVARIA, BUT IT DIDN'T DETER THE CROWDS.
Buttoned up in winter coats, they waited in long lines for entry, then
submitted to a body search—several, in fact, just to be sure. Security officials were on edge; February 26, 1924, was the first day of
Hitler's trial.[1]

He should have been tried in Leipzig at the Staatsgerichtshof, a court
for cases of high treason. That was the law. Of course, Bavaria didn't
much care for Weimar laws. Instead, the tribunal would be the People's
Court of Bavaria, in Munich, the verdict to be given by five judges—two
professional and three laypersons—without right of appeal. Their chosen location was the Reichswehr Infantry School, ironic in that its cadets
had joined Hitler in his attempt to overthrow the government.

Historian David King paints the scene: the "sprawling redbrick building" had become a mini-fortress with guards at the door, mounted state
police, barbed wire, and blocked traffic. Up went the crowds to a second-
floor dining hall with "winter sun casting an almost reddish glow" on
the wallpaper and oak beams. Fifty-three feet long and thirty-eight feet
wide, the hall offered standing room only, with journalists packed into
the gallery, and it was filled before eight o'clock that morning, leaving
lurkers outside the gates. At half past eight, officers escorted ten defen-
dants to tables at the front, and a *Chicago Daily* newsman caught sight
of Hitler for the first time: "Was this provincial dandy, with his slick
dark hair, his cutaway coat, his awkward gestures and glib tongue, the
terrible rebel? He seemed for the world like a traveling salesman for a
clothing firm." A reporter for the *Völkischer Kurier* described Hitler as
looking well-rested. And perhaps he was; in the courtroom were many

supporters. One of them was also presiding judge: fifty-three-year-old George Neithardt, the deeply right-wing Superior Court Director.

The prosecutor asked Neithardt to expel the audience from the room, since Hitler's case was "a threat to national security and public order." A debate ensued, but the prosecution lost its gambit. The trial, Neithardt announced, would be public and, writes King, Hitler would "exploit this situation with consummate skill." A public trial, with sixty international reporters, gave him exactly the platform he'd been looking for.

Hitler spoke for three hours that day, three hours of fervor and intensity, an absolutely flawless performance that any actor would envy. He wasn't speaking in his own defense; it was practically a stump speech. He used the time to explain why rebellions like his were necessary to cleanse Germany, that Jews were to blame for its hardships, and that Communism must be stamped out. He cited trouble in the Ruhr Valley as an example of how weak leadership "cut up and slashed" the country, then blamed the economic crisis on governmental mismanagement. Citizens were being robbed and kept down, he insisted, by the Weimar Republic and the left.

The partisan judge allowed him free rein, even when Hitler boasted about the Nazi party itself. "I refuse to be modest about something that I know that I can do," he said, telling the court he'd turned six like-minded men into millions. "I did not come into this courtroom to deny anything," Hitler told them, but he would not plead guilty because "there is no high treason against the traitors of 1918!" He repeated "stab-in-the-back" propaganda about the war having been stolen, and claimed that the Weimar government were the real criminals. Imagine the clicking typewriter keys and dazzling flashbulbs; as King so aptly puts it, the courtroom drama provided "publicity [Hitler] could never have hoped to purchase."

The court sentenced Hitler to five years in prison. He would only serve around nine months in minimum security at Landsberg, where he was permitted visitors (including forty attendees to his thirty-fifth birthday party),[2] and had time and means to write a book. Originally titled *4½ Years of Struggle against Lies, Stupidity and Cowardice: A Reckoning*, he would rename it *Mein Kampf* (*My Struggle*). The manifesto served up a taste of propaganda to come; in fact, it came with propaganda instructions: "The art of propaganda lies in understanding the emotional ideas of the great masses" through emotional appeal and psychology, not through science. Its task, he wrote, "is not to make an objective study of the truth," but "to serve our own right, always and unflinchingly."[3]

Hitler stepped out of Landsberg prison on December 20, 1924, just before Christmas, his sentence drastically commuted for reasons we can only assume were related to his popularity in Bavaria. A few months later, he relaunched himself into politics at the same beer hall where he'd attempted his putsch. By then, he had complete control of the Nazi party and turned his attention, almost immediately, to *Rassenhygiene*. Eugenicists and race hygienists would dub Hitler the "great doctor of the German people" for his recognition of "purely biological values." The Jews would be his principal, but by no means only, target. Physically and mentally disabled people, racial minorities, and homosexuals and transvestites would qualify as possessing "lives not worth living."[4]

A few years later, in 1928, Adolf Brand polled political parties about where they stood on the question of homosexuality. The Nazis sent him an extensive reply: Germany must be masculine, and it "can only maintain its masculinity if it exercises discipline, especially in matters of love. Free love and deviance are undisciplined. Therefore we reject you, as we reject anything which hurts our people. Anyone who even thinks of homosexual love is our enemy." The rest might almost be a veiled threat: "Might makes right. And the stronger will always win over the weak. . . . We therefore reject any form of lewdness, especially homosexuality, because it robs us of our last chance to free our people from the bondage which now enslaves it."[5] That bondage, they claimed, had been caused by Jews and by women—a Jewish conspiracy to feminize Germans so that they might fall to their rivals.

What began with Hans Blüher, the Wandervögel, and *Männerbund* ideology had been codified into the Nazi platform; in 1935, the same would be signed into law as the Nuremberg Race Laws. Jews would lose their citizenship and then their lives; women were pressured to leave the workforce and to have at least four children, while abortion of a healthy fetus became a "crime against the German body." The Gestapo orchestrated a grim manhunt for homosexuals and sent thousands to concentration camps. In 1939, Hitler introduced "mercy death" for supposedly incurable patients; some 70,000 people in mental institutions were killed in gas chambers that would later be repurposed for the Holocaust.[6]

At his trial, Hitler warned the prosecution that no sentence would hold him: "Our prisons will open [and] today's accused become the accusers!"[7] Even as Hirschfeld and the SHC prepared to make the biggest challenge yet to the penal code, the prison cell that had held Hitler was indeed empty, and "all the devils here."[8]

Hirschfeld's skull was fractured by the assault in Munich. Yet he continued to give lectures, in spite of bawdy, protesting youths wearing the swastika symbol at the fringe of every crowd.[9] The author Christopher Isherwood, befriended by Hirschfeld, wrote about his constant insecurity: "sometimes treated with official respect, sometimes threatened with death; to be alternately praised and lampooned by the press; to be helped by those who would later lose their nerve and betray him."

Dangerous, yes. But the political aims of Hirschfeld's design were never clearer, and he used the Institute's museum, its research, and its patients to woo lawmakers to his side. He had certainly wooed Christopher Isherwood, who described the Institute as a safe house. More than once, he peered from the upper windows to watch plainclothes detectives lurking at the park's edge, hoping "that one of their wanted victims [would] be tempted to venture out of Hirschfeld's sanctuary for a sniff of fresh air."[10] The Institute for Sexual Science never attained its goal of being a university research center, but it was, in many ways, much more: the hub from which gender affirmation surgeries could be enacted, a safe space with legal counseling, even a training center which attempted to place newly transitioned patients in suitable jobs.[11] And, through the newly formed Cartel for the Reform of the Sexual Penal Code, the Institute simultaneously became "the sexual reformist engine of the Weimar Republic" against an emerging Nazi party intent on stamping out homosexuality and all other intermediaries for good.[12]

A CARTEL RISES

After its 1923 defeat, the Action Committee all but dissolved. They had come so close to victory; that May, four of the five governing parties—the Social Democrats, the German Democratic Party (DDP), the Communists, and even the Republican Party of Germany—agreed in theory to a repeal of Paragraph 175.[13] However, Radbruch's replacement removed all liberal changes to the penal code, and even expanded Paragraph 175 before it came to a vote. In the new proposal, not only sodomy but also any "coital-like" acts—anal, oral, interfemoral, even possibly mutual masturbation—could be punished with up to five years in a penitentiary.[14] It exceeded Hirschfeld's worst expectations and fears.[15] There might be time to correct course (the changing government meant delays), but fixation on the anti-homosexual statute had so far doomed activists to failure.[16] Bias and hatred barred the way; they must expand their view and consider reforms not just for homosexuals but for all citizens regarding sexual life.

This, at least, was the position of younger members of the SHC such as Kurt Hiller and sexologist Richard Linsert. Would Hirschfeld, "more researcher than politician," balk at the new preferred strategy?[17] They needn't have worried. Hiller described Hirschfeld as "provoked by the brazen and dangerous idiocy of the opposition"—a force that now included former ally Adolf Brand and also the League for Human Rights. Brand's position wasn't a surprise; his masculinist ethos increasingly aligned with German nationalists and the right. Meanwhile, the League leaned into centrist "middle-class respectability," as opposed to the much broader sense of sexual freedom embraced by Linsert and Hiller (which included rights for sex workers).[18] The League penalized or refused membership to men they considered "effeminate" homosexuals, and though transvestites were ostensibly allowed to join, they were not permitted to serve in leadership roles.[19]

Some of the League's critiques were, however, valid enough; they attacked Brand's "self-owners" for having relations with minors, which they considered exploitative. They also considered Hirschfeld's work as a medical expert deeply hypocritical, and for good reason, as Hirschfeld exploited legal loopholes to save homosexuals from prison by claiming that homosexuality amounted to a "psychological impairment." This took advantage of the judicial practice of reducing a sentence for "compromised" states of mind—but it also promoted the idea of pathological homosexuality and even denial of rational accountability.[20] Hirschfeld had practical reasons for this, and continued to preach one thing and to practice another when it came to working within (and thwarting) the legal system—something the League refused to countenance.

So, neither Brand's masculinists nor the League for Human Rights would join Hiller and the SHC in their new 1925 campaign, especially as the plan championed sexual matters beyond Paragraph 175: namely, legalization of abortion and the support of mothers (including single mothers). The age-old divide resurfaced, and two of the largest homosexual groups ultimately chose misogyny over unity.

Hiller set the agenda. They would seek to win the favor of humanist reform groups dedicated to the principle of individual freedom. They already had a list of possible allies from participants in the First International Conference for Sexual Reform: Helene Stöcker's League for the Protection of Mothers, the Society for Sexual Reform, the Society for Sexual Science, the Association for Marital Law Reform, the Department of Sexual Reform at the Institute of Sexual Science, and finally the German League for Human Rights.[21]

This last should not be confused with the League for Human Rights mentioned above. The German League was a much larger and more wide-reaching group, boasting Albert Einstein and accomplished military historian Hans Delbrück as members.* With over 13,000 members, the German League maintained goals of pacifism, the abolition of violence, socialism, and the rights of the people. The Marital Law Reformers advocated no-fault divorce, the Society for Sexual Science desired national sex education, the Society for Sexual Reform fought

---

* Yes, if you are a fan of *Young Frankenstein, that* Hans Delbrück, or the disembodied brain thereof—though he was neither scientist nor saint.

for abortion rights and birth control, as did the League for the Protection of Mothers, which also promoted the legal rights of single mothers and illegitimate children (as well as their eugenics-influenced "new sexual ethic"). By widening the scope of reform, Hiller explained, the activists ceased to be a "clique of a maltreated minority that protested in exclusive self-interest" and instead rose as a supergroup fighting for self-government among free, rational, consenting people.[22] The law they sought to reform wasn't even called Paragraph 175 anymore, but Paragraphs 296, 184, 218, and 297 of the new penal code.

They named themselves the Cartel for the Reform of the Sexual Penal Code. The Reichstag would finalize the code and debate it in 1929. They had only a few years to change minds, and they needed to make them count. Their enemies, even imprisoned, had not been idle. This was their moon shot.

SEXUAL REFORM GOES GLOBAL

By all accounts, it was quite a celebration. On May 14, 1928, the Institute was hung with decorations, and a cocktail table had been erected for the pleasure of guests. Food, festivities, guests, alcohol: the expense gave even Karl Giese pause. The late-coming housekeeper Adelheid claimed people were still talking about the party months later, but the event was much more than a party.[23] Hirschfeld had used the occasion of his fiftieth birthday, in 1918, to set up his Dr. Magnus Hirschfeld Foundation, through which the Institute now operated. Now, about to turn sixty in the midst of Reichstag debates about the penal code, he and the SHC prepared their festivities with a political agenda.

The Cartel for the Reform of the Sexual Penal Code had published their counter-draft of the law a year earlier. In it, they demanded exemption from punishment for "medical abortion," "fornication between men," and "male prostitution."[24] Female prostitution had never been punished; the counter-draft merely demanded equity. The draft would also decriminalize adultery and provide for sex education, and Hirschfeld simultaneously released a small book on birth control. The

Cartel had managed to overcome its own (very significant) differences to bring the draft together, with compromises on all sides. The question now was whether the Reich would ever do the same.

The minutes of the 1928 SHC meeting make their position clear; this was the "last decisive phase" in their decades-long fight for legal reform. They had reached the now-or-never phase of the campaign and decided to use the birthday celebration to boost their cause. It started (perhaps not surprisingly, considering Hirschfeld's own predilection for surveys) with a questionnaire.

Linsert and Hiller took the lead. They sought the opinions of thirty impressive personalities, including Sigmund Freud, novelist Thomas Mann, and famed physician, eugenicist, and Marxist Max Hodann, along with allies such as Helene Stöcker and the recently retired Institute doctor Arthur Kronfeld. There were four questions:

Do you agree with Hirschfeld's idea that science is not a goal in itself, but is meant to serve humanity, and that the results of science should make mankind happier and be respected by the law?

Do you think it possible that his ideas, especially those on the sexual life, could be accepted in our time, and what means should be used to realize this?

Do you believe that Magnus Hirschfeld is sufficiently recognized?

Do you think it is necessary for the Reichstag to consult him before the law on sexual variants is worked out?[25]

The shortest, and perhaps least hopeful, response came from Kronfeld: "1. Yes. 2. No. 3. No. 4. Yes."[26] His hope that any sort of justice would be realized in Germany had evaporated some time before. Others were more sanguine; the president of the Reichstag, Paul Löbe, wrote that he had "always considered Magnus Hirschfeld to be a pioneer" and that he could "only wish the results of his investigations will, in future, be even more recognized and applied than now." Even Freud, who was certainly no friend to Hirschfeld, wrote that "the life and work of Dr. Magnus

Hirschfeld against the cruel and unjustifiable interference of the law in human sexual life deserves general recognition and support." Hodann claimed that a socialist government would have respected Hirschfeld, but that the "clerical and bourgeois circles" that persisted under the Weimar Republic maligned him. He was, very probably, correct.[27]

The comments were gathered together for publication in a volume, a means of demonstrating the respect that Hirschfeld ought to command with the Reichstag—but there existed a still more direct route. One of the respondents was Dr. Erich Frey, a well-known lawyer with a lucrative and high-profile career. He had worked on cases with Hirschfeld as an expert witness and agreed to petition the Reichstag commission on his behalf.[28]

There were, however, notable absentees from the respondents. Neither the League for Human Rights, run by Hirschfeld's rival Friedrich Radszuweit, nor Adolf Brand had been invited to reply. The two outsiders to the Cartel fumed at Hirschfeld's increasing popularity and support; Radszuweit even sent out his own survey to prove he was the more popular.* The mutual frustrations of these rivals resulted in a tenuous alliance between Radszuweit and Adolf Brand, mainly as a force against Hirschfeld and the Cartel.[29] Longtime Hirschfeld critic Dr. Albert Moll would soon join them, holding his own First International Congress for Sex Research in 1926, after the one held at the Institute; he refused to invite Hirschfeld on the grounds that Hirschfeld confused political agitation with science. A further reason for the snub was that many scientific minds refused to come if Hirschfeld was to attend. Some agreed with Moll that Hirschfeld was not an objective scientist; others were no doubt influenced by increasing anti-homosexual and anti-Semitic attitudes. Moll was one of the few scientists opposed to eugenics, another point on which he and Hirschfeld (as a monist

---

* Operating his own publishing house and putting out two homosexual magazines gave Radszuweit superlative media influence on the subject of homosexual rights. All the same, the race was a close one; Radszuweit received 1557 votes in his popularity contest; Hirschfeld 1491 (Herrn, *Der Liebe und dem Leid*, 341).

and Darwinist) disagreed—but though he was also Jewish by birth, his own conference included a lecture by a Catholic priest. Meanwhile, Moll called Hirschfeld's teachings "poison" and considered him a "danger to public safety."[30]

Hirschfeld had made powerful enemies among his fellow sexologists, with Moll ultimately proving the most dangerous. Even so, Linsert and Hiller intended their questionnaire to prove that Hirschfeld had many more—and more illustrious—friends. The celebration included nearly 100 articles in the press, 120 telegrams, and 600 congratulatory letters, and so many guests that additional tableware had to be purchased to serve them all.[31] Those friendships would be worth the expense.

From June 30 to July 6, 1928, Hirschfeld, with August Forel and the British sexologist and reformer Havelock Ellis, held their second international conference in Copenhagen, co-chaired by Dr. Hertha Riese Frankfurt, who directed the first marriage counseling service in the region, fashioned after Stöcker's League for the Protection of Mothers. Hirschfeld's first International Congress for Sexual Reform, the one held at the Institute before the dissolution of the Action Committee, had laid the foundation for something more—something greater than he or the SHC, or even the Cartel, had yet achieved: entrée to the world stage.

Delegates came to Copenhagen from the United States, France, Spain, England, Argentina, Chile, the Netherlands, Egypt, India, and the USSR—many of them celebrities in their own right.[32] There were also far more women at this meeting. Hirschfeld gave the first lecture, and admitted that he might not have given women their due. A product of masculinist-influenced Darwinism, he had habitually thought men superior. In this speech, he recognized women's equality, their ability in sports, business, economics, and more; "they can even be pilots!" he announced.[33] (A just-in-time recognition, given that a woman doctor had co-organized the conference.) Kurt Hiller wrote the defining lecture from the German perspective; he meant it as an international call for support and also as a petition to the Reichstag, titling it "Appeal in Favor of a Suppressed Variation of Man." Hirschfeld delivered it on Hiller's behalf. Same-sex sexual acts were not illegal in many of the represented nations; thus Paragraph 175 was, he concluded, "the shame of this century."

The conference was meant to be more than a meeting; it would serve as the platform for establishing a parent organization, the first truly international alliance for the purpose of sexual reform. In direct opposition to Albert Moll, the focus of the World League for Sexual Reform would be sexual-political as well as scientific; what good was philosophy if it didn't touch human lives in a practical and progressive manner? The founding committee gathered together many of Hirschfeld's birthday well-wishers: August Forel, Havelock Ellis, Helene Stöcker, and Hermann Rohleder (a urologist and sexologist), but also the American Harry Benjamin and the British archaeologist Francis Turville-Petre.

The World League for Sexual Reform drafted a resolution before the end of the conference.[34] Its principal goals were to "appeal to legislative bodies, the press and the people of all countries to help create a new social and legal attitude (based on scientific research in sexual biology, psychology and sociology) toward the sexual life of men and women." The happiness of many, they wrote, had been "sacrificed to false sexual standards, ignorance, and intolerance" about such diverse topics as marriage, divorce, contraception, prostitution, and sex education, as well as the role of women. Most especially, the League required "political, economic and sexual equality between men and women," which included the caveat that "procreation may be undertaken only voluntarily," and a "rational attitude toward sexually abnormal people and especially with regard to homosexuals both men and women." With the exception of language that regarded intermediaries as "abnormal," the WLSR's platform sounds almost as progressive today. Still embedded in their language, however, was the League for the Protection of Mothers' idea of eugenic procreation—"encouragement" for the "fit and gifted" and sterilization of the "unfit," a supposedly scientific model that remained popular internationally.[35]

The office of the WLSR would be, not surprisingly, at the Institute, but its reach would extend well beyond Germany. Members from different countries would set up their own branches and publish their own journals. The WLSR would hold a meeting in London in 1929, another in Vienna in 1930, and one in Brno, in what was then Czechoslovakia, in 1932, with meetings planned for Moscow, Paris, and Chicago. By then, the league had 190,000 members worldwide.[36]

Freshened and uplifted by this new international circle, Hirschfeld returned home to face Germany's Minister of Justice, who had invited him to an audience and further promised to send officials to the Institute before drafting final legislation.[37] For the first time, it seemed that real change was on the horizon, not only in Germany but well beyond.

THE LAST BATTLE

The Reich Minister of Justice was a somewhat difficult office to hold in the Weimar Republic. Dr. Erich Koch-Weser had been a founding member of the German Democratic Party in 1918, believed in liberal politics, and supported reform. On September 4, 1928, Hirschfeld and SHC board member Horst Kretschmann-Winckelmann sat before him. Hirschfeld pressed the need for quick action; the law had been in limbo much too long, subject to every vibration of political upheaval. If Koch-Weser agreed with their counter-draft, could a legal decision be made to protect the country from an even harsher penal code in future—as had happened last time?[38]

The minister made light of their concern, assuring them that he favored reform, even if he didn't agree with every point of the counter-draft. He promised, in addition, to personally learn more about the science of sexology. The published minutes of the SHC show guarded hope; the meeting had been "satisfactory," but they must now redouble their efforts, which involved inviting more members of the Reichstag to the Institute.[39] The politicians didn't come to see a museum, however; they came to see and hear from more patients.

Gerd Katter received his transvestite certificate in 1928, around the time of Hirschfeld's meeting with the justice minister. Hirschfeld had helped him attain it, and with deep gratitude, Katter returned after his surgeries to provide a living example to the Reichstag. In the spring of

1929, he told his story before the German Democratic Party, the Social Democrats, and Prussian Minister Otto Braun.[40] He arrived early, eagerly awaiting his turn. "The atmosphere at the Institute was positively charged with tension," he wrote. Standing before the politicians, he explained how he'd been "pre-programmed" a transvestite before birth, and that his life had been one of loneliness and misery until he came to the Institute. Here, he met others like himself, people whose birth sex didn't align with who they were. At last, he'd found a refuge, a home, and others who treated him "as if [he] were not a stranger."[41]

As before, personal testimony proved powerfully moving. Before the summer recess, the Reichstag announced that they would deliberate in October and vote by the end of the year. There was a problem, however; of the twenty-eight members of the Criminal Law Committee, fourteen were in favor of overturning the law against homosexuality and fourteen were against. On July 1, the Cartel met late into the night to discuss tactics for "the final battle." "The fate of the movement," they wrote, was "on a knife's edge. Nothing can be said yet about the outcome. It all depends on whether we can pull together all available forces at the last moment."[42] It had been three decades of constant struggle. Everything hung upon turning one more person to their cause.

The Cartel decided upon three strategies. First, they would publish short works debunking the myth that homosexuality arose from seduction. Second, they planned to have high-ranking and well-known personalities speak in favor of their cause before the issue was decided. The third strategy required some sleight of hand; Hirschfeld, for all of his achievements, was a divisive figure, and they couldn't chance having him as their spokesman at this crucial moment; much better to have less problematic experts represent their cause. Hiller drafted a letter to Wilhelm Kahl, chairman of the Criminal Law Committee, promising to provide the names of sexologists who would be more positively received.

The eighty-fifth session of the Criminal Law Committee met on October 16, 1929. The day's deliberations would solidify the penal code, meaning it would go from "draft" to "prospective" bill, up for a confirmation vote in the Reichstag. One by one, the members gave their votes and opinions. Fourteen voted to delete Paragraph 175, thirteen voted to retain it. The vote came down to the chairman, Wilhelm Kahl. In his notes he wrote that the paragraph had not a single "rational punitive purpose," and overturning it would end the "tragedies of blackmail"; most of all, however, he hoped that overturning Paragraph 175 would finally put an end to the Cartel's "rampant agitation and propaganda" in favor of homosexuality. Kahl believed that legalization would send homosexuals and transvestites back into the quiet fringes, where they could no longer offend or seduce; that is, he voted in favor of overturning the sodomy law so that Hirschfeld would finally shut up.[43] Whatever his reasons, the vote vindicated the Cartel, the SHC, the Institute—and, above all, the intermediaries themselves.

Germany awoke to bold headlines on the morning of October 17, 1929. The *Berliner Tageblatt* called the decision a "A Cultural Step Forward"; the conservative *Deutsche Zeitung* a "Victory for the Corrupters of the Volk."[44] Baskets of flowers arrived at the Institute in celebration, but the decision was anything but roses.[45] While removing Paragraph 175, the commission planned to approve Paragraph 297, which outlawed male–male sex if one partner was under the age of twenty-one and the other not, or if the act were "paid for" in either money or influence. Hiller, who had long supported sex workers, called the decision "useless" and "an illusion."[46]

The decision went against the primary tenet of Hirschfeld's beliefs, too; Kahl and others on the penal reform committee—even the Social Democrats—still considered homosexuality unnatural. When the reformed penal code was enacted, its strictures seemed to Kurt Hiller an "outburst of fury"[47] against his kind; members of the Cartel despaired, and it sparked a power struggle in the SHC—with devastating consequences. After more than thirty years at the helm of the Scientific Humanitarian Committee, Hirschfeld resigned.

An article written at the time by Karl Besser blamed the resignation on Hirschfeld's "poor health, his exhaustion from years of personal attacks," and his desire to concentrate "on the Institute and on his work as a sexologist."[48] In all probability, Hiller and Linsert forced him out.

First, we must remember that the Cartel was not fighting only to overturn Paragraph 175 but to make a more just penal code for many others, including male and female prostitutes. The 15–13 decision was predicated on absolving "respectable homosexual men" at the expense of those the government considered dangerous and criminal.[49] Would the SHC accept that bargain? It's more than a simple yes or no; a letter by Linsert and Max Hodann tells the story of clashing ideals and wounded egos. It returns us to why Linsert and Hiller wanted a list of experts other than Hirschfeld who supported the repeal and would be acceptable to the Criminal Law Committee.

Hiller had suggested approaching opinion leaders on the sodomy law and then, "discreetly, by word of mouth," relaying the names of those experts to Reichstag delegates most on their side. The plan wasn't precisely subterfuge, but it intended to manufacture the appearance of neutrality. Why such caution? Radszuweit, of the League for Human Rights, had potentially bungled the vote, having invited Wilhelm Kahl to a Berlin dance palace where a speaker demanded equal rights for homosexuals in an act that "spooked" the conservative chairman. They needed to move quickly to undo any damage, so Linsert and Hiller began the process of sharing (confidentially) their list of experts. Hirschfeld, however, had already sent the full list to Kahl—and because the names came from Hirschfeld, all appearance of objectivity was lost.[50]

Linsert considered this a betrayal and blamed Hirschfeld's ego; did he want to be the only expert named? Or was it an assertion of dominance over experts included by Hiller who did not endorse Hirschfeld's science? Either explanation is possible, but Hirschfeld's behavior may have more to do with his foundational belief that science, once presented, would plead its own case. He had always trusted, for better and for worse, that, when faced with scientific evidence, even his enemies would see the error of their ways. It wasn't true then, as it isn't true now. The argument from science works only on those who care to be changed by it.

Once Linsert and Hiller had the SHC well in hand, they abandoned the scientific angle altogether in favor of legal theory and the preservation of individual rights. Hiller, like Radszuweit, believed ardently that

Paragraph 175 ought to be struck down "on the grounds of rights and justice."[51] That was Brand's position, too, though the brief union between Radszuweit and Brand had reached its nadir. Radszuweit's commitment to "bourgeois respectability" meant that he aimed to tame—or "domesticate"—homosexuality so that it would be better accepted by society. As a result, he castigated Brand's "pederasty" as sexual and emotional abuse of boys and young men, and he flatly disagreed with Brand's belief in the fundamental bisexuality of all people.[52]

Radszuweit was a member of the Social Democratic Party, but he was also a savvy businessman and rightly surmised that the masculinist, *Männerbund* nature of the Nazi ethos would be attractive to certain homosexual communities. He polled 38,000 homosexuals and discovered that 12,000 belonged to right-wing parties: the German Nationalists, the German People's Party, and the ascendant Nazi party. As Robert Beachy writes in *Gay Berlin*, "blinded by the homoeroticism of the masculinist" propaganda, homosexuals failed to see how homosexuality threatened the "centrality of Nazi racialist doctrine."[53] Radszuweit's League and the SHC under Hiller and Linsert both pursued the image of respectable citizenship. This saved the fight for homosexual emancipation from eugenics, but it trusted in the power of nationality and of a government that respected homosexuals' role as good *völkisch* (as in "plain German folk") members of society. It was a trust misplaced.

After Hirschfeld's resignation, the SHC moved out of the Institute. The fight for homosexual emancipation in Germany would carry on without Hirschfeld, and he redirected his attention to giving lectures about the innate nature of sex and gender preferences. Hirschfeld, however, was tired. "I am no longer surprised at anyone who crosses over in the camp of my enemies," he wrote.[54] He held onto the one slim victory: that at the eleventh hour, he would at least see the overturn of Paragraph 175.

But this was not to be.

12

THE END OF EVERYTHING

WHY CAN'T YOU FIND A NICE GIRL, ASKED CHRISTOPHER ISHER-wood's mother.[1] She wanted him to settle down, to have children, and to stop messing about with other young men. Isherwood's characteristically wry reply is recorded in his memoir, *Christopher and His Kind*: "If boys didn't exist," he wrote, "I should have to invent them." Anglo-American, well-bred and well-heeled, Isherwood made up part of the literary circle surrounding the poet W. H. Auden. But despite his homosexuality (which he had in common with Auden), Isherwood preferred to think of male–male desire as "a private way of life discovered by himself and a few friends." He knew this was a pleasant fiction, a means of considering himself in a special class. He probably would have found kindred spirits among Brand's masculinists, but he didn't meet "his tribe" through *Der Eigene*. He met them at the Institute for Sexual Science, over lunch.

Christopher* arrived in Berlin in March 1929, a few months in advance of his friend Auden, who was planning to go there during his postgraduate gap year. He came to the Institute because the only English-speaking person he knew of in Germany, Francis Turville-Petre, was renting two rooms from Hirschfeld's sister, Recha Tobias, in the Institute's annex next door. A widow, she had moved from Berlin-Schöneberg to 9a In den Zelten in 1927. She'd also gathered an elite set of occasional guests, including cultural critic Walter Benjamin and Marxist philosopher Ernst Bloch.

---

* Isherwood refers to himself in third person as "Christopher" throughout his memoir, so I will do the same.

The rooms she let to Turville-Petre overlooked the park, she told Christopher, who briskly climbed the stairs—but their first meeting didn't go especially smoothly. Turville-Petre, robed in crimson silk, threw open the door and shouted curses in German—at least, until Christopher managed to introduce himself. Apparently, Turville-Petre mistook him for the male sex worker he'd brought home the night before, who had tried to rob him. Apologies made, he ushered Christopher into his rooms more genially. "This place is an awful mess," he said with a flourish, "I'm never up at the unearthly hour they want to clean it." ("They" would be the maids, including Dora and Toni.) To make up for his uncharitable greeting, he invited Christopher to lunch—and lunch at the Institute, by Hirschfeld's design, included the staff as well as patients and guests.

Lean and attractive, with a characteristic flop of bangs parted to the side, Christopher took a seat in the large dining room. He'd come for what he assumed would be amusement, and "pictured transvestites as loud, screaming, willfully unnatural creatures." Instead, he found himself unable to tell most of them apart from women assigned female at birth. They were, he wrote, "quietly natural" and "accepted by everyone else as a matter of course." It left him feeling like he was the unnatural outsider, and a tour through the facility unsettled him still more. He "giggled nervously" through the museum of fetishes, "embarrassed because, at last, he was being brought face to face with his tribe"—his "kind." The pleasant fantasy of being a privileged and selective elite vanished in the reality of community; he was not so different after all. His first reaction was one of anger, distaste, and blame, perhaps similar to Levy-Lenz's response to Fredy. Only when he heard the same scornful response from someone else, the French Nobel laureate André Gide, did he change his mind.

Hirschfeld had invited both literary men to see what he called "live exhibits"—a demonstration of hormonal preparations for male-to-female transvestites. A young patient kindly opened her shirt with a modest smile to show off "two perfectly formed female breasts." Gide pretended interest, but was internally "sneering"—just as Christopher himself had been. How dare he? Christopher suddenly felt a deep love and respect for Hirschfeld, the "silly solemn old professor with his doggy mustache, thick peering spectacles, and clumsy German-Jewish boots," and anger at the Nobel laureate. The doctor, the blushing transvestite, and Christopher himself were "on the same side," and that "tribe"—he later wrote—were "heroic leaders" worthy of all honor. He decided to stay among them.

Turville-Petre's rooms were spacious and airy; two windows looked out over the sprawling park of Tiergarten, now in early autumn colors. Christopher's room, by contrast, was "dark and cheap," with a view of the interior courtyard and a mostly, though not entirely, blank wall. On it, Hirschfeld had printed one of his many slogans; this time, the words came from Goethe: "Spirit of Man, how like thou to Water! Fate of Man, how like thou to Wind!" Christopher claimed to prefer it to the park view; "just as changes in the light make trees look different, so [his] varying moods made the poem speak in different tones . . . joyful, cynical, tragic." The Institute would soon experience them all.

MAKING NAZIS

Two hundred miles from Berlin lies the small town of Affinghausen. Home to Germans of the peasant class, it may have resembled Dora's town of Seifen far away to the south. Industrious, farming people with little to spare, they suffered more than most during the hyperinflation and hadn't enjoyed the recovery promised by the Social Democrats.

Starting in 1928, a young man from a neighboring community began turning up on the regular. He looked like them, he talked like them, and he'd been trying (and failing) to make ends meet just like them. Weren't they tired of the struggle, he wanted to know; didn't they long for a strong Germany that could feed its people? He knew just who to blame for that: the Weimar government. The villagers stopped, and they listened. The activist turned up more frequently, and now he brought party leaders, too, smartly clad men in uniform, all sporting the swastika. It didn't take long before a majority of the community joined as Nazi initiates.

At first, only a few joined the cause, but as the initiated repeated the claims, more and more were enticed. Then they, like the original activist, fanned out into neighboring towns to replicate the process. No political party had ever done such a thing; villages were outliers, considered beyond the fringe of politics. They existed off the radar. The Social Democrats, the Catholic Center Party, the Communists—none of them had the least idea that a groundswell of Nazi support had begun.[2]

The Weimar Republic was born amid division, and the gaps only widened with time. Splinter parties arose, robbing the larger political groups of power while remaining ineffectual on their own. The right had always been, writes historian Eric D. Weitz, the greatest threat to the republic—but it existed in hundreds of separate organizations. There were the monarchists, many of whom were still in positions of power as officers, businessmen, and civil servants, but there was also a ragtag band of government opponents from every echelon. The dissatisfied First World War veterans (some of whom joined the Storm Troops) felt cheated by the loss of the war, but so too did the "disgruntled teachers and shopkeepers, street-corner agitators, and lay Catholic and Protestants."

Then came the Nazis. They promised a "third empire," or *Drittes Reich*, with a strong leader to embody "the essence and destiny of the German people," a man who would take up the struggle against "all dissolute and degenerate people and ideas" and lead them to "prosperity, cultural achievement, and—not least—national grandeur." But that wasn't all. There is nothing so seductive as exoneration. It's not your fault, Hitler told the German people; Jews and immigrants were "growing rich off their misery" and "destroying the nation's purity."

How could such a heterogeneous collection of people, from day laborers to scholars to priests, fall victim to such rhetoric? Easy. It had been the language of the right for a very long time; the Nazis didn't invent, merely made devious use of key words and phrases already popular with conservatives: *Volkstum* (ethnicity), *Deutschtum* (Germanness), *Überfremdung* (foreign infiltration), *Schieberepublik* (thieves' republic). These terms, writes Weitz, were "thundered from the pulpit" and printed in press, leaflets, novels, film; little wonder they also turned up at dinner tables all across Germany.

Hitler didn't need to invent anti-Semitism, either; it had been simmering ominously since well before anthropologist Heinrich Schurtz's *Altersklassen und Männerbünde*, Blüher's *Wandervögel*, and Oswald Spengler's *Decline of the West* (from which Hitler borrowed heavily). Social Darwinism gave anti-Semitism a pseudoscientific pedigree; the Nazis weaponized it through propaganda. "Was there any form of filth or profligacy, particularly in cultural life, without at least one Jew involved in it?," Hitler asked in *Mein Kampf.* This is a rephrasing of work by Paul Althaus, an anti-Semitic theologian. When Hitler claimed that the Jews were getting rich off Germany, he merely repeated a common trope bandied about during the war about hyperinflation and profiteering.

Hitler's innovation came in his delivery. "You constantly saw the swastika painted on sidewalks or found them littered by pamphlets put out by Nazis," explained a German housewife. Nazis in uniform marched with banners while pamphlets literally rained down from the trucks following them, like ticker tape at a parade. "Serious people" joined, the housewife wrote; "there was a feeling of restless energy. . . . I was drawn to the feeling of strength about the party, even though there was much in it that was highly questionable." Somehow, in the sea of red and black, the pomp and circumstance, the endorsements from veteran military men and the stamp of approval from "serious people," the Nazi swastika and all it stood for had been normalized.

Yet the Nazis still needed an enemy. The Jews were scapegoats, yes, but Hitler required the visuals of conflict, of "heroic" Germans defeating their enemies (in pantomime if necessary). For that, he turned to the Communists of the far left.

The community of Wedding (pronounced *vedin*) in the borough of Mitte, Berlin, was a Communist stronghold, home to working-class and often militant members of the German Communist Party. In the years after the First World War, it earned the nickname Red Wedding. The Nazis knew this well, so they determined to hold a rally there as an intentional provocation. Nearly a thousand people turned up—around

800 Storm Troopers and 200 Communist protesters. To start, the Communists attempted to halt the meeting; failing that, they heckled the speakers. A beer mug was thrown, a chair seized as a weapon, and suddenly the meeting was a street brawl. The Nazis wounded 85 Communists and used their superior numbers to subdue the rest; they then boldly publicized that "Marxist terrorism has been bloodily suppressed."

They would replay this narrative again and again—causing disruption and then "restoring" law and order—to convince everyday Germans that without the Nazis, all would dissolve into chaos. But the Nazis excelled at more positive messaging, too. The Hitler Youth (a latter-day representation of the Wandervögel) offered camping, hiking, and group activities; at the same time, it dispensed with social distinctions. Political indoctrination was kept to a minimum—at least, at first. "I wanted to be in a boys' club where I could strive toward a national ideal," wrote one member. "For me this was the start of a completely new life," wrote another. "There was only one thing in the world for me and that was service to the movement."

By 1930, the Nazis had opened soup kitchens and charity drives funded by their wealthier supporters. Material aid to the unemployed helped keep numerous people fed and clothed; it also won the Nazis support— and made the government's own attempts to help the needy seem pitiful indeed. The Nazis played, writes Weitz, "a very nice game"; they caused disruption but presented themselves as "the party of law and order" protecting the *Volk* from Communists—but also from "alien elements" and the republic itself, which ever teetered on the edge of financial disaster.

DEMOCRACY DIES IN THE DARK*

When President Calvin Coolidge gave his final State of the Union address in January 1928, he reflected on the "pleasing prospect" before

---

* Now a slogan of the *Washington Post*, the phrase was coined by Judge Damon J. Keith, of the U.S. Court of Appeals for the 6th Circuit. He ruled on a Watergate-era case against wiretapping, and later, under the Bush administration, his ruling prohibited the secret deportations of Muslims following 9/11.

him: "In the domestic field there is tranquility and contentment. . . . In the foreign field there is peace, the goodwill which comes from mutual understanding." All could look to the future with optimism. Unlike Germany, which had been facing potential ruin even during the First World War, the United States had gone from strength to strength. Production and employment were high and rising, and Americans had a new taste for riches—and for getting rich quick. The best way to do that, it seemed, was to speculate on Wall Street.[3]

After an astonishing eight-year rise, the Dow Jones Industrial Average had increased sixfold and many economists predicted a "permanently high plateau."[4] Speculation, however, is no firm foundation. A real estate bubble had burgeoned and collapsed in Florida; that was a first sign. No one paid it much attention. Soon, an asset bubble followed; overconfidence on the part of average consumers and small investors alike inflated stock prices—the actual value of a stock separated from its price tag by a cavity of hot air.[5] In 1928, the market started bucking like a wild horse. A boom had begun. The meteoric rise in stock prices wasn't due to actual value so much as the instability of a market built on little more than the words of supposedly in-the-know luminaries. "There is no cause for worry," said Andrew Mellon, whose financial backing led to the creation of the Gulf Oil Company among others, "The high tide of prosperity will continue."[6] Banks were trading on margins, credit, and easily acquired loans. They had loaned a good deal of money to Germany, too, and sold the Weimar government (along with France and England) securities at a discount rate. All through 1928 and well into 1929, stocks went from strength to strength. But the market couldn't keep growing forever.

All seemed well until Thursday, October 24, 1929. The market opened 11 percent lower than it had closed the day before, inducing a wave of panicked selling. On Monday, stocks dropped again, and then, on Black Tuesday, October 28, the market crashed, and would keep on crashing for years—until 1932. By then, 90 percent of Dow wealth and value had been wiped out. America's Roaring Twenties, sparkling with glitz and glam, flapper fashion, mobsters, Prohibition, and jazz, came to a screaming halt. The economy went into a tailspin, but the wreckage wouldn't be limited to the United States. As the crisis deepened, American institutions demanded immediate repayment of loans—including those they had given so freely to German businesses and the German government itself.

In the first wave of the crash, Germany's capital essentially evaporated, halting production and creating a demand crisis—meaning that consumers couldn't get goods because industry didn't have the resources to make them. Factories shut down operations; small businesses closed their doors; unemployment soared. The depression marked the third major catastrophe (with the war and hyperinflation) to hit Germany in a single generation, and on a scale no one had ever experienced before. But things were about to get worse. The coalition government, still led by the Social Democrats, fell apart over what to do about unemployment and social benefits. Despite the cost, Social Democrats wanted to expand them. Conservatives wanted them cut. The acting president, conservative Paul von Hindenburg, tried to solve the problem by appointing a new chancellor even more to the right than himself: Heinrich Brüning. His plan? Extreme cutbacks, not only to individuals but to businesses, too. There would be no government aid granted; people must let their own financial management secure them. Brüning knew he didn't have the votes to put his plan into practice; there were still too many seats in the hands of the Social Democrats. His solution was to call for new elections on September 14, 1930.

Politics were about to reshuffle, all right—just not in his favor. The Nazi propaganda machine ensured that the party surged ahead. Of 577 seats, the Social Democrats held onto 143, but the Nazis won an astonishing 107 (they had previously held 12). The Social Democrats' chief rivals were no longer the Communists (77 seats) or the once-controlling Catholic Center Party (68 seats); the contest for Germany's soul would be fought by democrats on one side and Nazis on the other.

This should have been an obvious defeat for Brüning; he had lost a great deal of power to govern. But as an avid monarchist who wanted to reestablish an authoritarian government of his own, Brüning didn't much care for the parliamentary way of doing things. President Hindenburg was in his eighties; he'd taken office in 1925, a "massive, stolid presence," heavily-built and lumbering as a tank, but formidable in his military uniform.[7] With age, he'd become "impatient with the complexities of political events," and, in the words of British historian Richard J. Evans, "ever more susceptible to the influence of his inner circle of advisers." Brüning persuaded an increasingly confused and senile Hindenburg that a conservative dictatorship exercised in his name would save Germany from deepening crises. If he would just invoke Article 48, Brüning would take care of all that messy state business on his behalf.[8]

Article 48 had been written into the Weimar constitution as a safeguard, similar to the powers of a U.S. president during a declared national emergency. Under it, the chancellor, rather than the president, could acquire the power to rule by decree instead of by vote, and could use the army to enforce his decree or to restore law. The power had been used (and abused) by Hindenburg's predecessors, especially during the Ruhr crisis, and the street skirmishes provoked by the Nazis gave them plenty of reason to invoke it again. Hindenburg agreed, and Brüning had his power to issue decrees limiting everything from press freedom to unemployment and social welfare. Brüning still had to consult the Reichstag, but he wasn't bound by its authority.[9]

Thus, the civic freedoms of the Weimar democracy began disappearing long before the Nazis came to power.[10] In 1929, Germany became in effect a dictatorship.

This was the Germany Christopher Isherwood encountered, a "brew seething with unemployment, malnutrition, stock-market panic, hatred of the Versailles Treaty, and other potent ingredients."[11] Things had changed at the Institute as well, some of it solidifying in the months that Isherwood remained encamped next to Francis Turville-Petre on the upper floors. The Scientific Humanitarian Committee, to which Hirschfeld had given thirty years of his life, had changed both its address and its mission—and was now keen to distance itself from his beliefs.

"The constant connection of the homosexual phenomenon with effemination," wrote Kurt Hiller, "with hermaphroditism, transvestitism, and other more or less repulsive natural games," had served to harm "the enlightenment and liberation campaign for male–male love." He went on to reference aspects praised by Brand and Friedländer: "What made Sparta strong, and Michelangelo ardent, has nothing in common with bearded women, bosom men, or any other monstrosity." Abandoning and even attacking transgender people, Hiller decried any use of science or sexology; they had nothing to do with the "cult of the hero and the youth, the joy of man in man."[12]

Hirschfeld responded to this by shifting the focus of his Institute; policy work once dedicated to homosexual emancipation and Paragraph 175 would now be given over to the needs, rights, and freedoms of intermediaries. From 1930 onward, the Institute became a center for transgender people specifically, most especially those interested in transformative surgery. All of the transgender surgeries discussed in chapter 10 took place circa 1931; Dora had her penectomy performed early in the year, her vaginoplasty in June. Toni Ebel, Lili Elbe, and (probably) Charlotte Charlaque also transitioned in that year, but Hirschfeld was not there to witness this. Giving the Institute for Sexual Science its new mission would be Hirschfeld's last act while still under its roof. On November 15, 1930, he boarded the *Columbus* and decamped for America, already aware he might never be allowed to return.

THE WORLD TOUR BEGINS

Harry Benjamin first came to the Institute in the mid-1920s, following his interest in endocrinology and Steinach's surgeries. He had since established himself as a premier endocrinologist in the United States and remained on the founding committee for the World League for Sexual Reform, as did Francis Turville-Petre. The most recent meeting had been in Vienna, in September; Hirschfeld, one of three meeting presidents, had hoped to greet Benjamin there, but Benjamin hadn't been able to attend. His paper, detailing the use of testosterone injections, would be read in his absence.

When Hirschfeld returned to Berlin from the conference, he wrote the younger man a letter saying that it had been a long and frustrating year and he could use a change of scene. Perhaps he had advance knowledge of an invitation. The president of the American Society of Medical History contacted him in early November, asking if he would speak on December 4 and attend a dinner in his honor at the Astoria Hotel. He graciously accepted.[13]

American newspapers were only too happy to write about the "prophet of the scientific roots of love and sex," and Hirschfeld was only too happy to lap up the praise. His lectures focused on the Institute's marriage counseling service—neutral territory for the public forum. Benjamin gave Hirschfeld the use of his apartment; he was supposed to be recovering from the past years' strain, which had exacerbated his diabetes. Instead, Hirschfeld used that private space to meet with doctors about more specialized and controversial subjects, namely the treatment of sexual intermediaries. Soon, other speaking invitations arrived, from as far away as California. Hirschfeld accepted every one, blazing a trail across the country for forty-eight talks in three and a half months, speaking in German and in English and featuring in headlines in over forty newspapers. It was not the holiday Karl Giese had envisioned for him, and it didn't stop at the U.S. border. A Japanese professor, Keijo Dohi, invited Hirschfeld to a Tokyo medical conference.

"I am glad that my old dream of circling the globe once seems to be coming true after all," he wrote in March 1931, "doubly glad, since it is clear from Hauptstein's reports that the Institute seems to be passing the dress rehearsal of my nonexistence quite well."[14] Hirschfeld trusted Friedrich Hauptstein, who served as secretary of the Institute-based office of the International Conferences on Sexologically-Based Sexual Reform and would later become administrative head of the Institute, to ensure continuity. As his health continued to deteriorate, however, he worried about the future. For the time being, sales of his hormone preparation Testifortan, or Titus Pearls, was providing financial support, but what would happen to the Institute in the event of his death? Even before leaving Berlin, Hirschfeld admitted, "I can hardly have full confidence in any of my coworkers after the experiences I have had . . . who will continue the work in my spirit?" [15] He relied on Karl Giese, absolutely. But Karl was neither a scientist nor a doctor, and Hirschfeld wanted "a student whom I can educate and form in my own sense." [16] No longer directing the Institute or the Scientific Humanitarian Committee, a sixty-three-year-old man facing the specter of mortality, Hirschfeld wanted nothing more than a young man to be apprentice, student, and successor.

Hirschfeld found exactly that while in Shanghai, where he went after the Tokyo conference in March 1931. Li Shiu Tong, known familiarly as Tao Li, was a well-to-do Chinese student of philosophy and medicine. Hirschfeld admired his "noble character," his "intelligence," but also his "unshakable loyalty and devotion." He agreed to travel with Hirschfeld and dedicate himself to sexology back in Germany—and should Hirschfeld die before they reached Berlin, he bequeathed to Tao Li everything he had with him, asking only that his ashes be returned to Karl Giese at the Institute. [17]

Hirschfeld hoped to settle the matter of succession at Christmas, 1931. But he wouldn't make it back to Berlin; Giese warned him away. Between the Nazi surge and "dictator Brüning," Germany had "fallen into madness," he wrote, and "in Prussia almost every second voter [is] a Nazi." [18] So Hirschfeld remained abroad, deferring his reunion with Giese for another year. In the meantime, Hirschfeld and Tao Li became lovers—a relationship, somewhat ironically, that Adolf Brand would have approved of, as mentor and ephebe.

As for Brand, his society of self-owners—never as large or robust as the SHC or Radszuweit's League for Human Rights—began to collapse. Many couldn't pay their dues in the worsening depression, and few had pocket money to buy its two publications. *Der Eigene* ceased publication in 1931, *Eros* in 1932. "Events of the last year have thinned the ranks dramatically," Brand complained. "The former members have now given their trust and support to the very person who marches at the apex of reaction, and whose own publication publicly declares that if the [Nazi] Party comes to power, all homosexuals will be strung up from the gallows." That Brand's devotees would find Nazism enticing should not have been a surprise, since his group had been at the fore of misogynistic and anti-Semitic attacks and engaged in a rhetoric of genetic, economic, and cultural superiority. But Brand would never admit his complicity. In the wake of the Nazis' ascendance, he followed Hans Blüher's example and prudently married, retiring from the public eye.[19]

The Nazis had plenty of homosexuals in their ranks, with or without him.

Thick-waisted and round-faced, with a short-clipped mustache over bulldog jowls, Ernst Röhm believed in war's power to strip away "all that was inessential" from life, until "only the real, the true, the masculine held its value."[20] As chief of the SA, or Storm Troops, Röhm had provided the muscle for the Beer Hall Putsch; referred to as Hitler's "loyal dog," he continued to direct the Führer's military might.[21] Each of his Brownshirts would be trained in *Manneszucht*, or masculine discipline, to counteract the "chaos" of femininity. As historian Eleanor Hancock describes it, Röhm's ideal German state was "one in which women had no say," were silent in public and denied the freedoms provided by the Weimar government. These were old-fashioned ideas; he aspired to an "all-male political brotherhood," an elite set of men who would rule together in *Männerbund* solidarity. In addition, Ernst Röhm was a homosexual, which put him at odds with the party he helped create—at least as far as sexuality was concerned. And yet, as he wrote to sexologist Karl-Günther Heimsoth, "I make no secret of my inclinations. From this you can gather that even National Socialist circles have had to get used to this criminal peculiarity of mine."[22]

Röhm was already a member of Radszuweit's splinter homosexual group, the League for Human Rights. "I pride myself on being homosexual," he explained to Heimsoth, even if it caused him occasional difficulties.[23] The League, both *völkisch* and anti-Semitic, agreed with his principles—and with his desire to see Paragraph 175 overturned. That doesn't mean Röhm lived as a publicly open homosexual. He was "outed" but not "out"; he wanted to keep his private life behind closed doors. His lovers, however, did not always adhere to the same discretion.

In 1929, Ludwig Levy-Lenz treated a young man who had been Röhm's frequent sexual partner. This was not, perhaps, as surprising as it first sounds. As Levy-Lenz put it, "sexual disorders" obey no party lines; the Institute "thus had a great many Nazis under treatment." "It would be against medical principles to provide a list of the Nazi leaders and their perversions," wrote Levy-Lenz, but he could have done. While no one of national repute would ever darken the Institute's doors as a patient, plenty of their partners did. Levy-Lenz treated a serious rectal lesion in a thirteen-year-old boy who had been sodomized by a senior Nazi party official in Breslau; he likewise treated a young girl who had been scratched all over with pins by a prominent Nuremberg Nazi sadist. Many more were consenting homosexual men seeking treatment for sexually transmitted diseases, such as rectal gonorrhea. In this case, Röhm's lover gave into a bit of gossip about the Führer: "Adi," he said, referring to Adolf Hitler, "is the most perverted of us all, but at the moment he is acting the heroic male."[24] (Levy-Lenz would later write that Hitler was a "hypotrophic" or under-developed sexual person with feminine and masochistic bias.)[25] It would be Röhm, however, who ended up in the scandal papers.

In April 1931, distressed at the growing support for Nazis in the Reichstag, the Social Democratic paper *Münchener Post* began a campaign against Röhm.[26] He'd only just returned from Bolivia, summoned home by Hitler to bring the SA more completely under his control. As the SA chief of staff, however, the line between public and private life that kept Röhm in the clear began to dissolve. An attack upon him was an attack on the party; following the tactics of Maximilian Harden, the Social Democrats hoped to hobble Hitler. Prosecutors brought Röhm to court five times between 1931 and 1932 on accusations of homosexuality; they also seized his letters. Dr. Helmut Klotz, a Social Democrat and former Nazi, editor of the *Münchener Post*, published them ahead of the next presidential election.

Like Harden before him, Klotz didn't just attack the SA chief of staff; he attacked all homosexuals, accusing them of "corruption of morals" and "depravity." Klotz asserted that homosexuals should not have leadership roles and called Hitler's retention of Röhm an "unparalleled irresponsibility." The allegations appeared on election posters and pamphlets, made the rounds in newspapers, and threatened to upend the Nazis' electoral support. For the second time, in a bid to bring down their political opponents, even progressives willingly sacrificed homosexuals. This time, however, they did so in vain. The Nazis might be embarrassed, but the scandal "did not cause any electoral damage to the party" nor "slow its rise to power."

Röhm relied on Hitler's influence to keep him out of trouble. "I stick to my job, following him blindly," he told a friend who suspected that Hitler enjoyed the man's utter dependency. Hitler took different positions on the matter depending on the audience: denying it to some, admitting to others that Röhm had a sickness, but ultimately intimating that "his private life does not interest me as long as he maintains the necessary discretion." And yet, it's also possible that the attacks on Röhm failed (where the attacks on the Eulenburg Round Table succeeded) because in the two decades since, Hirschfeld and the Institute had so valiantly fought to create space for homosexuals.

Meanwhile, the Social Democrats' foray into propaganda and scandal backfired; homosexual rights groups that had formerly supported the SDP denounced them as hypocrites. Radszuweit assured his followers in the League that Nazi attacks against homosexuality were only directed against the Jewish Hirschfeld and his Institute—not upstanding Aryan gay men. In fact, he believed that homosexuals were "indirectly making propaganda for our goals within the Hitler camp" and, because of Röhm, expected to meet with "some success." After all, Radszuweit told his followers, the Nazi party valued "love among friends" and "that intimate friendship between leader and led." In reality, Nazism only provided, as historian and former diplomat Eleanor Hancock so aptly puts it, the "precarious status of exception homosexuals."

That status would be revoked the moment it became inconvenient to Hitler's ascension.

THE ENEMY RISES

Dora Richter grew up on one side of the Ore Mountain's Hercynian block, the steep escarpment rising over its coinciding trench. Together, the formations are *Horst* and *Graben*, mountain and valley, signs of tectonic tension and upheaval.[27] Beneath the green fields and black rock, the crust strained against fault lines to generate thermal springs. Goethe traveled to the West Bohemian spa triangle of Karlovy Vary, Franztiskovy Lazne, and Marianske Lazne to take the waters; so did Russian tsar Peter the Great and King Edward VII of England.[28]

At the end of the First World War, the German-speaking population of Bohemia was incorporated into the new state of Czechoslovakia. This change in political geography proved an unexpected blessing for Hirschfeld; he could follow in Goethe's footsteps for the second time, seeking the rest and respite of health spas that were no longer on German soil.* He was, in 1932, truly in exile and knew he would never again see the land of his birth.

Hirschfeld's letters make mention of malaria, high fevers, and heart trouble, always without specifics, but it can be said with certainty that his health remained poor. Convalescent, he made a tour of the three resorts, nestled among greenery in the shadow of mountain ridges. Karlovy Vary, the largest of the resort towns, stood some 21 miles from the German border, around 250 miles from Berlin—tantalizingly close, impossibly far. "I long for Berlin, Berg, the Institute, the Tiergarten, my coworkers," he wrote; it was May, and the grand park would be in bloom, spring flowers bending over the pond's edges.[29] But as he couldn't go to the Institute, the Institute (in part) came to him. Sexologist Felix Abraham, head of radiology Bernhard Schapiro, and Arthur Röser, manager

---

* In 1939, Hitler would retake the region, naming it the German Protectorate of Bohemia and Moravia. It was returned to Czechoslovakia in 1945, after the Second World War, and remained part of the country until 1992. What was once Bohemia now makes up much of the central and western parts of the Czech Republic, or Czechia.

of the Ernst-Haeckel-Hall, were among those who made the trip—and with them, Hirschfeld's little Dorchen.

The long road to becoming herself was nearly at its end; Dora had almost everything she required. She had attempted in 1924 to get a passport under the name Dora Richter, but the request was denied. Researcher Clara Hartmann has uncovered records in the Ministry of Foreign Affairs of the Czech Republic, showing that[30] Dora presented the local office with her original passport (awarded in May 1921, before she traveled to Berlin), in the name of Rudolf Richter, along with her transvestite certificate (which Hirschfeld helped to procure). At the time, she sought a German passport in the name of Dora Richter, while retaining her Czech passport as Rudolf Richter. This was impossible, the officials explained; she would be permitted only one name, and it had to match the name in the registry of her birth: Rudolf Richter. To change the passport, Dora would first have to change the name in the registry.

Whether this rejection had a bearing on her decision to undergo additional feminizing surgeries we have no way to determine. We do know that she began the process of seeking the name change not long after meeting Hirschfeld in the valley not far from her hometown. When she returned to Berlin with the others, she had said goodbye to Hirschfeld for the last time.

In March 1932, German president Paul von Hindenburg found himself unexpectedly reapplying for his job.* At eighty-four years old, he had not planned to run again, but Social Democrats and Catholic Center Party members believed that he offered the best chance of defeating Hitler, who was running on the Nazi ticket. Ernst Thälmann had also entered the race, for the Communists. The popular vote went to Hindenburg by a good margin—53 percent to Hitler's 36 percent. The result

---

* Weimar government structure included a president, a chancellor, and a parliament (Reichstag). The president was elected by popular vote to a seven-year term. Reichstag members were also elected by popular vote, but the president had the power to call for new parliamentary elections at any time and also appointed the chancellor. The chancellor (usually from a majority party) appointed the cabinet and handled most basic operations of government on behalf of the president.

was the least of three evils, but the moderate left did not have much to celebrate. Hindenburg plodded along as before, with a difference; a group of advisors convinced him to get rid of Brüning. At the end of May, a Catholic noble from Westphalia, Franz von Papen, was appointed chancellor. As an aristocrat, Papen wanted nothing more than to overthrow the republic; he started by dismissing the elected officials of Prussia and installing his own candidates. But Papen was as alienated from the German people as his predecessor, and just as foolishly overconfident. Only two months later, he called for new elections to legitimize his position. Germans went to the polls on July 31, 1932—and voted for Nazis.[31]

The Nazi party received 37.3 percent of the vote, enough to make it the largest party in the Reichstag. As their leader, Hitler made a bid for the chancellorship, but Hindenburg refused him. When Papen convened the assembly in September, the Nazis responded with a no-confidence vote. His newly appointed government dissolved before the end of the month and everything once more came to a halt. The Nazis hadn't won; they had just prevented others from winning—and at considerable cost. Their funds were exhausted. New elections would be called in November and a new chancellor appointed, an army general named Kurt von Schleicher who wanted to bring the right and left together, but it was far too little and much too late. The parties were now separated by a bottomless chasm. No one had faith in the government, certainly, but faith had been shaken among the Nazi ranks, too, as they had thought their success was assured. The stalemate stretched, threatening to spill into the new year.

Hirschfeld could see the storm gathering. He'd made some provisions already; should the Institute be closed or worse, taken over, he wrote, then "the World League for Sexual Reform on the basis of sexual science will take its place as universal heir."[32] This wasn't to be, either.

As 1932 wound to a close, catastrophe struck. "All the foundations of my previous effectiveness," Hirschfeld wrote, "were thrown overboard, above all my sole right of disposal within the Foundation's nonprofit status, etc." An official inspection had determined that the last time annual statements were filed was in 1923; therefore, nonprofit status was summarily revoked, leaving the foundation at the mercy of taxes it could not pay. Hirschfeld responded by changing his will, entrusting Karl Giese alone with any income (largely from Titus Pearls). Giese would dispose of the inheritance as he saw fit. Tao Li would benefit, too; Hirschfeld ultimately bequeathed his collections and the income from his publications to both men, with a condition. As Ralf Dose, head of the Hirschfeld Archive in Berlin, explains, his successors were enriched only on "the condition that it be used not for themselves but to found a new institute or, if that should not be possible, for the purposes of 'our movement.'" Hirschfeld signed the testament in Switzerland on January 14, 1933. That winter had already been the "hardest and worst of my life so far," Hirschfeld wrote. Being struck with rheumatism, heart spasms, worsening diabetes, and the "economic collapse of our institute and my foundation" was enough to shake any constitution.[33] And the winter was not yet over.

In early January, while the new chancellor struggled to find his feet, the recently ousted Papen held a secret meeting with Adolf Hitler. Conservatives believed they could use the Nazis to overthrow the republic from within. And why not? Both Nazis and conservatives clamored for the return of authoritarian government and the revival of Germany's great-power status abroad. Both felt that achieving this required stamping out trade unions, socialist groups, modern art, and any sex reform—and the simultaneous introduction of restrictions against non-Aryan races (most especially the Jews). That the Nazis and the conservatives formed a coalition should not surprise us. The right disapproved of the Nazis' manners, not their politics.[34]

On January 30, 1933, Hindenburg named Hitler the new chancellor and Papen vice-chancellor. The Nazis still did not control the majority of parliamentary seats; at best, they occupied a third. But Brüning had already established a means of sidestepping majority rule. All the Nazis needed was a reason to declare a national emergency. They had already proven their effectiveness at creating disruption and then turning up to quell it. Hitler's loyalists knew exactly what to do—and who to blame.

Christopher Isherwood did not, at first, despair. Hitler would "now have to cope with the economic mess," he wrote, and "reveal himself as an incompetent windbag"; Christopher expected him to resign in defeat before long. Instead, on the night of February 27, disguised Nazis set the Reichstag building on fire, then claimed the blaze had been set by Communists as a signal for an uprising. Hindenburg declared a state of emergency, and Hitler began to make mass arrests. As chancellor, Hitler urged the president to dissolve the Reichstag and order brand-new elections. The Nazis would not win a majority in the March 5 election either, but they did capture 288 seats, 44 percent of the Reichstag to the Social Democrats' shrinking 18 percent. Hitler formed a coalition government with the German National People's Party, which gave him the votes he needed for the next step of his plan. Using the panic of an imaginary Communist threat, Hitler introduced the Enabling Act on March 23, which would give him the power to make laws without parliamentary approval for the next four years. It passed by a two-thirds vote, effectively making him dictator.

"In a mad, meaningless way," Isherwood wrote, "[Hitler's] successive steps toward absolute power had all been legal." Streets hung red with swastika flags, and uniformed Storm Troops walked the pavements. These stern-faced extortionists demanded funds for the party from every business they entered, and it was unwise to refuse them. Meanwhile, out on the Nollendorfplatz and other public squares, loudspeakers played incessant propaganda speeches. Isherwood wandered among the cafés and described blank-faced people cowed into complacency, "accepting what had happened but not the responsibility for it. Many of them hadn't even voted—how could they be responsible?"

No one spoke up, but everyone spoke about it; rumors swirled in the quiet doorframes of private abodes. Political prisoners had been taken to the Storm Troop barracks—Communists, mostly. What happened to them remained a matter of speculation; "it was said that some were made to spit on Lenin's picture, swallow castor oil, eat old socks; that some were tortured; that many were already dead." The government denied anything of the sort; they also deemed that repeating the rumors amounted to treason.

Isherwood knew he'd been listed on the roster of what he called "Hirschfeld Homosexuals," yet there were homosexuals who joined the Nazi side. "Misled by their own erotic vision of a New Sparta," he wrote, "they fondly supposed Germany was entering an era of military man-love"—the erotic *Männerbund* of Blüher and Brand. Isherwood knew that Germany wasn't his homeland; as for the homosexual Nazis, they learned too late that it "wasn't their homeland either."[35] The end was coming. It had been, for three years, a steady creep of intensity that everyone ignored until it threw open their doors and demanded tribute.

From March 1933 onward, Hitler had full control. The man who had been ignored as unimportant, laughed at as a clown, a buffoon, a salesman, now determined the future of Germany and enforced his power with every violence. The Weimar era was over, and in place of the republic rose a dictatorship intent on ruling the individual lives of its people—and on determining which of those lives were worth living.

WHO DECIDES THE VALUE OF A LIFE?

The word *Rassenhygiene* had been coined in 1895 by Alfred Ploetz, one year before a patient's suicide changed the course of Magnus Hirschfeld's life and career. Ploetz considered racial hygiene a means of genetic cleansing, a way of "improving the white race."[36] In 1904, he founded the first Society for Racial Hygiene.[37] His primary goal was to "avert a civilization-induced reversal" of survival of the fittest, which he wished to enact through marriage and reproductive licensing so that "degenerative" hereditary material could be weeded out.[38] One of Ploetz's geneticist colleagues, Heinrich Poll, described how the process would create a "more pure" race: "Just as the organism ruthlessly sacrifices degenerate cells, just as the surgeon ruthlessly removes a diseased organ, both, in order to save the whole," so too should the state intervene "in personal liberty to prevent the bearers of diseased hereditary traits from continuing to spread harmful genes throughout the generations."[39] Both men admired Charles Davenport for his ruthlessness in carting away those considered inferior to his Virginia State Colony for Epileptics and

Feebleminded; both likewise lauded his sterilization programs. By the 1920s, German universities already promoted courses and professorships on "race biology," and racism and anti-Semitism fueled the ardor of students and scholars alike.

Rassenhygiene appealed to Germans for other reasons, too. As a Nazi-era textbook would make plain, "You are sharing the load! A hereditarily ill person costs 50,000 Reichsmarks on average up to the age of sixty." In other words, care for inferior people strapped the state for cash. So-called mental defectives would be targeted as an especially burdensome financial liability. The depression brought about by the 1929 crash rendered six million Germans unemployed, and industry demanded that the government trim the welfare budget. If limits were to be placed on the work-willing, should those who did not contribute at all to the German economy be provided for? Biologist Hermann Muckermann reported that mental illness alone cost 185 million marks a year, while healthy people starved; another eugenics supporter put it more baldly still: "We can protect our position in the world . . . only through a wise human economy" by "limit[ing] the number of those who consume." Eugenics, they argued, offered a way out; the state could institute its own form of natural selection, stated a writer for the journal *Eugenik*. Only then could Germany shed the "ever-growing burden of useless individuals unworthy of life."[40]

Discovered and named in the same year, 1905, genes and hormones had carried scientific inquiry in Germany since the turn of the century. Hormones continued to be examined, used, developed—but they had not moved the needle politically, for all of Hirschfeld's efforts. The gene, interpreted by Nazi eugenics, would be another matter entirely.

During his brief imprisonment for the Beer Hall Putsch, Hitler read Ploetz, and later the work of Davenport. His rhetoric already encompassed the failures of masculinity and the weakening of the state; he already blamed Jews and other minorities for Germany's failures. The concept of race hygiene didn't just agree with his natural bias, it provided a seemingly scientific veneer and a means of implementation. Hitler introduced the Sterilization Law only five months after taking

over as chancellor, largely borrowing its tenets from American eugenics (where forced sterilization had been legal since 1907). Anyone suffering "hereditary disease" could be surgically rendered sterile—and
this applied to the deaf and blind, the depressed, the epileptic, those
with physical abnormalities, and anyone labeled "mentally deficient."
The procedure would be carried out against the patient's will. New laws
then permitted the forced sterilization of criminals, including political
prisoners, and the Nuremberg Laws for the Protection of the Hereditary
Health of the German People outlawed couplings between ethnic Germans and Jews.

The National Socialist ideology wound itself around the central concept of applied biology; eugenics and racial politics merged under the
Third Reich. By 1934, 5,000 adults were sterilized every month, with
200 Genetic Courts in operation to hear appeals (which were almost universally denied).[41] By 1935, Hitler was already toying with the idea of
doing much more, and in 1939 he had his first opportunity to legalize
Rassenhygiene euthanasia.

It was summer in Germany's capital when two parents appealed to
Hitler: would he permit them to kill their child? At eight months old,
baby Gerhard was blind and had malformed limbs. The couple were
devoted Nazis who desired to support their nation by eliminating their
own child from the gene pool. The horror we feel at such a request
scarcely prepares us for ensuing events. Hitler agreed and immediately
acted to expand the program to any disabled child under three years of
age. By September, adolescents made the list, and then otherwise abled
and healthy "delinquents" were added to the roster. In October, adults.

The policy would become known as Aktion T4, named after Tiergar-
tenstrasse, home of the euthanasia headquarters. It presented a stately
façade for murder happening in other quarters, such as the Hadamar
Hospital and the Brandenburg Welfare Institute. There, the basements
had been cleared out and refitted with airtight chambers. Patients
would be led inside, locked in, and gassed with carbon monoxide before
being dissected for "science."[42] We don't have all the numbers; we can't
be sure exactly how many met their end this way. Records indicate that

100,000 people (labeled "useless eaters") died between 1939 and 1941, but we know the extermination campaign began earlier and continued much later than the written evidence provides.[43] When Hitler at last initiated the "final solution," killing six million Jews, the gas chambers were already in operation and waiting to receive them.

The principal claim of eugenics, before and after Hitler came to power, centered on the centrality and permanence of biology. A Jew was always a Jew—and the Nazis believed that even a drop of Jewish blood rendered a citizen unfit. Hirschfeld had been targeted for this even more than for his sexuality, but he had also introduced and fought for the idea that homosexuality was congenital. You were born with your sexual and gender preferences, and no amount of counseling or medication or surgery would change that. He had hoped to bring justice through science; instead, the very core of his argument would be used by the Nazis to round up homosexuals, too, as genetically tainted—as *Lebensunwertes*, lives unworthy of living.

THE FALL OF RÖHM

Two soldiers walked the hall to a cell in Munich's Stadelheim prison, expecting to find a dead man, slain by his own hand. But the Browning pistol remained where they had left it, and the battle-scarred Ernst Röhm stood before them, defiant. He unbuttoned his shirt and spread it wide; if they wanted him dead, they would have to do it themselves. The soldiers executed him on the spot with a bullet to the chest.[44]

Röhm was the last to fall. The evening before, Hitler had ordered an internal purge of the party, sanctioning the murder of approximately ninety people, many of them Röhm's friends.[45] Hitler accused the Storm Troop leaders of plotting to overthrow him, in collusion with France and with the former chancellor General Kurt von Schleicher (also killed), but in his speech justifying the event he refers to Röhm's sexuality. "The life which the Chief of Staff and a certain circle around him began to lead was intolerable from any National Socialist viewpoint," Hitler explained; a "circle" this time and not a round table, but the words echo those of the Eulenburg affair. Röhm stood accused of hand-picking other homosexuals, a "clique" that monopolized promotions.[46] Whether or not it was true hardly mattered.

Hitler needed to consolidate power, and more than anything to join the Storm Troops with the military in support of his own ascendancy. He desired the military to be his tool, whereas Röhm held that soldiers should have primacy over politicians.[47] Röhm had become an obstacle, and therefore he was obsolete. Where once his position had given hope to homosexuals that they would be tolerated under Nazi rule, he now served as the catalyst for Hitler to accuse and remove anyone who opposed him.

The hours between dusk on June 30 and dawn on July 1 are remembered as the Night of the Long Knives, but the night didn't end with dawn. Fifty thousand homosexuals would be convicted during the Third Reich, with as many as 15,000 ultimately sent to concentration camps.[48] Heinrich Himmler, who had partly instigated the purge of Röhm and his followers, advocated for stricter laws, and in 1935, Paragraph 175—so nearly abolished only a few years before—was expanded to include even homosexual feelings.[49] Gay panic had returned, and the SS newspaper *Das Schwarze Korps*—Himmler's mouthpiece—declared homosexual men to be enemies of the state.[50]

The SHC, headed now by Kurt Hiller, had no illusions about where the Nazis stood regarding homosexuality. Many of its remaining members and Institute staff, including Levy-Lenz, were Jewish leftists with every reason to oppose Nazism. It's possible that they had possession or knowledge of Röhm's letters as early as 1931, and may have used them as a bargaining tool against Nazi threats.[51] They never leaked the documents, however, and denounced those who did. They still maintained that homosexuality was inborn, congenital, a natural variation—with the addition of the insistence by Hiller and Linsert that the private lives of citizens were no one's business. But despite all of their efforts, and those of the previous thirty-odd years, sexual science had reversed course.

For Himmler and other Nazi leaders, a distinction could be drawn between inborn and acquired homosexuality. They didn't deny the former, but they appended to it the old fear of moral contagion. Himmler's speeches warned about homosexual contamination in the same manner that epidemiologists warned of the flu pandemic. All men, Nazis included, might "succumb" to this "disease," and racial laws, penalties, concentration camps, castration, even murder of the offenders could not wholly contain the epidemic. The Hitler Youth handbook for "Combating Same-Sex Acts" states that "one individual seduces ten or more youths or infects an entire group. Many who have been seduced later become seducers so that often . . . an endless chain of infection occurs." Nazi propaganda called it the "homosexual conspiracy" to bring down the state and replace it with one of "sick individuals"; in fact, their propaganda introduced an atmosphere of terrified vigilance and constant threat.[52] Any SS officer found guilty of homosexuality, Himmler declared, would first serve a sentence in the camps—and then be "shot dead while trying to escape."[53]

Hitler and Himmler described homosexuals as weak and cowardly, feminine; at the same time, they feared them as having "special intuitions and aptitudes" that allowed them to organize and grow in number, making them a threat to those in power.[54] The distinction between inferior and superior races might have been at the core of Nazi eugenics and race hygiene, but so too was the difference between masculine and feminine nature. Homosexuals and women, too, would be purged from all public and political life. There is, as author, biologist, and physician Siddhartha Mukherjee writes, a reason why "genocide" shares a root word with "gene"; the language of science would be used not to emancipate but to exterminate.[55]

13

INCENDIARY MATTERS

THE GERMAN STUDENT UNION, NOW THOROUGHLY WITHIN THE NAZI
camp, declared an "action against the un-German spirit" on April 8,
1933, and determined to cleanse the Institute of Sexual Science by
fire.[1] They would make good on that threat the morning of May 6. The
intention is clear upon reflection—they wanted to close the Institute
not only for what it was and did, but for what it embodied. It was a place
of safety, a place where differences were honored, where diversity was
encouraged—and so it was among the first victims of the Nazi purge.
The students vandalized the institute, overturned bookcases, tore
down artwork and photographs, and threw ink on walls and carpets.
This was but the first insult; later that night, Storm Troops arrived
in force to take away the Institute's treasures. Anything of material
value, including the scientific instruments, were sold at auction. Some
of the books (those not deemed pornography, and those that might be
but would fetch a profit) went into private Nazi hands. The rest would
be burned four days later near the opera house: thousands of books and
case histories, a lifetime of work for sexual justice, all of it lost forever
and rendered to ashes.

The flames on the Opernplatz rose high into the night sky; film footage reveals a carnival scene, revelers ecstatic in the destruction. The
students who raided the Institute paraded about the fire with Nazi flags
on tall standards. Black-and-white technology mutes the effect, but the
flames would have burned hot and cast their glow on the bright red
banners. The band that played outside 10 In den Zelten during the raid
on the Institute struck up again at the book burning—a backdrop of
brass horns, shouting, cheers. Speeches painted the destruction as civic

duty. Singing drowned out the crackle of burning paper. In the crowd, watching in horror, was Christopher Isherwood. "Shame!" he said to the participants, "shame"—but he spoke in a whisper, out of fear.[2]

"Whence [came] this hatred . . . this haste and thoroughness?" asked chief surgeon Ludwig Levy-Lenz. "The answer to this is simple and straightforward—we knew too much." According to his account, "our knowledge of such intimate secrets regarding members of the Nazi Party and our other documentary material"—he mentioned 40,000 confessional letters—"was the cause of the complete and utter destruction of the Institute for Sexual Science."[3] In fact, it's unlikely that the psychobiological questionnaires of Nazis and Nazi associates were still there at the time of the raid.

Günter Maeder, a secretary at the Institute about three months before the raid, claimed that the librarian, Arthur Röser, turned against Hirschfeld and acted as a Nazi spy. He had easy access to documents and could hand over anything he pleased. Maeder claims that he himself was locked inside Richard Linsert's old rooms, presumably to prevent him from interfering. From this vantage, he claims to have seen Karl Giese creeping along the courtyard of the Institute before breaking into the library and making away with books and papers, despite police surveillance outside. Isherwood's account supports this, saying that the "really important papers and books had been removed by friends of Hirschfeld and sent abroad."[4]

Both stories—Levy-Lenz's claim that the Institute had information that could destabilize the Nazis, and Maeder's claim that the trusted librarian acted as a double agent—were recorded many years after the events, and without corroborating evidence. However, Röser's betrayal is seemingly supported by a letter he wrote to Hirschfeld. He described the Nazis as "correct" and "polite" when they raided the Institute, despite clear evidence to the contrary. The letter was co-signed, with "love for our fatherland," by administrative secretary Hauptstein and Ewald Lausch, who managed the archive after Giese joined Hirschfeld in exile.[5] It would be sent in duplicate to a Nazi official, so it's likely that the three men were attempting to secure clemency for the Institute under the Nazi regime, but Lausch had always been an enthusiastic Nazi supporter and Röser pledged allegiance to the party after the raid.[6] The Institute would remain in the building until 1934, when the Nazis abolished it and rented the storied halls to anti-Semitic organizations.

Additionally, despite accounts that violence and murder accompanied the raid on the Institute, no one was injured. (Dora Richter, sometimes listed as a casualty, was not present.) Instead, the Nazis attempted a ritual murder by proxy. The SA had removed a bronze bust of Hirschfeld from the Institute during the raid. On the night of May 10, they carried it through the chanting crowds on the Opernplatz, intending to burn him in effigy; the footage of this macabre parade can still be viewed today. And yet, even Hirschfeld's likeness proved resistant to the last; the bust ultimately survived the flames. Historian Rainer Herrn suggests that it was probably too heavy to throw and that the fire was too hot to approach for the purpose of more casual placement, while Heike Bauer asserts that the bust would not have burned anyway (the melting point of bronze is 1,675 degrees Fahrenheit, far higher than the heat of burning wood and paper). Hirschfeld's books, however, were reduced to ashes.

Hirschfeld's library wasn't the only one burned—there were four raiding parties and over seven hundred libraries which had to be "cleansed" with fire—but only the Institute of Sexual Science was ever named in the Nazi propaganda or in the news headlines that followed. Hitler had made Hirschfeld the face of the international Jewish conspiracy, the primary representation of everything the Nazis stood against; his Institute was an engine of sexual reform, a center of transgender science, a safe space for homosexuals and trans persons, Jews, and women. They burned his words, his collections, and his image as a means of eliminating "the un-German spirit." As one official wrote, "I read with sincere satisfaction that you . . . have at last thoroughly smoked out the pigsty of the perverted Doctor Hirschfeld."[7]

Hirschfeld, then living in France with Tao Li and Karl Giese, who had joined them before the persecution began, watched the Institute burn via newsreel in a Paris cinema. He'd hoped, with Giese and Tao, to rebuild the Institute in France. He wouldn't get the chance. Giese would be arrested for "immorality"—for being a homosexual—and despite Hirschfeld's attempts to intervene, Giese would be exiled from France. To make matters worse, Hirschfeld's old adversary, sexologist Albert Moll, wrote a letter to the University of Paris denouncing Hirschfeld for medical misconduct and claiming that he had been run out of Germany for his immorality. Moll sent a copy to the German foreign secretary, too, who replied with "most profound thanks, Heil Hitler!"[8] Perhaps it was out of spite. Perhaps he meant to curry Nazi favor. (If the latter, it didn't end well. In 1938, the Nazis revoked Moll's medical license because of his Jewish heritage; he died a year later.) Hirschfeld gave up on Paris and moved with Tao Li to Nice. He would die there on his sixty-seventh birthday, of a stroke.

Karl Giese, who loved him, had risked his life for him, and who had carried many of the books and documents to safety, was able to return for the funeral. It was a last act of loyalty. Following his return to Brno, in Czechoslovakia, he ended his own life.[9]

Only eight people still worked at the Institute for Sexual Science in May 1933. Most of them had already made preparations to flee. Some succeeded; others disappeared into the Nazi machinery. Felix Abraham worked until he was deprived of his medical license for being Jewish; he fled to Italy where he, like Karl Giese, committed suicide. Arthur Kronfeld fled to Moscow with his wife; they committed suicide together when the Germans invaded. Wilhelm Kauffmann poisoned himself with a dish of mushrooms, and Institute radiologist August Bessunger ended his days in Auschwitz.[10] Ludwig Levy-Lenz, also Jewish, escaped under cover of darkness with his wife just hours before the Gestapo arrived to arrest him. Finding him flown, they treated his personal library to the same fate as the Institute's; "they burned all my books," he wrote. "Be still, O my soul."[11]

He would emigrate to the United States—while his colleague Erwin Gohrbandt, who had performed both Dora's and Lili's vaginoplasties, joined the Nazi Luftwaffe as chief medical adviser.[12] Gohrbandt contributed to grim experiments in the Dachau concentration camp, where Jewish people were forced naked into tanks of ice water to study hypothermia, and published the results in a surgical journal.[13] He would be awarded the War Merit Cross Second Class by Hitler's decree, for services rendered.[14]

Science hadn't led to justice at all; it was, like every other tool of human improvement, subject to those who wielded its power.

RELIVING HISTORY

The Nazi ideal was based on white, heterosexual, and normative (that is, cisgender) masculinity masquerading as genetic superiority. Any who strayed were considered depraved, immoral, and worthy of eradication. What began as a project of "protecting" German youth and raising healthy families became, under Hitler, a mechanism for genocide. The world saw these horrors and said, "Never again." But the future doesn't guarantee progress.

Current attacks upon trans people bear a striking resemblance to those terrible campaigns against so-labeled aberrant lives. We who continue to fight for rights and representation as homosexual, transgender, and other intermediary identities are heirs to Hirschfeld's hopes—and we have inherited the struggle in a world with its own rising tide of hatred and abuse. Long before the Nazis came to power, the German conservative right banned books; they denounced homosexual and transgender people as immoral criminals; they refused women reproductive rights; they attacked and disenfranchised Jews, immigrants, and refugees; they attempted to overwrite science with politically and racially motivated pseudoscience. They courted the dangerous ideal of toxic white masculinity while chasing a myth of past triumphs. It does not take much imagination to see the parallels today. On television and social media, pundits like Matt Walsh claim that modern life destroys masculinity and that transgender people are groomers and pedophiles.*[15] At the Conservative Political Action Conference in 2023, Michael Knowles called

---

* A charge echoed by Representative Marjorie Taylor Greene.

for the "eradication" of "transgenderism,"[16] and Charlie Kirk called for men to "take care of" trans people like they did in the fifties and sixties, in what has been broadly denounced as courting mob lynching.[17]

In 2023, there were 550 legislative bills targeting trans people nationwide. And these are only those policies directed most ardently against transgender people; we have witnessed the overturning of abortion and reproductive rights, the rise of literal bounty hunters chasing women across borders, and renewed attacks even on legal birth control. Incidents of anti-Semitism reached their highest level ever recorded in the United States in March 2023, and renewed fervor against ethnic minorities and immigrants in particular has gripped the right.[18] In 2024, ahead of the presidential election, candidate Donald Trump gave an interview to *Time* in which he outlined his intention to invoke the 1798 Alien Enemies Act, which allows for summary deportation of any noncitizen from a foreign enemy country. Despite the fact that undocumented immigrants have equal protection under the Constitution, Trump has hinted at the construction of mass detention camps—yes, camps.[19] "These aren't civilians," Trump told *Time*—though a civilian is anyone not engaged in military action; you need not be a citizen to be a civilian, and civilians are protected under the Geneva Convention on Human Rights.[20] Meanwhile, Trump's legal team argued that as president he had and will continue to have total immunity, even suggesting that the ordered killing of a political rival would be immune to prosecution; the Supreme Court, occupied by three justices appointed by Trump, granted that immunity.[21] This may be so much posturing from a former president facing trial and consequence, but the claims echo those of fascist leaders who wished to rule with impunity. The political climate has not been so divisive—with polarities skirting dangerous edges—in nearly a hundred years. The books may not yet be burning, but they are already being banned. Then has become now.

Looking back on the story of Hirschfeld's Institute for Sexual Science—his protocols not only for surgery but for a trans-supportive community of care, for mental and physical healing, and for social change—it's hard not to imagine a world history that might have been.

What future might have been built from a platform where sexual intermediaries were indeed thought of in more just terms? Still, these everyday people serve as transgender pioneers; they provided a modern articulation of what it means to feel at odds with one's assigned sex and gender. Moreover, the Institute honored a plurality of identities that many believe were impossible before the 1960s. This history helps to deepen a sense of pride—and extend the legacy—for LGBTQ+ communities worldwide.

The story of the Institute ends in 1933, but the story of homosexual and transgender rights does not. Harry Benjamin, who invited Hirschfeld to the United States, would go on to write *The Transsexual Phenomenon* in 1952 after seeing a patient referred by sexologist Alfred Kinsey. He would ultimately treat Christine Jorgensen, a former Second World War pilot who underwent gender affirmation surgery in 1952 (and became a bombshell celebrity). Kinsey would found an Institute for Sex Research at Indiana University—now known as the Kinsey Institute—where some of Hirschfeld's surviving papers reside to this day. Many of the first gay rights organizations in the United States, including the Society for Human Rights in Chicago and the Mattachine Society, founded in Los Angeles in 1950, owed their genesis to Hirschfeld's Institute and to early pioneers like Dora Richter.[22] We are all heirs to their bravery and their sacrifice. We cannot, any of us, sit idle in cafés while hatred plays on loudspeakers. We must speak now, act now—while there is still time.

EPILOGUE

ON APRIL 23, 1934, A LETTER CAME FROM PRAGUE TO THE BERLIN address of a forty-two-year-old flower-seller. The subject: change of name and gender, approved. Dora Rudolfine Richter—Rudolfa Richterová in Czech—had permission from the state president of Prague to change both her name and her gender, in an order that extended to the provincial register of births. With the documentation came a report, dated a decade earlier, from the Institute for Sexual Science. It identified Dora as a "hermaphrodite," the so-useful term Hirschfeld broadened to make legal transition possible. In the baptismal records of Seifen parish, Dora's old name and gender were crossed out, her chosen name written in. A pasted-in record mentions the Institute, and over it all is stamped the purple seal of approval.[1]

Dora had waited her whole life for this; the last vestige of assigned gender at last fell away. She didn't apply for a German passport, however; she was leaving Germany behind. Charlotte Charlaque, who escaped the Nazis by fleeing to Brno and later to Prague with Toni Ebel, said that Dora moved to Karlovy Vary, in the spa triangle, to work as a cook. Evidence has surfaced, however, that tells us a bit more. Census records in the Czech national archive in Prague, discovered by researcher Clara Hartmann, show that Dora returned to the village of her birth. Her father had died in 1931; her mother—who first taught her to work the bobbin—died in 1938. Perhaps Dora returned during the last illness of her mother; we cannot be sure, though it's the sort of thing Dora would have done.

The family home then belonged to her sister Ida and her growing family. Dora had her own home, at no. 61 Seifen, which was previously

the home of her uncle, a master baker—perhaps the baker Dora apprenticed with so many years before. She registered now as a lacemaker—
and though she remained unmarried, she wasn't alone. Her younger
brother Hermann lived under her roof.[2] Dora had achieved peace and
domesticity, but she would not be permitted to rest for long.

Hitler had claimed the Sudetenland—the German-speaking part of
Bohemia that included border towns like Seifen—in 1938, and in 1946
political boundaries shifted once again. The easternmost parts of the
Nazi empire fell under Soviet rule, and the restored state of Czechoslovakia deported three million ethnic-German Bohemians.[3] The order came
on May 1, 1946. Once more, Dora was on the move; she was no longer
welcome on her side of the mountain. The German Red Cross archive
holds the certificate of Dora's passage back into Germany: Dora Richter, single, Catholic, to reside at 377 in Allersberg, a small town south
of Nuremberg where many other refugees from the Czech region had
settled. There is some evidence that Hermann may have been with her
there as well; he never married.[4]

The twentieth-century expansion of Allersberg has taken place outside
the city center; the Bavarian architecture, crooked little streets, and city
wall that greet us today would have been there to welcome Dora, too. She
would live the next twenty years in the charming little town. We don't
know much about her time there, other than a few anecdotes recalled
by now-elderly Allersbergers. There was a woman, they said. She lived
in barrack-like buildings on the outskirts of town with her brother and
a handful of other Bohemian refugees. They remembered her because
of her jolly disposition, and because of her handbag. It seems Dora never
gave up her beloved birds; seated inside on a makeshift nest was a pigeon
that she would feed by dropping it crumbs. That she is remembered in
the end as the "lady with pigeons" would, I think, have pleased her.

LILI ELBE LIES BENEATH a dark gray stone at Trinitatis Cemetery in
Dresden, Germany. Her grave attracts visitors; they travel to the mossy,
tree-shadowed grounds to leave stones as tribute. She has been immor-

talized in film and even in street names: a transgender icon in life and in death. We still don't know as much about Dora Richter, and what I have reconstructed comes from ephemeral traces and long-forgotten case histories. Dora died on April 26, 1966, at age seventy-four, and was laid to rest in the oldest part of the Allersberg cemetery, though the grave no longer exists. According to records, the plot was returned to the municipality sometime after 1998. The places where Dora lived—and even where she died—no longer exist. As Hartmann writes, "I have been to Berlin. I have been to Seifen. And I have been to Allersberg. Nothing remains to remember Dora Richter."[5] She lived as a mostly anonymous Czech-German woman, and she died a mostly anonymous Czech-German woman—but a *woman*, through and through. Dora outlived two wars; she outlived displacement; she outlived hate. Hers is a private success, the intimate journey of a woman to find herself and to be accepted on her own terms.

ACKNOWLEDGMENTS _____

This book would not exist without the time, input, and aid provided by numerous colleagues, scholars, activists, editors, and friends, especially in the LGBTQ+ community. I would like to mention specifically Ralf Dose of the Magnus Hirschfeld Archive, Berlin, and Erin Reed, American journalist and transgender rights activist, for serving as consultant readers. I also want to thank queer and transgender historian Laurie Marhoefer (University of Washington), associate professor of German and gender studies Katie Sutton (Australian National University), and English and gender studies lecturer Heike Bauer (Birkbeck College, University of London) for their incredible input, especially in the early stages of my work. I am also deeply indebted to historian, filmmaker, and formative theorist Susan Stryker for her feedback, scholarship, and encouragement all along the way, as well as those who read drafts and snippets and otherwise listened to me think out loud, including Mark Schillace, Lance Parkin, and Mya Byrne. Much of the work in any project begins before pen touches paper, so I want to lift up Laura Helmuth, editor of *Scientific American*, whose enthusiasm for a short article helped bring the book into being; Anja Katharina Peters, who shepherded me around Dresden and to the grave of Lili Elbe; the fine people at Humboldt University, Berlin, which housed an important piece of my research; Ulrike Walter-Lipow, my esteemed translator, who translated that research and double-checked my own less-than-perfect attempts. Many thanks, too, to my amazing editors at W. W. Norton, Jill Bialosky and Laura Mucha, to the production team and cover designers, and to Allegra Huston, who spent many hours in line edits with me. Finally, Clara Hartmann, whose diligence has brought so much more of Dora's later life into focus. So many LGBTQ+ historians, archivists, librarians, and activists made the work possible that its publication testifies to the power of the queer community and its dedication to preserving and celebrating history. Thank you, all.

GLOSSARY

Terms and persons with their own entry in the glossary and "Characters of Note" are shown in bold on first appearance.

Adaptation therapy (also known as psychological milieu therapy): A therapeutic technique for homosexual, transvestite, and other intermediaries introduced in 1914 by Magnus Hirschfeld. In order to support people "according to their nature," Hirschfeld suggested helping them build community so as to gain access to other "intellectually sophisticated" people who felt and lived like themselves.

Anders als die Andern (Different from the Others): A silent black-and-white film produced in Weimar Germany in 1919. Co-written by Richard Oswald and **Magnus Hirschfeld**, it was intended to strike a blow to **Paragraph 175**, the prohibition of homosexuality. The film explores a doomed homosexual relationship between a violinist, played by silent film star Conrad Veidt (*The Cabinet of Dr. Caligari*), and his student, with extensive flashback scenes showing both characters' early sexual experiences, their failed attempts to change their sexual orientation (including treatment with bogus "ex-gay" therapies), and their eventual self-acceptance. The violinist is ruined by blackmail. The film includes a lecture by Hirschfeld explaining that homosexuality is natural and should not be criminalized. The sympathetic portrayal affected many who saw themselves represented for the first time. However, the film's release was short-lived due to backlash and censorship.

Der Eigene: **Adolf Brand** launched his own publishing endeavor, a journal he called *Der Eigene*, "self-owner" or "Ego." "Egoists unite," Brand wrote, and "we will make our own empire, our own earth." The inaugural issue of *Der Eigene* appeared in 1896, and the title, not wholly translatable to English, provides layers of meaning, vacillating among "own," "self," and "same"; this was Brand's way of expressing homosexuality in a non-pathologizing, non-medical manner. It was a masculinist publication and rejected everything feminine; Brand's supporters were noted for their misogyny.

Dolchstosslegende: Literally translated as "stab in the back," *Dolchstosslegende* was a conspiracy theory promoted by anti-Semites and misogynists who blamed Germany's defeat in the First World War on Jews, women, Marxists, and socialists. Adolf Hitler would make use of this myth in his propaganda, claiming that the leaders of the Weimar Republic were criminals for signing the Armistice of 1918, though shifting blame increasingly upon Jews.

Endocrinology: The study of the secretions known as hormones, the entire endocrine system and its glands, as well as its diseases. Today we know there are nine types of glands in the human body: hypothalamus, pineal, and pituitary, located in the brain; thyroid and parathyroids; the islets of Langerhans, located in the pancreas; the adrenals; the ovaries; and the testes.

Eugenics: At its most basic, eugenics was a philosophy of "improving" human genetic material, through selective breeding practices. In practice, it helped to fuel genocide. First developed by Francis Galton, who believed that some humans were inherently better than others (along race and class lines), eugenics suggested a means of rooting out disease but also difference. Galton's ideas about heredity aligned neatly with a concept that would become popular in interwar Germany: *Rassenhygiene*, or race hygiene (a term coined by German biologist Alfred Ploetz).

Gender: The word "gender" was first used in our modern sense by a controversial sexologist named John Money in 1955. Gender refers to socially constructed characteristics and norms of behavior associated with men or women. Since these characteristics and behaviors (and expectations for both) are socially constructed, they vary throughout history and from one culture to another. As pointed out by the World Health Organization, gender is hierarchical and produces inequalities via gender discrimination. Gender concerns and interacts with biological and physiological differences in chromosomes, hormones, and reproductive organs—but gender and sex are not the same. Gender identity refers to a person's internal and individual experience of gender (the characteristics and behaviors of being a man or woman or neither or both), and it need not align with one's sex at birth.

Gene: A unit of hereditary material passed from parent to offspring. Discovered through Gregor Mendel's hybridization of peas and later rediscovered and expanded by Hugo de Vries, originally known as "pangenes." In 1905, William Bateson suggested in a private letter that the field should be called "genetics," meaning "study of genes." Credit for coining the word, however, usually goes to Danish botanist Wilhelm Johannsen, who shortened Bateson's "genetics" to "gene" in a published article four years later.

Genetics: The study of how genes and traits are passed between parents and offspring.

Geschlechtsübergänge (roughly, Sexual Transitions): A pamphlet written by Magnus Hirschfeld in which he introduced the idea that the "absolute man" and "absolute woman" are fantasies, abstractions. All human beings, he wrote, exist on a continuum.

Hermaphrodite: An antiquated term for intersex, meaning persons with both male and female reproductive organs, or reproductive anatomy that doesn't fit into strict categories of male and female. However, the term took on new meaning in the work of Magnus Hirschfeld. For Hirschfeld, a person could be psychologically or emotionally hermaphroditic; he would frequently assign the term "hermaphrodite" to those we today consider transgender, partly because this allowed them to legally change their names.

Heterosexuality: A term coined by Karl Maria Kertbeny, a friend of **Karl Heinrich Ulrichs**, in 1868. The Greek root *hetero* means "different." Kertbeny used the term to describe those who loved or desired those of the opposite sex.

Homosexuality: A term coined by Karl Maria Kertbeny, a friend of Karl Heinrich Ulrichs, in 1868. The Greek root *homo* means "same." Kertbeny used the term to describe those who loved or desired those of the same sex. Ulrichs had already begun to consider sexual orientation as an identity, not merely a practice, so even in its earliest formulation, "homosexual" carried with it the understanding of a being—an identity and not a choice.

Hormone: The term coined by **Ernest Starling** in 1905 for the chemical messengers of the body and their importance, from a Greek word meaning "to arouse" or "set into motion." Whether adrenal, pancreatic, or based in the sex glands, hormones were seen to impact the brain rather than being ruled by it.

Institute for Sexual Science: Housed in a mansion in the Tiergarten district, the Institute served as a center for sexology, broadly conceived. In addition to providing services such as marriage and fertility counseling, the Institute explored surgical and hormonal treatments for homosexuals and transgender patients. It became the hub of the era's homosexual rights movement, supported the women's rights movement, and treated sexual nonconformists both physically and psychologically. It was founded by Magnus Hirschfeld as the practical component of his Scientific Humanitarian Committee, to further homosexual rights and acceptance.

Intermediaries: The term, coined by Magnus Hirschfeld, suggested transitional states, but also offered an in-between state of being, the closest approximation of nonbinary identity at this time in history. Hirschfeld suggested there might be, mathematically speaking, 43 million possible combinations for sex/sexuality/sexual identity. "Intermediaries" became an umbrella term for those who existed between, alongside, or outside the male/female binary and its gender expectations. By joining those we would today consider transgender with homosexuals and other gender nonconformists, Hirschfeld did away with divisions between, for instance, masculinist and feminist ideals.

Intersex: persons with both male and female reproductive organs, or reproductive anatomy that doesn't fit into strict categories of male and female.

Inversion: A term used in the nineteenth century to mean homosexuality. **Albert Moll** wrote *Sexual Inversion (Conträre Sexualempfindung)* in 1897. The term referred to a possibly inborn reversal of traits considered male or female; for example, male inverts were thought to be inclined toward traditionally female pursuits. This could extend to how they dressed or their sexual desire. The term went out of fashion in the early twentieth century.

Jahrbuch für sexuelle Zwischenstufen (Yearbook for Sexual Intermediaries): The annual publication of the **Scientific Humanitarian Committee**. It ran from 1899 to 1923 and is a unique record of research on sexual and gender minorities through history, ethnology, medicine, politics, law, biology, emancipation struggle, literature, art, religion and biography.

Liebenberg Round Table: Kaiser Wilhelm II surrounded himself with a group led by the wealthy aristocrat **Prince Philipp Fürst zu Eulenburg**. This privileged inner ring included Eulenburg's closest friend, **Lieutenant General Kuno von Moltke**, municipal commandant of Berlin. To its critics, the Round Table was a byzantine "camarilla," a group of irresponsible and self-serving advisors. They held seances; they wrote homoerotic poetry; they represented, in fact, just the kind of homosocial masculinist ideals that appealed to Adolf Brand (but went against the traditional idea of German masculinity).

Männerbund: Described by German anthropologist Heinrich Schurtz in 1902, it meant the free association of "male bands," the power of male bonding and masculine rites of passage. Integral to the term was the idea that men were inherently superior, acting as the "masculine engine of all human culture and social evolution." This misogynistic theory would be embraced by the boys' clubs and youth group movement, fostered in part by **Hans Blüher**.

Memoirs of a Man's Maiden Years: Published in 1907, *Memoirs of a Man's Maiden Years* describes the young womanhood of a man named Karl M. Baer. Born with ambiguous genitalia, he was assigned female at birth and would later be diagnosed with a form of born "pseudohermaphroditism" called hypospadias, in which the opening of the urethra is not located on the tip of the penis (in Karl's case, it was located on the underside). Baer described the social restrictions on those raised as women, and after changing his birth certificate in 1904 published the book.

Monism: The single-origin theory of zoologist and evolutionary biologist Ernst Haeckel, monism sought to answer a deep-time question: where did life originate? What was the originary cell? Haeckel believed that all of us evolved from a single egg. The theory abolished the sex binary through its singularity; since all beings must have begun as "hermaphroditic" cells, the male would have a bit of female and the female a bit of male (with plenty in between). Hirschfeld embraced the concept and joined the Monist Society. Haeckel's theories would be embraced by social Darwinists and Nazi eugenicists.

Paragraph 175: "Unnatural fornication, which is committed between male persons or between people with animals, is to be punished with imprisonment. Loss of civil rights can also be recognized." The law, a version of a Prussian law, extended to all of Germany with unification in 1871, criminalized homosexuality; it would be gradually expanded in its application.

Pederast: A term meaning pedophile or child sex predator, the slur was thrown at homosexuals as a means of criminalizing their behavior. The same tactic continues to be used today, when those who wish to attack homosexual or transgender people accuse them of being "groomers." The slur was leveled at Oscar Wilde after his trial, despite his relationships being with consenting adults, and led to the banning of his books.

Primary sex characteristics: The reproductive organs and sexual anatomy present at birth, which include the penis, scrotum, testicles, uterus, ovaries, and vagina.

Putsch: A coup. The Beer Hall Putsch refers to Hitler's failed coup in 1923, when he attempted to overthrow the sitting government.

Reichstag: The governing body, or parliament, established in Berlin after the independent German states united in 1871. The body moved into the Reichstag building in 1894; the word may refer to either the body or the building. Under imperial electoral law at that time, 397 members were elected for five-year terms, and all male Germans over the age of twenty-five were eligible to vote. There were roughly five parties before the First World War, including the German Progress Party, the German Liberal Party, the Liberal People's Party, the Progressive People's Party, and the Socialist Workers' Party, which was renamed the Social Democratic Party of Germany (SPD). The Reichstag amended the constitution after the war and in 1918 the empire became a parliamentary monarchy, and then, under the Social Democrats, a republic.

Scientific Humanitarian Committee (SHC, *Wissenschaftlich-humanitäres Komitee*): Founded by Magnus Hirschfeld with Eduard Oberg and **Max Spohr**, the SHC existed for the furtherance of sexual science, the emancipation of the **homosexual**, and above all the overturning of **Paragraph 175**. The SHC held together through written communications, with the ***Jahrbuch für sexuelle Zwischenstufen*** acting as a critical outlet for promotion and organization. The core messages were Hirschfeld's utter conviction that biology determined sexual orientation, and that the congenital argument was the most effective means of changing the law. The argument from biology eventually made allies (if not friends) of Dr. Richard von Krafft-Ebing, Dr. Albert Eulenberg, and even Albert Moll, whose theory of homosexuality was ever at odds with Hirschfeld's own.

Secondary sex characteristics: Physical features that usually appear during puberty, such as breasts and facial hair. They are the "bodily signs," as Susan Stryker wrote in *Transgender History*, that others use to attribute gender, and "the aspect of our bodies that we all manipulate in an attempt to communicate to others our own sense of who we feel we are."

Secretions: The original term for the chemical messengers traveling through the bloodstream. They would later be renamed hormones.

Sex: The definition of this word changes over time. It can mean sexual acts; it can mean the differentiation of reproductive organs. In the nineteenth century, scientists like **Adolf Berthold** meant the distinction between and operation of the genitals.

Sexuality: The term first entered the English language in 1879, meaning the "possession of sexual powers, or capability of sexual feelings." It became increasingly central to individual identity, while the terms themselves exploded: "sex" and "sexuality" might mean biological sex, gender identity, or sexual orientation.

Sexualwissenschaft (sexology or sexual science): *Wissenschaft*, the German word for "science," is more inclusive than the Anglo-American idea of science, broad enough to also encompass aspects of the humanities and social sciences as classifiable forms of knowledge. At the time of its emergence, *Sexualwissenschaft* interlinked other professions, such as human psychology, psychoanalysis, ethnography, anthropology, criminology, physiology, social activism, and the still nascent field of endocrinology.

Sodomite: A common derogatory term used to mean homosexual, it emphasized the sex act, most especially anal penetration. The Marquess of Queensberry accused Oscar Wilde of being a sodomite when he discovered Wilde's affair with his son, Lord Alfred Douglas. Wilde would be convicted not of sodomy but of gross indecency, which carried much the same connotations.

"Third sex": A term used by Karl Heinrich Ulrichs as well as Magnus Hirschfeld in his book *Berlin's Third Sex*, later replaced by "intermediaries." Based upon extensive questionnaires completed in 1903–04, Hirschfeld estimated the gay population of Berlin to be something over 50,000 people. *Berlin's Third Sex* is less a scientific philosophy than a grand invitation to see with fresh eyes; Hirschfeld had already understood that "homosexual" as a term didn't cover all the diversity he encountered. As a group, these people were not easily identifiable, did not fit into categories, and spent much of their time concealing their "true" selves.

Transgender: The term presently used to describe people who do not align with the gender assigned to them at birth. The word was first coined by psychiatrist John F. Oliven in 1965 and has come to replace earlier terminology such as "transsexual," Magnus Hirschfeld's term "intermediary," and the early-twentieth-century "transvestite." Transgender became the word chosen by trans people in the 1990s, and Susan Stryker's *Transgender History* defines it further as "people who cross over (trans-) the boundaries constructed by their culture to define and contain the gender." It may include trans women (a space between; the words are not elided), trans men, nonbinary persons, agender persons, and all others for whom prescribed gender roles do not fit.

Transvestite: The word means, literally, one who "dresses across" or cross-dresses. For Hirschfeld, it meant something much closer to our concept of transgender. Hirschfeld wrote *Die Transvestiten* in 1910. The majority of the case studies included were heterosexual (that is, many still considered themselves male in sexual terms, and desired women sexually);

as a result, Hirschfeld separates "transvestites" from homosexuals for the first time. Clothing, he writes, is an "unconscious projection of the soul," evidence of male and female psyches expressing themselves in contrary physical bodies.

Transvestite certificate (*Transvestitenschein*): Hirschfeld successfully petitioned for this in 1909. Transvestites carrying the certificate had proof of professional medical permission to dress as they wished and could not be arrested on these grounds.

Übermensch: The concept of the *Übermensch*, or superman, comes from the work of philosopher Friedrich Nietzsche. The *Übermensch* rises above the masses by thinking only of himself. He resists the social order and strives above all for individualism. Similar to and conversant with the super-individual characterized by Max Stirner's egoist in *Der Einzige und sein Eigentum* (translated variously as *The Ego and his Own*, *The Ego and Its Own*, and *The Unique and Its Property*), it formed an essential part of the masculinist ideals of Adolf Brand, his *Der Eigene* publication, and his followers.

Urning (uranian, uranism): A word coined by Karl Ulrichs after the myth of Aphrodite's birth by Uranus—a male god who plays both the male and female part in her creation. The term referred not to same-sex acts but to same-sex-desiring identities. Ulrichs referred to "lasting covenants of love" among the ancients, and also to scientific and medical studies of *zwitter*, the German word for hermaphroditism or intersex.

Volk: Originally and literally meaning crowd or mass of the population—similar to the English word "folk"—after 1800 it came to mean the German people, particularly in the context of German nationalism.

Wandervögel: Literally "wandering bird," the Wandervögel became a powerful youth movement under German nationalism. Facing a crisis of masculinity over the **Eulenburg** scandal, Germany sought to indoctrinate boys into ideal white, German, heterosexual male society as a matter of national security.

Weimar Republic: From November 9, 1918, to March 23, 1933, Germany dispensed with its imperial monarchy and operated as a constitutional federal republic for the first time in history. The Weimar Republic, also known as the German Reich, permitted its citizens, men and women, to vote for president and for the parliamentary body (the Reichstag). The period was known for progressive attitudes. It fell when Hitler took over as chancellor and initiated passage of the Enabling Act, effectively making him dictator.

World League for Sexual Reform: Founded in 1928 by Magnus Hirschfeld, August Forel, and Havelock Ellis, the WLSR was an outgrowth of the First International Conference for Sexual Reform on a Scientific Basis, organized by Hirschfeld in 1921. Like the **Scientific Humanitarian Committee** before it, the League focused on reforms to sex legislation, but broadened the scope and reach. The records and books of the League were destroyed by Nazi forces during the raid on the **Institute for Sexual Science** in 1933; by 1935, it had dissolved.

Zwitter: The German word for hermaphroditism or intersex. However, the term did not always refer to the physical body; Karl Ulrichs used it to refer to men with a "female soul." We would not, today, consider homosexual, transgender, or intersex persons the same, but Ulrichs's thinking was influenced by strictly enforced gender roles. Because in nineteenth-century Germany only women loved men, Ulrichs assumed that his desire for other men must be due to an internal "womanly" quality. Though not physically intersex, he believed he was psychically feminine, and what he called **uranism** was a new kind of *zwitter*.

Terms and persons with their own entry in the glossary and "Characters of Note" are shown in bold on first appearance.

William Bateson: English biologist who coined the term "genetics" for the study of genes and championed the principles of heredity discovered by Gregor Mendel. His work resulted in the popularization of genetics among other scientists and the public, without which Mendel's work might have been forgotten.

William Bayliss: British physiologist and Nobel Prize winner, who, along with Ernest Starling, first studied pressures in the veins and capillaries. In 1897 they radically changed direction to work on the control of the motility of the gut. They would ultimately do experiments that led to the discovery of hormones as chemical messengers of the body.

Harry Benjamin: A German American physician with an interest in endocrinology, Benjamin came to the **Institute for Sexual Science** in the mid-1920s, participated in congresses of the World League for Sexual Reform, and ultimately would carry Hirschfeld's mantle. He would become famous for clinical work with transgender people, and took referrals from Alfred Kinsey (author of the classic investigation of sexuality *The Kinsey Report*). He published *The Transsexual Phenomenon* in 1952.

Arnold Adolph Berthold: A German scientist, physiologist, and zoologist, best known for his pioneering experiments in the field of endocrinology. He removed and re-transplanted the testicles of roosters to show that vital information about puberty and sex characteristics are transferred through the body without the involvement of nerves.

Hans Blüher: A German philosopher who popularized the masculinist *Wandervögel* movement. At first identifying as a homosexual and befriending **Magnus Hirschfeld**, Blüher would ultimately side with **Adolf Brand** and **Benedict Friedländer** against women and what he considered "feminine" homosexuality. Blüher would ultimately marry a woman and turn against both homosexuals and Jewish people, making the argument that both groups emasculated the German nation. His works were used by Nazi propagandists.

Adolf Brand: At first an ally of Hirschfeld and a member of the **Scientific Humanitarian Committee**, Brand supported masculinist "Greek" ideals of homosexuality, decried anything feminine, and did not support those who wished to change their gender to be women. In 1906 he and Benedict Friedländer broke from the SHC for good. Hirschfeld considered them misogynists; the two would found a masculinist society, which ultimately became hypernationalistic and anti-Semitic. Brand turned against Hirschfeld and sought to bring him down as the Nazis rose to power.

Charles-Édouard Brown-Séquard: The "father of endocrinology," Brown-Séquard is generally heralded as an eccentric genius. A prominent neurophysiologist, his interest in hormone replacement theory led to the creation of an "elixir" made of crushed dog testicles. He injected this into himself and claimed to have been rejuvenated. He is best known for his description in 1850–51 of what became known as Brown-Séquard syndrome, which results from lateral hemisection of the spinal cord.

Toni Ebel: A painter, she joined the staff of the Institute for Sexual Science at the same time as **Dora Richter**, but paid for her surgery through sale of her paintings. Born Hugo Otto Arno Ebel, she had lived as a woman off and on while painting in Munich. She married in 1911 and had a son, but the role of husband and father made Toni consider taking her own life.

After the death of her spouse, Olga, she came to the clinic to seek consultation. Toni began her transition after Dora, but completed it in a more compressed timeframe.

Lili Elbe: A glamorous and well-known trans woman with a largely supportive spouse, she was a painter and the subject of the book and film *The Danish Girl*. Elbe also wrote an autobiography, *Man into Woman*. Her consultations begin at the Institute for Sexual Science, though her surgery would ultimately be finished in Dresden by **Erwin Gohrbandt**. She died after an attempted womb transplant.

Prince Philipp Fürst zu Eulenburg: Chief confidant, friend, and supervisor of Kaiser **Wilhelm II**'s inner circle, Eulenburg would be accused of homosexuality and of leaking state secrets to a French homosexual. The trial to clear his name—involving himself, **Lieutenant General Kuno von Moltke**, and **Maximilian Harden**—would lead to a national scandal, a nationwide panic about homosexuality and the weakening of the nation, and a crisis of masculinity.

Benedict Friedländer: With Adolf Brand and others, Friedländer helped to found the organization called *Gemeinschaft der Eigenen* (GdE), usually translated as Community of the Special, in 1903. It advocated the "Greek" masculine ideal and homosocial networks, and countenanced homosexuality among men as a choice—but only so long as it was "masculinized." A misogynist who believed that women were inferior in every way, he broke with Hirschfeld over Hirschfeld's support of women and his understanding of sexuality as a spectrum.

Karl Giese: Head of the archives at the Institute of Sexual Science, Giese served as secretary, lecturer, and tour guide. He was, quietly, Hirschfeld's lover for over a decade, and was referred to by those visiting the Institute as the "woman of the house." He was a favorite with trans patients and with Christopher Isherwood, who found him charming and attractive—and a bit of a gossip.

Erwin Gohrbandt: Gohrbandt studied medicine at the Military Medical Academy and graduated in 1917. He performed the initial transgender operations with **Ludwig Levy-Lenz**, including those on Dora Richter and **Lili Elbe**. When the Nazis came to power, he did not flee as Levy-Lenz was forced to do, but became medical chief and later a general in the Luftwaffe. He also participated in the grim and lethal hypothermia experiments at Dachau concentration camp. He turned on his Institute colleagues and was considered a traitor and a Nazi by Levy-Lenz.

Maximilian Harden: A journalist and former supporter of the monarchy, Harden became a fierce critic of Kaiser Wilhelm II and his entourage, especially Prince Eulenburg and General Kuno von Moltke. His public accusations of homosexuality led to numerous trials and deeply damaged the reputation of the Kaiser, weakening Germany's position among other nations.

Kurt Hiller: A lawyer, author, pacifist, and ardent supporter of homosexual rights. After the publication of his law dissertation "The Right over One's Self" in 1908, he joined the Scientific Humanitarian Committee. Hiller was critical, if not dismissive, of Magnus Hirschfeld's theories on sexual intermediaries, but they worked together until Hirschfeld left the SHC. Hiller succeeded him as chairman.

Magnus Hirschfeld: German Jewish doctor and sexologist who championed the rights of homosexuals and intermediaries. Founder of the Institute for Sexual Science and also of its forebear, the Scientific Humanitarian Committee, which in 1897 set the foundations of his research and also his social justice agenda, what he called the "high holy fight" for equality. Hirschfeld published many works of sexual science and philosophy, as well as some of the more definitive volumes of his day. His work on "transvestites" offers up the first sensitive portrayal of transgender people. He would ultimately support surgical and hormonal affirmation practices for transgender patients, as well as provide for transvestite certificates to allow them to appear publicly in the gender of their choice.

Christopher Isherwood: Among the literati and artists who broadly supported the Institute for Sexual Science, homosexuals, trans persons, and gender nonconformists, were English writers W. H. Auden and Christopher Isherwood. Isherwood's extensive diaries provide a window into the provocative, daring, and joyous occasions at the Institute and the Eldorado, a club frequented by its members.

Gerd Katter: A carpenter, artist, amateur sexologist, and trans man. As Eva Katter, he sought aid and refuge at the Institute for Sexual Science in the mid-1920s, considered Hirschfeld like a father, and described the years he spent at the Institute as "among the most interesting of my life." Like Dora Richter, Gerd realized that he wasn't "like the others" at an early age. Unlike Dora, Gerd was supported by his parents; his mother even accompanied him to the Institute. He would spend the next year attaining a transvestite license through Hirschfeld's expert diagnosis, and then attempted to change his name: the "patient," wrote Hirschfeld, suffered "difficulties in [his] professional life" because the name Eva contradicted his masculine qualities and appearance. Sometime after this, Gerd requested breast removal and was denied. Gerd then attempted to do the surgery himself. One case in the notebooks of Dr. Ludwig Levy-Lenz describes a sixteen-year-old who did this, but the two cases cannot be considered the same person as there is some discrepancy in the dates.

Richard von Krafft-Ebing: A German neuropsychiatrist, Krafft-Ebing was a pioneering student of sexual psychopathology, or the study of mental disorders. He is best known today for his *Psychopathia Sexualis* (1886), a groundbreaking examination of sexual aberrations. Hirschfeld acknowledged his debt to Krafft-Ebing's work, but their views did not align.

Ludwig Levy-Lenz: Like Hirschfeld a Jewish physician, Levy-Lenz began practice as a gynecologist and would go on to be a plastic surgeon. Levy-Lenz would pioneer the first gender affiramation and transition surgeries and oversee transitions at the clinic. He was also a researcher, and a collector of books and patient records.

Richard Linsert: Originally a commercial clerk, Linsert joined the Institute for Sexual Science on the recommendation of the jurist Kurt Hiller in 1923, and became secretary of the Scientific Humanitarian Committee. From 1926, he was head of the Department of Sexual Reform at the Institute and organized public question-and-answer evenings on sexual matters in the Institute's lecture hall.

Franziska Mann: Magnus Hirschfeld's sister, with whom he co-wrote the pamphlet *Was jede Frau vom Wahlrecht wissen muß!* ("What every woman needs to know about the right to vote!")

Albert Moll: A fellow Jewish physician (though converted to Lutheran Protestantism), Moll was one of the earliest signatories of the petition against **Paragraph 175**. He wrote a monograph on homosexuality, *Sexual Inversion (Conträre Sexualempfindung)*, in 1897, and published an extensive work on heterosexuality (*Untersuchungen über die Libido sexualis*) the same year from which Sigmund Freud likely borrowed. His differences with Hirschfeld led to a split and animosity; Moll eventually wrote a letter to the University of Paris denouncing Hirschfeld for medical misconduct and claiming he had been run out of Germany for his immorality.

Lieutenant General Kuno von Moltke: Lieutenant General Kuno von Moltke, municipal commandant of Berlin, was a member of the **Liebenberg Round Table**, a close-knit group around Kaiser Wilhelm II led by **Prince Philipp Fürst zu Eulenburg**. Maximilian Harden accused Moltke and Eulenburg in print of being lovers and therefore a threat to the nation. This led to a scandal, which led to a panic over homosexuality, a purge of homosexuals in government, and renewed attacks against those who did not conform to normative sexuality or gender constructs.

Friedrich Radszuweit: A German publisher and author, he published two homosexual magazines and had a great deal of media influence on the subject of homosexual rights. He was also president of the League for

Human Rights and a "masculinist" who aligned more with Adolf Brand than with Magnus Hirschfeld.

Dora Richter: Dora was a lacemaker and apprenticed to a baker. Born in Seifen in the kingdom of Bohemia, she was assigned male at birth and christened Rudolf. She would live most of her life as a woman, taking on male clothing only when forced by necessity. Despite a great deal of suffering, Dora remained gentle, well liked, "dreamy," and friendly. Dora didn't hear of the Institute until adulthood. Hirschfeld called her *Dorchen*, "little Dora," and she helped reframe his understanding of transgender sexuality. She was the first to undergo gender affirmation surgeries, including vaginoplasty.

Ernst Röhm: A close friend and ally of Adolf Hitler, and from 1931 leader of the Storm Troops (*Sturmabteilung* or SA), the Nazi Party's paramilitary soldiers. Röhm was also a homosexual whose lifestyle was semi-public knowledge and whose lovers were occasional visitors to Hirschfeld's Institute. Hitler countenanced his homosexuality until he felt his usefulness had come to an end, and ordered his murder during the Night of the Long Knives, June 30–July 2, 1934.

Max Spohr: Co-founder of the Scientific Humanitarian Committee, a publisher who risked his career to publish not only Hirschfeld's work but the works of other homosexual and nonconforming people. He would be loyal until his death, following which his son undertook to publish for the cause.

Heinrich Stabel: A surgeon and gynecologist, Stabel performed testicle transplants and was a leader in sexual reform. He spoke out for decriminalization of homosexuality and abortion, and carried out artificial inseminations.

Ernest Henry Starling: A British physiologist who contributed many fundamental ideas to endocrinology and coined the term "hormone" in

1905. He participated with William Bayliss in experiments on motility of the gut that proved chemical messengers, and not the nervous system, were responsible for many bodily processes.

Eugen Steinach: A proponent of hormone research and the first to try implanting male sex organs into female test animals. The namesake of the Steinach procedure for male rejuvenation, he would be one among several endocrinologists closely acquainted with Hirschfeld (and one of the more colorful).

Nettie Maria Stevens: American geneticist who discovered sex chromosomes. In 1905, after the rediscovery of Mendel's paper on genetics, she noted that male mealworms produced two kinds of sperm, one with a large chromosome and one with a small chromosome. Sperm with the large chromosome produced female offspring and sperm from the small one produced males. These would later be named the X and Y chromosomes.

Max Stirner: Johann Kaspar Schmidt, known professionally as Max Stirner, was a German post-Hegelian philosopher. He is considered one of the principal forerunners of nihilism, existentialism, postmodernism, anarchism, and egoism. His work *Der Einzige und sein Eigentum* (translated variously as *The Ego and his Own*, *The Ego and Its Own*, and *The Unique and Its Property*), published in 1844, had an impact on Adolf Brand.

Helene Stöcker: A feminist and founder of the League for the Protection of Mothers and Sexual Reform (later shortened to the League for the Protection of Mothers), Stöcker was a member of the Scientific Humanitarian Committee and joined its board of directors. Stöcker was opinionated and outspoken and often disagreed with Hirschfeld, who clung to the idea that there were mental differences between men and women. Known for wearing green and for her wide-brimmed feathered hat, she championed women's rights, the right to abortion, and sex education. Several other notable feminists became important to the SHC and shared its causes, including Margaret Sanger, champion of birth control.

Tao Li (formally, Li Shiu Tong): One of Hirschfeld's later acolytes and his second lover; he and Karl Giese and Hirschfeld lived together in Paris. Li, from Hong Kong, had hoped to open the first Institute for Sexual Science in his country.

Karl Heinrich Ulrichs: A German jurist and writer, Ulrichs openly declared himself homosexual in an attempt to foster understanding and gain rights for those like himself. He is regarded today as a pioneer of sexology and the modern gay rights movement; his work deeply influenced Magnus Hirschfeld.

Oscar Wilde: Irish poet and playwright, author of *The Picture of Dorian Gray* and *The Importance of Being Earnest*, Wilde was a cultural icon and advocate of art for art's sake. He became the object of civil and criminal suits regarding his homosexuality which ended in a prison sentence (1895–97) and censorship of his work. He became an important figure in the movement for gay rights, especially in Germany, both before and especially after his untimely death.

Wilhelm II: The last German Emperor (Kaiser) and King of Prussia, Friedrich Wilhelm Viktor Albert reigned from 1888 until his abdication in 1918. This marked the beginning of the Weimar Republic and the end of the German Empire. His rule was marked with controversy, from his dismissal of longtime chancellor Otto von Bismarck to his problematic foreign policy leading to the First World War.

TIMELINE

Terms and persons with their own entry in the glossary and "Characters of Note" are shown in bold on first appearance.

1848

Arnold Berthold experiments with rooster testicles.

1867

Lawyer **Karl Heinrich Ulrichs** approaches the Odeon in Munich to speak before the Association of German Jurists, the government establishment of the nascent German Empire, against anti-sodomy laws, supporting his case by declaring himself homosexual.

1868

Magnus Hirschfeld is born in Kolberg, Pomerania (present-day Kolobrzeg, Poland), the sixth of seven children.

1871

The German Empire is declared, and adopts the Prussian anti-sodomy law known as **Paragraph 175**.

1877

Richard von Krafft-Ebing, an Austrian who became the leading nineteenth-century sexologist, cites Ulrichs in writing about same-sex love. In 1886 he will publish *Psychopathia Sexualis*.

1889

Charles-Édouard Brown-Séquard, the "father of endocrinology," gives a lecture recommending a serum made of dog testicles for increased vitality.

1891

Hirschfeld starts his studies in Strasbourg (then in Germany).

1892

Hirschfeld graduates from Friedrich-Wilhelms-Univerität, now Humboldt University, Berlin, with a doctorate in medicine, specializing in illnesses of the nervous system following influenza.

Dora Richter is born (April 16).

1893

Hirschfeld becomes a journalist in Hamburg and travels to the Chicago World's Fair. His brother, practicing medicine in Milwaukee, invites him to give a lecture on the "natural way of living" in New York; its success leads to lectures in Boston and Washington, DC.

1894

Hirschfeld settles in Magdeburg and works for two years as an obstetrician before moving to Berlin.

1896

Hirschfeld moves to Berlin to begin work in hydrotherapy and natural cures.

The suicide of one of Hirschfeld's patients changes his career direction. He publishes *Sappho and Socrates* and describes homosexuality as inborn and congenital.

Adolf Brand publishes the journal ***Der Eigene*** in support of masculinist "Greek" ideals of homosexuality, in opposition to Hirschfeld's more feminine ideas of homosexuality.

1897

In May, Hirschfeld invites a group of like-minded associates to his Berlin apartment to found the **Scientific Humanitarian Committee**, which would target Paragraph 175 and ultimately find a home at the **Institute for Sexual Science**. Their petition against Paragraph 175 would be heavily supported by artists and literary greats.

1898

Hirschfeld and publisher **Max Spohr** republish all of Karl Ulrichs's works. Hirschfeld brings forward a petition to revoke Paragraph 175, though the attempt is unsuccessful.

1899

Hirschfeld launches the *Jahrbuch für sexuelle Zwischenstufen* (Yearbook for Sexual Intermediaries), the first journal dedicated to same-sex sexuality. It will become the mouthpiece for the Scientific Humanitarian Committee.

1902

Ernest Henry Starling and **William Bayliss** perform their dog experiments in London, which result in an anti-vivisection court case. They discover peptide secretions—introducing the concept of body secretions—which will lead to the identification of hormones.

1903

Hirschfeld publishes *Der urnische Mensch* (The Uranian Person).

Hirschfeld establishes the Scientific Humanitarian Committee "propaganda" commission for "public education."

1904

Hirschfeld publishes *Berlin's Third Sex*.

1905

The word "genetics" (study of genes) is coined by English biologist **William Bateson**. (The first published use of the shortened "gene" will occur in 1909.)

The word "hormone" is coined by English physiologist Ernest Henry Starling in a lecture titled "The Chemical Correlation of the Functions of the Body."

Sex chromosomes are discovered by **Nettie Maria Stevens**.

Hirschfeld supports, with **Helene Stöcker**, the progressive League for the Protection of Mothers and Sexual Reform. He will later agitate for decriminalization of abortion.

Dora Richter tries to remove her penis with a string, attempts suicide at the age of thirteen.

1906

The Scientific Humanitarian Committee splits between the masculinist group, led by Adolf Brand and **Benedict Friedländer**, and the more inclusive group represented by Hirschfeld.

1907

Hirschfeld's involvement in the **Eulenburg** libel case causes trouble for the Scientific Humanitarian Committee.

Memoirs of a Man's Maiden Years by Karl M.[artha] Baer is published.

1908

Hirschfeld publishes a pamphlet on homophobia, *Sexualpsychologie und Volkspsychologie*, asserting that anti-homosexual attitudes are generated by "mass suggestion," or the production and perpetuation of anti-homosexuality discourse in the media.

1910

Hirschfeld publishes *The Transvestites*, coining the term "transvestite" and explaining that sexual preference is not necessarily connected to the desire for a different gender identity. He develops the term and theory for sexual intermediaries: a spectrum with 43 million variations.

Hirschfeld begins providing diagnoses that allow individuals to get a **transvestite certificate**, or a license to cross-dress.

Eugen Steinach begins research on rats.

Dora Richter leaves her apprenticeship as a baker and gets a job as a waitress.

1912

Eugen Steinach publishes *Arbitrary Transformation* suggesting that "pure woman" and "pure man" are only concepts, though he is still attempting to "cure" homosexuals.

Hirschfeld and Helene Stöcker argue against the extension of Paragraph 175 to lesbians and win.

Dora Richter takes a job as a performer of women's roles in a traveling theater.

1913

Albert Eulenburg, Iwan Bloch, and Hirschfeld found the Medical Society for Sexual Sciences in Eugenics in Berlin.

Hirschfeld goes to London for the 14th International Medical Conference to present his theory of intermediaries, bringing with him 150 photographs from his clinical practice to demonstrate sexual variation from homosexuals to "transvestites" to intersex people.

1914

Hirschfeld publishes *The Homosexuality of Men and Women*, on the results of his "Psychobiological Questionnaire." He opposes the idea that homosexuality was pathological, pitting him against **Albert Moll**.

Hirschfeld introduces **adaptation therapy**.

1916

Max Marcuse, a Berlin doctor and psychotherapist, gives an "ovarian preparation" to Herr A., who wishes to have his testicles removed.

Dora Richter is sent to military service, then discharged; she falls in love with a soldier and is estranged from her family.

1917

Eugen Steinach publishes a sensational report claiming that by transplanting the testicle of a heterosexual man into a homosexual he has cured him of his homosexuality. This is later disproven.

1918

Hirschfeld is appointed to the Hygiene Council of Germany in the new **Weimar Republic**. He begins working on a film, *Anders als die Andern*.

Hirschfeld meets the young Karl Giese after one of his lectures.

1919

Anders als die Andern is released.

The **Institute for Sexual Science** is opened.

1920

Anders als die Andern is banned.

Hirschfeld is attacked in Munich and beaten badly. After this, a pamphlet attacks him directly with anti-Semitic threats.

Adolf Hitler singles out Hirschfeld as the "Jewish swine" and calls for him to be attacked and killed.

The Scientific Humanitarian Committee sets up the Action Board against Paragraph 175.

Hirschfeld publishes *Sexual Pathology* and a second volume of *Sexual Intermediaries*.

Dr. Ludwig Levy-Lenz meets Hirschfeld. He will later work at the Institute.

A primitive sex change operation is attempted in Dresden by Dr. Kronfeld and completed by Richard Mühsam, who did not remove the penis but hid it from view by tucking it into a wound. The patient will later demand to have the surgery reversed and abandon his cross-dressing.

1921

Richard Mühsam performs a female-to-male surgery by removing the ovaries of a patient who had breasts removed in 1912. He will go on to attempt to transplant sex organs.

Dr. Arthur Weil receives an award from the Berlin Physicians' Society for Sexual Science and Eugenics for his study of physical measurements of homosexuals, aiming to provide evidence of a specifically homosexual body type.

Hirschfeld approves a gonad transplant based on Steinach's work; it has disappointing results.

The Institute for Sexual Science buys the building next door, which will house the Scientific Humanitarian Committee and other political activities as well as rental apartments.

The first International Conference for Sexual Reform Based on Sexual Science is held at the Institute. Among those present are Helene Stöcker and Dr. Mathilde Vaerting, who asserts that masculine and feminine were social terms and not based in reality.

The Scientific Humanitarian Committee renews attempts to overthrow Paragraph 175, this time in collaboration with Adolf Brand.

1922

The Institute practices adaptation therapy, later to be known as psychological milieu therapy.

Together with the lawyer Walther Niemann, Hirschfeld makes efforts to get name changes approved for "transvestite" patients. Male and female transvestites were permitted to change their first names to gender-neutral names, e.g., Alex, Toni, or Gert.

The wall of photographs titled "Sexual Transitions" is shown publicly for the first time at the Hundred-Year Celebration of German Natural Scientists and Physicians in Leipzig.

In March, Hirschfeld sends the petition against Paragraph 175 to the government, and minister of justice Gustav Radbruch suggests that the law criminalizing homosexuality may be overturned. By the time the petition arrives, Radbruch has resigned.

1923

Dora Richter arrives at the Institute for Sexual Science.

The Great Inflation makes the Weimar Republic unstable. Hirschfeld struggles to keep the Institute solvent.

On February 4, Hirschfeld speaks on "Sexual Crises" in Vienna. A group of young Nazis throw stink bombs and fire shots; some audience members are beaten.

1924

Inflation wipes out Hirschfeld's charitable foundation, forcing the Institute to rely on donations. The *Jahrbuch* ceases publication.

To bring in funds, Hirschfeld allows his Titus Pearls, a hormone concoction, to be mass-produced. It contained testosterone, pituitary gland hormones, and a proprietary blend of other items.

1925

Hirschfeld helps to found the Cartel for Reform of the Law against Sexual Offenses (with **Kurt Hiller** and **Richard Linsert**), to fight for human rights for all, not just intermediaries. Seven organizations joined the Cartel: the Department for Sexual Reform at the Institute, the League for the Protection of Mothers and Sexual Reform, Deutsche Liga für Menschenrecht, Gesellschaft für Geschlechtskunde, Gesellschaft für Sexualreform, Verband Eherechtsreform, and the Scientific Humanitarian Committee.

1926

Dr. Ludwig Levy-Lenz joins the Institute for Sexual Science full-time as primary surgeon, performing the new gender affirmation or transition surgeries.

Hirschfeld tours the USSR.

1927

Fred C. Koch, Professor of Physiological Chemistry at the University of Chicago, and his student Lemuel McGee extract pure testosterone from bull testicles.

1928

Hirschfeld turns sixty.

The second International Congress for Sexual Reform takes place in Copenhagen June 30–July 6. Hirschfeld's paper "Sexual Reform in the Light of Sexual Science" outlines the difference between theological and biological, and asserts that religion is to blame for suffering. The **World League for Sexual Reform** is founded at this congress.

Hirschfeld meets with the Minister of Justice about proposed new laws banning homosexual publications.

1929

In March, **Christopher Isherwood** joins W. H. Auden in Berlin. He is "brought face to face with his tribe" at the Institute for Sexual Science.

The **Reichstag** commission formally recommends decriminalizing sex between men over twenty-one. Newspapers claim that this cancels Paragraph 175. Unfortunately, in the political disorder as the Weimar government falters, the law is not brought forward for a vote.

Hirschfeld resigns from the Scientific Humanitarian Committee.

The second congress of the World League for Sexual Reform takes place in London, September 8–14. Hirschfeld gives the presidential address.

Estrone (later renamed estrogen) is isolated as a hormone

The third International Conference for Sexual Reform (of the World League for Sexual Reform) takes place in London.

1930

The fourth International Conference for Sexual Reform (of the World League for Sexual Reform) convenes in Vienna.

Steinach's student Walter Holweg suggests that the hypothalamus is where sex orientation evolved.

German geneticist Theo Lang publishes a study suggesting that homosexual men are chromosomal females.

Lili Elbe goes for her initial surgery in Dresden.

Hirschfeld commences a world tour.

1931

Dora Richter asks Dr. Ludwig Levy-Lenz to remove her penis. The next two years of surgeries will be detailed in two case studies. Her penis is removed in June.

Hirschfeld goes to Tokyo, then to China where he meets **Tao Li** (Li Shiu Tong), who will become his lover.

Hirschfeld goes to India.

Dora Richter's external vagina surgery is completed by **Erwin Gohrbandt**, who also performed a vaginoplasty on Lili Elbe a few weeks later.

1932

The fifth International Conference for Sexual Reform (of the World League for Sexual Reform) convenes in Brno.

1933

The National Socialist (Nazi) party rises. Hirschfeld is listed as "enemy number 1."

Karl Giese leaves Berlin for France.

Ludwig Levy-Lenz flees Germany before he can be arrested.

Christopher Isherwood flees Germany with his lover Heinz Neddermeyer, who is denied entry to England and will ultimately be arrested by the Gestapo in 1937.

The Institute for Sexual Science is raided and its archive and library are burned.

1934

Ernst Röhm is killed during the Night of the Long Knives; and the war on homosexuals begins. By 1945, 50,000 people will be convicted of homosexuality.

1935

The testicular hormone is named testosterone by biologist Ernst Laqueur.

Hirschfeld dies of a stroke on May 14, his birthday, in Nice on the French Riviera.

1938

Synthetic estrogen is developed.

1952

The *New York Daily News* breaks the story of Christine Jorgensen, an ex-GI who has undergone transition surgery. As a result, patients are referred to **Harry Benjamin**, Hirschfeld's one-time pupil. Benjamin will go on to write *The Transexual Phenomenon* in 1966 and the introduction to Jorgensen's autobiography in 1967.

NOTES

INTRODUCTION

1. Elena Mancini, *Magnus Hirschfeld and the Quest for Sexual Freedom* (Palgrave Macmillan, 2010), 140.
2. Rainer Herrn, *Der Liebe und dem Leid: Das Institut für Sexualwissenschaft 1919–1933* (Suhrkamp, 2022), 471.
3. Heike Bauer, *The Hirschfeld Archives: Violence, Death, and Modern Queer Culture* (Temple University Press, 2017), 98–99.
4. Herrn, *Der Liebe und dem Leid*, 465.
5. Susan Stryker, *Transgender History: The Roots of Today's Revolution*, 2nd ed. (Seal Press, 2017), 40.
6. Véronique Mottier, "The Invention of Sexuality," in *Chic, chèque, choc*, edited by Françoise Grange Omokaro and Fenneke Reysoo (Graduate Institute Publications, 2012), 25.
7. Victoria Harris, "Histories of 'Sex,' Histories of 'Sexuality,'" *Contemporary European History* 22, no. 2 (2013): 295–301.
8. Jonathan Ned Katz, *The Invention of Heterosexuality* (University of Chicago Press, 2007), 20.
9. Katz, *The Invention of Heterosexuality*, 20.
10. Katz, *The Invention of Heterosexuality*, 88–89.

CHAPTER 1: **THE SCIENCE OF SMALL THINGS**

1. Randi Hutter Epstein, *Aroused: The History of Hormones and How They Control Just About Everything* (W. W. Norton, 2018), 8.
2. German E. Berrios, "Historical Epistemology of the Body–Mind Interaction in Psychiatry," *Dialogues in Clinical Neuroscience* 20, no. 1 (2018): 9.
3. Berrios, "Historical Epistemology," 10.
4. K. K. Soma, "Testosterone and Aggression: Berthold, Birds and Beyond," *Journal of Neuroendocrinology* 18, no. 7 (July 2006): 543–51.
5. As was the case for Gaspare Pacchierotti (one of the most famous). Alberto Zanatta et al., "Occupational Markers and Pathology of the Castrato Singer Gaspare Pacchierotti (1740–1821)," *Scientific Reports* 6, no. 1 (September 2016): 28463.
6. Randy Joe Nelson and Lance J. Kriegsfeld, *An Introduction to Behavioral Endocrinology*, 5th ed. (Sinauer Associates, 2017), 7.

7. Homer P. Rush, "A Biographic Sketch of Arnold Adolf Berthold: An Early Experimenter with Ductless Glands," *Annals of Medical History* 1, no. 2 (1929): 208–14.

8. Ralph Matthew Leck, *Vita Sexualis: Karl Ulrichs and the Origins of Sexual Science* (University of Illinois Press, 2016), 37.

9. James Cowles Prichard, "A Treatise on Insanity and Other Disorders Affecting the Mind," in *Embodied Selves*, edited by Jenny Bourne Taylor and Sally Shuttleworth (Oxford University Press, 1998).

10. Karl Heinrich Ulrichs, *The Correspondence of Karl Heinrich Ulrichs, 1846–1894* (Palgrave Macmillan, 2020), 184.

11. Ulrichs, *Correspondence*, 189.

12. Ulrichs, *Correspondence*, 187.

13. Robert Beachy, *Gay Berlin: Birthplace of a Modern Identity* (Vintage, 2015), 17–18.

14. Ulrichs, *Correspondence*, 199.

15. Ulrichs, *Correspondence*, 187.

16. Ulrichs, *Correspondence*, 191.

17. Ulrichs, *Correspondence*, 228.

18. Beachy, *Gay Berlin*, 4.

19. Ulrichs, *Correspondence*, 262.

20. Ulrichs, *Correspondence*, 29.

21. Yongsheng Liu and Qi Chen, "150 Years of Darwin's Theory of Intercellular Flow of Hereditary Information," *Nature Reviews Molecular Cell Biology* 19 (2018): 749–50.

22. Siddhartha Mukherjee, *The Gene: An Intimate History* (Scribner, 2017), 75.

23. Mukherjee, *The Gene*, 61.

24. Mukherjee, *The Gene*, 58.

25. Jamshed R. Tata, "One Hundred Years of Hormones," *EMBO Reports* 6, no. 6 (2005): 490–96.

26. Amy Koerber, *From Hysteria to Hormones: A Rhetorical History* (Pennsylvania State University Press, 2018), 79.

27. Charles-Édouard Brown-Séquard, *Elixir of Life* (Boston: J. G. Cupples, 1889), 39.

28. Brown-Séquard, *Elixir of Life*, 25.

29. Brown-Séquard, *Elixir of Life*, 30–31.

30. Koerber, *From Hysteria to Hormones*, 79–81.

31. Magnus Hirschfeld, in *Literarische Welt*, May 25, 1928, quoted in Charlotte Wolff, *Magnus Hirschfeld: A Portrait of a Pioneer in Sexology* (Quartet, 1986), 27.

32. There is uncertainty about the exact date; Hirschfeld gives it as both the evening before and the evening after the wedding.

33. Magnus Hirschfeld, *Sappho and Socrates: How Does One Explain the Love of Men and Women to Persons of Their Own Sex?*, trans. Michael A. Lombardi-Nash (Urania Manuscripts, 2019), Kindle ebook location 79.

34. Hirschfeld, *Sappho and Socrates*, Kindle ebook location 79.

CHAPTER 2: **TROUBLED ALLIANCES**

1. Patrick Nobbs, *The Story of the British and Their Weather* (Amberley, 2015), 26.

2. Yvonne Ivory, "The Trouble with Oskar: Wilde's Legacy for the Early Homosexual Rights Movement in Germany," in Joseph Bristow, ed., *Oscar Wilde and Modern Culture: The Making of a Legend* (Ohio University Press, 2009).

3. Douglas Murray, *Bosie: A Biography of Lord Alfred Douglas* (Hyperion, 2000), 51.

4. Richard Davenport, review of *The Marquess of Queensberry: Wilde's Nemesis* by Linda Stratmann, *Guardian*, April 7, 2013.

5. Murray, *Bosie*, 56–57.

6. Murray, *Bosie*, 73.

7. Murray, *Bosie*, 74.

8. "A Scandal in High Life," *Yorkshire Herald*, March 4, 1895, 5.

9. Joseph Bristow, "The Blackmailer and the Sodomite: Oscar Wilde on Trial," *Feminist Theory* 17, no. 1 (April 2016): 41–62.

10. Bénédicte Coste, "Autonomy in the Dock: Oscar Wilde's First Trial, " *Cahiers victoriens et édouardiens* 79 (Spring 2014).

11. Heike Bauer, *The Hirschfeld Archives: Violence, Death, and Modern Queer Culture* (Temple University Press, 2017), 55.

12. R. J. V. Lenman, "Art, Society, and the Law in Wilhelmine Germany: The Lex Heinze," *Oxford German Studies* 8, no. 1 (January 1973): 86.

13. Gary D. Stark, "Pornography, Society, and the Law in Imperial Germany," *Central European History* 14, no. 3 (1981): 216.

14. Robert Beachy, *Gay Berlin: Birthplace of a Modern Identity* (Vintage, 2015), 91.

15. Beachy, *Gay Berlin*, 91.

16. Ivory, "The Trouble with Oskar."

17. Charlotte Wolff, *Magnus Hirschfeld: A Portrait of a Pioneer in Sexology* (Quartet, 1986), 33.

18. Bauer, *The Hirschfeld Archives*, 55.

19. Magnus Hirschfeld, *Sappho and Socrates: How Does One Explain the Love of Men and Women to Persons of Their Own Sex?*, trans. Michael A. Lombardi-Nash (Urania Manuscripts, 2019), Kindle ebook location 116.

20. Hirschfeld, *Sappho and Socrates*, Kindle ebook location 525.

21. Benjamin L. S. Furman et al., "Sex Chromosome Evolution: So Many Exceptions to the Rules," *Genome Biology and Evolution* 12, no. 6 (June 1, 2020): 750–63.

22. Rudolfo Rey, Nathalie Josso, and Chrystele Racine, "Sexual Differentiation" (Endotext, 2020).

23. Hirschfeld, *Sappho and Socrates*, Kindle ebook location 183.

24. Hanne Blank, *Straight* (Beacon Press, 2012), 16–17.

25. Hirschfeld, *Sappho and Socrates*, Kindle ebook location 214.

26. Hirschfeld, *Sappho and Socrates*, Kindle ebook location 273.

27. Ivory, "The Trouble with Oskar."

28. Wolff, *Magnus Hirschfeld*, 42.

29. Carolin Kosuch, *Anarchism and the Avant-Garde: Radical Arts and Politics in Perspective* (Brill, 2020), 153.

30. Yvonne Ivory, "The Urning and His Own: Individualism and the Fin-de-Siècle Invert," *German Studies Review* 26, no. 2 (May 2003): 338.

31. Beachy, *Gay Berlin*, 101.

32. Beachy, *Gay Berlin*, 116.

33. Harry Oosterhuis, ed., *Homosexuality and Male Bonding in Pre-Nazi Germany: The Youth Movement, the Gay Movement, and Male Bonding before Hitler's Rise* (Harrington Park Press, 1991), 102.

34. Benedict Friedländer, "Male and Female Culture: A Causal-Historical View," in Oosterhuis, ed., *Homosexuality and Male Bonding in Pre-Nazi Germany*, 187.

35. Ivory, "The Urning and His Own," 339.

36. Beachy, *Gay Berlin*, 103.

37. Jonathan Ned Katz, *The Invention of Heterosexuality* (University of Chicago Press, 2007), 182.

38. Ivory, "The Urning and His Own," 144.

39. Oosterhuis, *Homosexuality and Male Bonding in Pre-Nazi Germany*, 31.

40. My account of Moll is drawn from Volkmar Sigusch, "The Sexologist Albert Moll— Between Sigmund Freud and Magnus Hirschfeld," *Medical History* 56, no. 2 (April 2012): 193–95.

41. My account of the Reichstag commission and the SHC meeting is drawn from Beachy, *Gay Berlin*, 90, 94, 114.

42. "Friedrich Alfred Krupp, Margarethe Krupp," Thyssen Krupp website, updated 2024.

43. Elena Mancini, *Magnus Hirschfeld and the Quest for Sexual Freedom* (Palgrave Macmillan, 2010), 18.

44. Beachy, *Gay Berlin*, 72.

45. Material about Krupp is drawn from Clayton John Whisnant, *Queer Identities and Politics in Germany: A History, 1880–1945* (Harrington Park Press, 2016), 61–62.

46. Beachy, *Gay Berlin*, 95.

47. Beachy, *Gay Berlin*, 96.

48. Beachy, *Gay Berlin*, 114.

49. Beachy, *Gay Berlin*, 116.

50. Mancini, *Magnus Hirschfeld and the Quest for Sexual Freedom*, 109.

51. Beachy, *Gay Berlin*, 117.

CHAPTER 3: **THE THIRD SEX ON TRIAL**

1. My account of this period of Dora Richter's life is drawn from her intake interview as recounted in Werner Holz, *Kasuistischer Beitrag zum sogenannten Transvestismus (erotischen Verkleidungstrieb) mit besonderer Berücksichtigung der Ätiologie dieser Erscheinung. Inaugural-Dissertation*, trans. Ulrike Walter-Lipow (Humboldt University, n.d.), 5–10.

2. Clara Hartmann, "A Puzzle Piece for the Trans* History — Dora Richter's Baptism Record Found," *Lili-Elbe-Bibliothek Trans* Bücher Und Filme* (blog), accessed June 13, 2023.

3. The story of this Christmas Eve is told in Magnus Hirschfeld, *Berlin's Third Sex*, trans. James Conway (Rixdorf Editions, 2017), 43–46.

4. Hirschfeld, *Berlin's Third Sex*, frontispiece.

5. Veronika Fuechtner, Douglas E. Haynes, and Ryan M. Jones, eds., *A Global History of Sexual Science, 1880–1960* (University of California Press, 2018), 5.

6. Ethel Spector Person, "As the Wheel Turns: A Centennial Reflection on Freud's Three Essays on the Theory of Sexuality," *Journal of the American Psychoanalytic Association* 53, no. 4 (December 2005): 1257–82.

7. Sigmund Freud, *Three Essays on the Theory of Sexuality* (Nervous and Mental Health Diseases Publishing, 1920), 35: A. A. Brill translates this phrase as "the roots of all perversions" but I prefer "seeds" as more exact. In the original: "Wir werden uns aber ferner sagen, daß die angenommene Konstitution, welche die Keime zu allen Perversionen aufweist, nur beim Kinde aufzeigbar sein wird, wenngleich bei ihm alle Triebe nur in bescheidenen Intensitäten auftreten können."

8. Hirschfeld, *Berlin's Third Sex*, 14.

9. Robert Beachy, *Gay Berlin: Birthplace of a Modern Identity* (Vintage, 2015), 87.

10. Hirschfeld, *Berlin's Third Sex*, 21.

11. Hirschfeld, *Berlin's Third Sex*, 86.

12. Beachy, *Gay Berlin*, 56.

13. Ulrike Brunotte, "Queering Judaism and Masculinist Inventions: German Homonation-alism Around 1900," in Marco Derks and Mariecke van den Berg, eds., *Public Discourses About Homosexuality and Religion in Europe and Beyond* (Springer, 2020), 127–28.

14. Hirschfeld, *Berlin's Third Sex*, 58–60.

15. Hirschfeld, *Berlin's Third Sex*, 35.

16. Hirschfeld, *Berlin's Third Sex*, 85.

17. The "power of moral interpretation by journalists," writes historian Norman Domeier, ultimately "proved mightier than the traditional, authoritarian power of the monarchy." Norman Domeier, "The Homosexual Scare and the Masculinization of German Politics before World War I," *Central European History* 47, no. 4 (December 2014): 743.

18. Elena Mancini, *Magnus Hirschfeld and the Quest for Sexual Freedom* (Palgrave Macmillan, 2010), 94.

19. Beachy, *Gay Berlin*, 121.

20. Harry F. Young, *Maximilian Harden, Censor Germaniae: The Critic in Opposition from Bismarck to the Rise of Nazism* (M. Nijhoff, 1959), 104.

21. Domeier, "The Homosexual Scare," 740.

22. Historian George L. Mosse quoted in Mancini, *Magnus Hirschfeld and the Quest for Sexual Freedom*, 94.

23. Raymond J. Sontag, "German Foreign Policy, 1904–1906," *American Historical Review* 33, no. 2 (January 1928): 278.

24. Sontag, "German Foreign Policy," 301.

25. Robert Beachy, "The German Invention of Homosexuality," *Journal of Modern History* 82, no. 4 (December 2010), 813.

26. Domeier, "The Homosexual Scare," 747.

27. Young, *Maximilian Harden*, 96.

28. Quoted in Young, *Maximilian Harden*, 96.

29. Mancini, *Magnus Hirschfeld and the Quest for Sexual Freedom*, 96.

30. My account of the Harden trial is drawn from Young, *Maximilian Harden*, 102, and Beachy, "The German Invention of Homosexuality," 830–33.

31. Domeier, "The Homosexual Scare," 741.

32. Quoted in Domeier, "The Homosexual Scare," 745.

33. Beachy, "The German Invention of Homosexuality," 129.

34. My account of the Brand trial is drawn from Beachy, "The German Invention of Homosexuality," 130–31.

35. Quoted in Beachy, "The German Invention of Homosexuality," 138.

36. Young, *Maximilian Harden*, 106.

37. Charlotte Wolff, *Magnus Hirschfeld: A Portrait of a Pioneer in Sexology* (Quartet, 1986), 71.

38. Young, *Maximilian Harden*, 107.

39. Domeier, "The Homosexual Scare," 739–45, 754.

40. Brunotte, "Queering Judaism," 140.

41. Domeier, "The Homosexual Scare," 739.

42. Brunotte, "Queering Judaism," 130.

43. Brunotte, "Queering Judaism," 128.

44. Beachy, "The German Invention of Homosexuality," 139.

45. Heike Bauer, *The Hirschfeld Archives: Violence, Death, and Modern Queer Culture* (Temple University Press, 2017), 27.

46. Magnus Hirschfeld, *The Homosexuality of Men and Women* (Prometheus, 2000), 365–67.
47. Wolff, *Magnus Hirschfeld*, 80.
48. Wolff, *Magnus Hirschfeld*, 84–85.
49. Wolff, *Magnus Hirschfeld*, 80.
50. Bauer, *The Hirschfeld Archives*, 26.
51. Bauer, *The Hirschfeld Archives*, 26.
52. Mancini, *Magnus Hirschfeld and the Quest for Sexual Freedom*, 101.
53. Bauer, *The Hirschfeld Archives*, 26.
54. Bauer, *The Hirschfeld Archives*, 26.

CHAPTER 4: **UNBRIDGEABLE DISTANCE**

1. Matthew Immanuel Wiencke, "Johann Winckelmann," *Encyclopedia Britannica* online.
2. Charlotte Wolff, *Magnus Hirschfeld: A Portrait of a Pioneer in Sexology* (Quartet, 1986), 80.
3. Magnus Hirschfeld, *Sexualpsychologie und Volkspsychologie* (Georg H. Wigand Verlag, 1908), 29. In the original: "Wir sahen, wie Vorkommnisse, die das Grundproblem der Homosexualität kaum berühren, Beleidigungsprozesse, Fälle von Mißbrauch der militärischen Dienstgewalt, von Verleumdung ausreichen, um die wissenschaftliche-Arbeit vieler Männer und vieler Jahre zu gefährden."
4. Robert Aldrich, *The Seduction of the Mediterranean: Writing, Art, and Homosexual Fantasy* (Taylor and Francis, 2002), 69.
5. Quoted in Wolff, *Magnus Hirschfeld*, 80.
6. Hirschfeld, *Sexualpsychologie und Volkspsychologie*, 37.
7. Hirschfeld, *Sexualpsychologie und Volkspsychologie*, 12.
8. Heike Bauer, *The Hirschfeld Archives: Violence, Death, and Modern Queer Culture* (Temple University Press, 2017), 42.
9. Robert Beachy, *Gay Berlin: Birthplace of a Modern Identity* (Vintage, 2015), 151.
10. Daniel Boyarin, *Unheroic Conduct: The Rise of Heterosexuality and the Invention of the Jewish Man* (University of California Press, 1997), 217–24.
11. My account of this period of Dora Richter's life is drawn from her intake interview as recounted in Werner Holz, *Kasuistischer Beitrag zum sogenannten Transvestismus (erotischen Verkleidungstrieb) mit besonderer Berücksichtigung der Ätiologie dieser Erscheinung. Inaugural-Dissertation*, trans. Ulrike Walter-Lipow (Humboldt University, n.d.), 9.
12. Rainer Herrn, *Schnittmuster des Geschlechts: Transvestitismus und Transsexualität in Der Frühen Sexualwissenschaft* (Psychosozial-Verlag, 2005), 73.
13. Magnus Hirschfeld, *The Transvestites*, translated by Michael Lombardi-Nash (Urania, 2020), 1:10–11.
14. Hirschfeld, *The Transvestites*, 1:11.
15. Hirschfeld, *The Transvestites*, 1:124.
16. Holz, *Kasuistischer Beitrag zum Transvestismus*, 8.
17. Hirschfeld, *The Transvestites*, 2:11.
18. Hirschfeld, *The Transvestites*, 2:176.
19. Hirschfeld, *The Transvestites*, 2:191.
20. Hirschfeld, *The Transvestites*, 2:20.
21. Hirschfeld, *The Transvestites*, 2:42.
22. Hirschfeld, *The Transvestites*, 2:114.

23. Zavier Nunn, "Trans Liminality and the Nazi State," *Past and Present* 260, no. 1 (August 2023): 123–57.

24. Beachy, *Gay Berlin*, 88.

25. Hirschfeld, *The Transvestites*, 2:121, 127.

26. Wolff, *Magnus Hirschfeld*, 211.

27. Hirschfeld, *The Transvestites*, 2:127.

28. Hirschfeld, *The Transvestites*, 2:132.

29. Hirschfeld, *The Transvestites*, 2:141–42.

30. Rainer Herrn, *Der Liebe und dem Leid: Das Institut für Sexualwissenschaft 1919–1933* (Suhrkamp, 2022), 40.

31. Quoted in Ulrike Brunotte, "Queering Judaism and Masculinist Inventions: German Homonationalism Around 1900," in Marco Derks and Mariecke van den Berg, eds., *Public Discourses About Homosexuality and Religion in Europe and Beyond* (Springer, 2020), 13.

32. Quoted in Beachy, *Gay Berlin*, 147.

33. Charlotte Alt, " 'Steel Their Bodies and Minds'—How the Wandervögel Reconciled Nature with Modernity," *Doing History in Public*, March 2022.

34. Beachy, *Gay Berlin*, 142.

35. Quoted in Beachy, *Gay Berlin*, 142.

36. Brunotte, "Queering Judaism," 131.

37. Brunotte, "Queering Judaism," 131.

38. Beachy, *Gay Berlin*, 154.

39. Quoted in Beachy, *Gay Berlin*, 156.

40. Robert D. Tobin, "Queer German Roots of the Alt-Right: Ulrichs, Weininger, Blüher—and Evola," *Monatshefte* 114, no. 3 (2022): 470–88.

41. Beachy, *Gay Berlin*, 158.

42. Harry Oosterhuis, ed., *Homosexuality and Male Bonding in Pre-Nazi Germany: The Youth Movement, the Gay Movement, and Male Bonding before Hitler's Rise* (Harrington Park Press, 1991), 123.

43. Tobin, "Queer German Roots of the Alt-Right."

44. My account of this period of Dora Richter's life is drawn from her intake interview as recounted in Holz, *Kasuistischer Beitrag*, 10–11.

CHAPTER 5: **POWDER KEG AND PLUCKED STRING**

1. My account of the assassination of Archduke Ferdinand is drawn from Lindsey Fitzharris, *The Facemaker: One Surgeon's Battle to Mend the Disfigured Soldiers of World War I* (Allen Lane, 2022), 29; Luigi Albertini, ed. and trans., *The Origins of the War of 1914*, vol. 2, *The Crisis of July 1914. From the Sarajevo Outrage to the Austro-Hungarian General Mobilization* (Enigma Books, 2005); and "How Bad Directions (and a Sandwich?) Started World War I," *All Things Considered*. NPR, March 6, 2014.

2. Vjosa Hamiti and Milote Sadiku, "Wahrnehmung Und Evaluierung Des Balkan Als Pulverfass Im Deutschsprachigen Pressediskurs," *Alman Dili ve Edebiyatı Dergisi—Studien zur Deutschen Sprache und Literatur*, June 22, 2020.

3. Emperor Franz Josef, *The Imperial Rescript and Manifesto*, July 28, 1914, reprinted in *Viereck's: The American Weekly* (later *American Monthly*) 7 (1917).

4. "A Published Interview Explaining the 'Scrap of Paper' Phrase by German Chancellor Theobald von Bethmann-Hollweg," *Source Records of the Great War*, vol. 1, edited by Charles F. Horne (National Alumni, 1923).

5. Norman Domeier, "The Homosexual Scare and the Masculinization of German Politics before World War I," *Central European History* 47, no. 4 (December 2014), 754.

6. Elena Mancini, *Magnus Hirschfeld and the Quest for Sexual Freedom* (Palgrave Macmillan, 2010), 111.

7. "Armistice Day: World War I Ends," *This Day in History*, History Channel, n.d.

8. Robert Weldon Whalen, "War Losses (Germany)," *International Encyclopedia of the First World War*, October 2014.

9. Magnus Hirschfeld, *The Sexual History of the World War* (University Press of the Pacific, 2006), 127–28.

10. Hirschfeld, *The Sexual History of the World War*, 122.

11. Mancini, *Magnus Hirschfeld and the Quest for Sexual Freedom*, 112.

12. Hirschfeld, *The Sexual History of the World War*, 11.

13. Peter Gay, *Weimar Culture: The Outsider as Insider* (W. W. Norton, 2001), 17.

14. Charlotte Wolff, *Magnus Hirschfeld: A Portrait of a Pioneer in Sexology* (Quartet, 1986), 167–68.

15. Wolff, *Magnus Hirschfeld*, 175.

16. Hirschfeld, *The Sexual History of the World War*, 13.

17. Wolff, *Magnus Hirschfeld*, 190.

18. Mancini, *Magnus Hirschfeld and the Quest for Sexual Freedom*, 100.

19. Ina Linge, "Sexology, Popular Science and Queer History in *Anders Als Die Andern* (*Different from the Others*)," *Gender and History* 30, no. 3 (October 2018): 595–610.

20. Thomas Elsaesser, *Weimar Cinema and After: Germany's Historical Imaginary* (Routledge, 2000), 19.

21. James D. Steakley, "Cinema and Censorship in the Weimar Republic: The Case of Anders Als Die Andern," *Film History* 11, no. 2 (1999): 185.

22. Steakley, "Cinema and Censorship," 182.

23. Quoted in Steakley, "Cinema and Censorship," 182.

24. Steakley, "Cinema and Censorship," 22.

25. "National Affairs: Object Lesson," *Time*, December 25, 1950; Mark Cornwall, "Conflating Treason and Homosexuality: The Queer History of Colonel Redl," *Proceedings of the European Social Science History Conference*, April 23, 2014.

26. Hirschfeld, *The Sexual History of the World War*, 125.

27. My account of *Alders als die Andern* is drawn from Steakley, "Cinema and Censorship," 187–92.

28. Wolff, *Magnus Hirschfeld*, 191.

29. My account of the ruling against *Alders als die Andern* is drawn from Steakley, "Cinema and Censorship," 192.

30. Laurie Marhoefer, *Sex and the Weimar Republic: German Homosexual Emancipation and the Rise of the Nazis* (University of Toronto Press, 2015), 3–4.

31. Wolff, *Magnus Hirschfeld*, 178.

32. Marhoefer, *Sex and the Weimar Republic*, 6, 14.

33. Ralf Dose, *Magnus Hirschfeld: The Origins of the Gay Liberation Movement*, trans. Edward H. Willis (Monthly Review Press, 2014), 47.

34. Marhoefer, *Sex and the Weimar Republic*, 16.

35. Quoted in Katie Sutton, *Sex between Body and Mind: Psychoanalysis and Sexology in the German-Speaking World, 1890s–1930s* (University of Michigan Press, 2019), 118.

36. Hirschfeld, *Geschlechtskunde* (J. Püttmann, 1926), 1:206.

CHAPTER 6: **THE ENDOCRINOLOGIST'S GAMBLE**

1. Chelsea Wald, "Austria's Ahead-of-Its-Time Institute That Was Lost to Nazis," *Nautilus*, April 22, 2014.
2. Chandak Sengoopta, *The Most Secret Quintessence of Life: Sex, Glands, and Hormones, 1850–1950* (University of Chicago Press, 2006), 58.
3. Charles Edwards, "The Vienna Institution for Experimental Biology," *Popular Science Monthly*, June 1911.
4. Katie Sutton, *Sex between Body and Mind: Psychoanalysis and Sexology in the German-Speaking World, 1890s–1930s* (University of Michigan Press, 2019), 134.
5. Hirschfeld, *Geschlechtkunde*, quoted in Sutton, *Sex between Body and Mind*, 119.
6. Rainer Herrn, *Der Liebe und dem Leid: Das Institut für Sexualwissenschaft 1919–1933* (Suhrkamp, 2022), 40.
7. Charlotte Wolff, *Magnus Hirschfeld: A Portrait of a Pioneer in Sexology* (Quartet, 1986), 101.
8. Amy Koerber, *From Hysteria to Hormones: A Rhetorical History* (Pennsylvania State University Press, 2018), 84.
9. My account of the brown dog experiment and the ensuing lawsuit is drawn from Randi Hutter Epstein, *Aroused: The History of Hormones and How They Control Just About Everything* (W. W. Norton, 2018), 18–26.
10. "The Croonian Lectures on the Chemical Correlation of the Functions of the Body," *Lancet* 166, no. 4275 (August 1905): 339–41.
11. Koerber, *From Hysteria to Hormones*, 83.
12. "Croonian Lectures."
13. Epstein, *Aroused*, 79.
14. My account of Steinach's experiments is drawn from Sengoopta, *The Most Secret Quintessence of Life*, 58–65.
15. Epstein, *Aroused*, 80.
16. Claire Ainsworth, "Sex Redefined: The Idea of 2 Sexes Is Overly Simplistic; Biologists Now Think There Is a Larger Spectrum than Just Binary Female and Male," *Scientific American*, October 22, 2018.
17. Andrea Ford, "Sex Biology Redefined: Genes Don't Indicate Binary Sexes," *Scope: Stanford Medicine*, February 24, 2015.
18. Ainsworth, "Sex Redefined." This is also the source for Achermann's quote above.
19. Goran Štrkalj and Nalini Pather, "Beyond the Sex Binary: Toward the Inclusive Anatomical Sciences Education," *Anatomical Sciences Education* 14, no. 4 (July 2021): 513–18.
20. Claire Ainsworth, Twitter post, July 7, 2017.
21. Quoted in Epstein, *Aroused*, 82.
22. Sengoopta, *The Most Secret Quintessence of Life*, 65.
23. Sutton, *Sex Between Body and Mind*, 123.
24. Sengoopta, *The Most Secret Quintessence of Life*, 79.
25. Quoted in Sutton, *Sex Between Body and Mind*, 128.
26. Sengoopta, *The Most Secret Quintessence of Life*, 79–80.
27. Simon LeVay, *Queer Science: The Use and Abuse of Research into Homosexuality* (MIT Press, 1996), 31.
28. Herrn, *Der Liebe und dem Leid*, 43.
29. Quoted in Sutton, *Sex Between Body and Mind*, 135.
30. My account of this period of Dora Richter's life is drawn from her intake interview as recounted in Werner Holz, *Kasuistischer Beitrag zum sogenannten Transvestismus*

(erotischen Verkleidungstrieb) mit besonderer Berücksichtigung der Ätiologie dieser Erscheinung. Inaugural-Dissertation, trans. Ulrike Walter-Lipow (Humboldt University, n.d.), 14–15.

31. Hirschfeld, *The Homosexuality of Men and Women* (Prometheus, 2000), 488.

32. Hirschfeld, *The Homosexuality of Men and Women*, 31.

33. LeVay, *Queer Science*, 32.

34. Sengoopta, *The Most Secret Quintessence of Life*, 80.

35. Herrn, *Der Liebe und dem Leid*, 58–59.

36. Herrn, *Der Liebe und dem Leid*, 60.

37. Quoted in Sengoopta, *The Most Secret Quintessence of Life*, 86.

38. Ralf Dose, *Magnus Hirschfeld: And the Origins of the Gay Liberation Movement*, trans. Edward H. Willis (Monthly Review Press, 2014), 95–100.

39. Rainer Herrn, *Schnittmuster des Geschlechts: Transvestitismus und Transsexualität in Der Frühen Sexualwissenschaft* (Psychosozial-Verlag, 2005), 114.

40. Quoted in Robert Beachy, *Gay Berlin: Birthplace of a Modern Identity* (Vintage, 2015), 175.

CHAPTER 7: **THE LOVE AND THE SORROW**

1. My account of this period of Dora Richter's life is drawn from her intake interview as recounted in Werner Holz, *Kasuistischer Beitrag zum sogenannten Transvestismus (erotischen Verkleidungstrieb) mit besonderer Berücksichtigung der Ätiologie dieser Erscheinung. Inaugural-Dissertation*, trans. Ulrike Walter-Lipow (Humboldt University, n.d.), 16–20.

2. Heike Bauer, *The Hirschfeld Archives: Violence, Death, and Modern Queer Culture* (Temple University Press, 2017), 7.

3. Charlotte Wolff, *Magnus Hirschfeld: A Portrait of a Pioneer in Sexology* (Quartet, 1986), 198.

4. Robert Beachy, *Gay Berlin: Birthplace of a Modern Identity* (Vintage, 2015), 169.

5. David Conradt, "Social Democratic Party of Germany," *Encyclopedia Britannica*, May 24, 2023.

6. My account of the Freikorps is drawn from Robert M. Citino, "Meet the *Freikorps*: Vanguard of Terror 1918–1923," National World War II Museum, June 7, 2018.

7. Conradt, "Social Democratic Party of Germany."

8. Chandak Sengoopta, *The Most Secret Quintessence of Life: Sex, Glands, and Hormones, 1850–1950* (University of Chicago Press, 2006), 78.

9. "Comparative Embryology: The Vertebrate Body," WGBH Educational Foundation and Clear Blue Sky Productions, PBS Library.

10. "Comparative Embryology: The Vertebrate Body."

11. Elizabeth Barnes, "Ernst Haeckel's Biogenetic Law (1866)," *The Embryo Project Encyclopedia*, Autumn 2014.

12. Quoted in Rainer Herrn, *Der Liebe und dem Leid: Das Institut für Sexualwissenschaft 1919–1933* (Suhrkamp, 2022), 38. My translation.

13. Peter Davies, "Transforming Utopia: The 'League for the Protection of Mothers and Sexual Reform' in the First World War," in Alison S. Fell and Ingrid Sharp, eds., *The Women's Movement in Wartime* (Palgrave Macmillan, 2007), 217.

14. Davies, "Transforming Utopia," 211.

15. Darwin, *Descent of Man and Selection in Relation to Sex* (Barnes & Noble Books, 2004), chapter 5.

16. Richard Weikart, "Progress through Racial Extermination: Social Darwinism, Eugenics, and Pacifism in Germany, 1860–1918." *German Studies Review* 26, no. 2 (May 2003): 273.

17. Davies, "Transforming Utopia," 211.

18. Laurie Marhoefer, *Sex and the Weimar Republic: German Homosexual Emancipation and the Rise of the Nazis* (University of Toronto Press, 2015), 204.

19. Bauer, *The Hirschfeld Archives*, 8.

20. Bauer, *The Hirschfeld Archives*, 79.

21. Marhoefer, *Sex and the Weimar Republic*, 203–4.

22. Weikart, "Progress through Racial Extermination," 275.

23. Weikart, "The Role of Darwinism in Nazi Racial Thought," *German Studies Review* 36, no. 3 (2013): 538.

24. Weikart, "The Role of Darwinism in Nazi Racial Thought," 541.

25. Weikart, "Progress through Racial Extermination," 273.

26. Siddhartha Mukherjee, *The Gene: An Intimate History* (Scribner, 2017), 95.

27. Marhoefer, *Sex and the Weimar Republic*, 204.

28. Adolf Hitler, *Mein Kampf* (Houghton Mifflin, 1999), 285.

29. Lily Rothman, "How a Speech Helped Hitler Take Power," *Time*, February 24, 2020.

30. Wolff, *Magnus Hirschfeld*, 196.

31. Wolff, *Magnus Hirschfeld*, 197.

32. Susan Stryker, *Transgender History: The Roots of Today's Revolution*, 2nd ed. (Seal Press, 2017), 40.

33. Bauer, *The Hirschfeld Archives*, 97.

34. Ralf Dose, *Magnus Hirschfeld: And the Origins of the Gay Liberation Movement*, trans. Edward H. Willis (Monthly Review Press, 2014), 28–29.

35. Dose, *Magnus Hirschfeld*, 37.

36. Herrn, *Der Liebe und dem Leid*, 198.

37. Dose, *Magnus Hirschfeld*, 24.

38. Mel Gordon, *Voluptuous Panic: The Erotic World of Weimar Berlin* (Feral House, 2006), 176.

CHAPTER 8: **THE DOCTOR WILL SEE YOU NOW**

1. Quoted in Rainer Herrn, *Der Liebe und dem Leid: Das Institut für Sexualwissenschaft 1919–1933* (Suhrkamp, 2022), 123–24.

2. Rainer Herrn, "Arthur Kronfeld," in *Institute of the History of Medicine of the Charité*, n.d.

3. Herrn, *Der Liebe und dem Leid*, 124.

4. Rainer Herrn, *Schnittmuster des Geschlechts: Transvestitismus und Transsexualität in Der Frühen Sexualwissenschaft* (Psychosozial-Verlag, 2005), 103.

5. Kit Heyam, *Before We Were Trans: A New History of Gender* (Basic Books, 2023), 14.

6. Harry Oosterhuis, "Sexual Modernity in the Works of Richard von Krafft-Ebing and Albert Moll," *Medical History* 56, no. 2 (April 2012): 133–55.

7. Oosterhuis, "Sexual Modernity."

8. Herrn, *Schnittmuster des Geschlechts*, 104.

9. Jana Funke, "The Case of Karl M.[artha] Baer: Narrating 'Uncertain' Sex," in Ben Davies and Jana Funke, eds., *Sex, Gender and Time in Fiction and Culture* (Palgrave Macmillan, 2011), 136.

10. Funke, "The Case of Karl M.[artha] Baer," 144.

11. N. O. Body, *Memoirs of a Man's Maiden Years* (University of Pennsylvania Press, 2009), 5.

12. Herrn, *Der Liebe und dem Leid*, 276.

13. Quoted in Herrn, *Der Liebe und dem Leid*, 276. My translation.

14. Magnus Hirschfeld, *Geschlechts-Umwandlungen: (Irrtümer in Der Geschlechtsbestimmung); Sechs Fälle Aus Der Forensischen Praxis* (Alder-Verlag, 1912), 12.

15. The story, as reported by Strasburg sexologist Eugen Wilhelm in 1914, is told in Herrn, *Der Liebe und dem Leid*, 276.

16. Magnus Hirschfeld, epilogue to Body, *Memoirs of a Man's Maiden Years.*

17. Robert Beachy, *Gay Berlin: Birthplace of a Modern Identity* (Vintage, 2015), 177.

18. Herrn, *Schnittmuster des Geschlechts*, 172.

19. Herrn, *Der Liebe und dem Leid*, 270.

20. Michael Taylor, Annette Timm, and Rainer Herrn, eds., *Not Straight from Germany: Sexual Publics and Sexual Citizenship since Magnus Hirschfeld* (University of Michigan Press, 2017), 42.

21. Quoted in Herrn, *Der Liebe und dem Leid*, 271.

22. Quoted in Herrn, *Der Liebe und dem Leid*, 277.

23. Quoted in Herrn, *Der Liebe und dem Leid*, 277.

24. This has been remarked upon by Rainer Herrn, Ralf Dose, and numerous other scholars, but the power of Wikipedia persists.

25. Charlotte Wolff, *Magnus Hirschfeld: A Portrait of a Pioneer in Sexology* (Quartet, 1986), 182–84.

26. Herrn, *Schnittmuster des Geschlechts*, 115.

27. Christopher Isherwood, *Christopher and His Kind: 1929–1939* (Farrar, Straus and Giroux, 2015), 25.

28. Magnus Hirschfeld, *The Homosexuality of Men and Women* (Prometheus, 2000), 506.

29. The details appear in a 1991 interview with Dr. Grafe by filmmaker Rosa von Praunheim, published in the German magazine *Capri: Zeitschrift für schwule Geschichte*, 1991.

30. Beachy, *Gay Berlin*, 179.

31. Herrn, *Der Liebe und dem Leid*, 415.

32. Magnus Hirschfeld, *Berlin's Third Sex*, trans. James Conway (Rixdorf Editions, 2017), 72–73.

33. Beachy, *Gay Berlin*, 179.

34. Isherwood, *Christopher and His Kind*, 29.

35. Isherwood, *Christopher and His Kind*, 34.

36. Herrn, *Der Liebe und dem Leid*, 417.

37. Katie Sutton, " 'We Too Deserve a Place in the Sun': The Politics of Transvestite Identity in Weimar Germany," *German Studies Review* 35, no. 2 (2012): 336.

38. Katie Sutton, *Sex Between Body and Mind: Psychoanalysis and Sexology in the German-Speaking World, 1890s–1930s* (University of Michigan Press, 2019), 146.

39. Laurie Marhoefer, *Sex and the Weimar Republic: German Homosexual Emancipation and the Rise of the Nazis* (University of Toronto Press, 2015), 54–57.

40. Marhoefer, *Sex and the Weimar Republic*, 58.

41. Sutton, " 'We Too Deserve a Place in the Sun'," 340.

42. Herrn, *Schnittmuster des Geschlechts*, 101.

43. Sutton, " 'We Too Deserve a Place in the Sun'," 342–43.

44. Sutton, " 'We Too Deserve a Place in the Sun'," 345.

45. Herrn, *Der Liebe und dem Leid*, 423–24.

CHAPTER 9: **1923 IN FOUR ACTS**

1. Wolfgang Sternstein, "The Ruhrkampf of 1923: Economic Problems of Civilian Defence," in Adam Roberts, ed., *The Strategy of Civilian Defence: Non-Violent Resistance to Aggression* (Faber and Faber, 1967), 107.

2. The French suspected that Germany intentionally devalued the mark and went bankrupt on purpose. See Sally Marks, "The Myths of Reparations," *Central European History* 11, no. 3 (1978): 231–55.

3. Gunther Birkenstock, "The Rise of the Krupp Steel Empire," *DW* (blog), April 10, 2012.

4. My account of the Ruhr crisis is drawn from Sternstein, "The Ruhrkampf of 1923," 110–27.

5. Adam Bisno, "How Hyperinflation Heralded the Fall of German Democracy," *Smithsonian History* online, May 23, 2023.

6. Adam Smith, "The German Hyperinflation, 1923," *Paper Money* (Summit, 1981).

7. Detlev Clemens, "The 'Bavarian Mussolini' and His 'Beerhall Putsch': British Images of Adolf Hitler, 1920–24," *English Historical Review* 114, no. 455 (February 1999): 77.

8. Sternstein, "The Ruhrkampf of 1923," 127.

9. Sternstein, "The Ruhrkampf of 1923," 128.

10. Clemens, "The 'Bavarian Mussolini'," 77.

11. "Gustav, Ritter von Kahr," *Britannica*, June 26, 2023.

12. My account of the Beer Hall Putsch is mostly drawn from Harold J. Gordon, *Hitler and the Beer Hall Putsch* (Princeton: Princeton University Press, 2016), 281–88. Though first published decades ago, the book remains a key text for the sheer amount of documented evidence it contains. The review by Allan Mitchell (*Central European History* 6, no. 4 [1973]) is also useful, as is "The Rise of Hitler," History Place, 1996.

13. "The S.A.," Holocaust Encyclopedia, n.d.

14. Clemens, "The 'Bavarian Mussolini'," 67–68.

15. Alan Bullock, Wilfrid Knapp, and John Lukacs, "Adolf Hitler," *Britannica: History and Society*, June 30, 2023.

16. Clemens, "The 'Bavarian Mussolini'," 71.

17. Clemens, "The 'Bavarian Mussolini'," 68.

18. Clemens, "The 'Bavarian Mussolini'," 76.

19. Gordon, *Hitler and the Beer Hall Putsch*, 429–33.

20. Rainer Herrn, *Der Liebe und dem Leid: Das Institut für Sexualwissenschaft 1919–1933* (Suhrkamp, 2022), 149.

21. Glenn Ramsey, "The Rites of Artgenossen: Contesting Homosexual Political Culture in Weimar Germany," *Journal of the History of Sexuality* 17, no. 1 (2007): 94–95.

22. Herrn, *Der Liebe und dem Leid*, 150.

23. Ramsey, "The Rites of Artgenossen," 92.

24. Herrn, *Der Liebe und dem Leid*, 151–52.

25. Ramsey, "The Rites of Artgenossen," 95.

26. Herrn, *Der Liebe und dem Leid*, 153.

27. Ramsey, "The Rites of Artgenossen," 95.

28. Herrn, *Der Liebe und dem Leid*, 154.

29. Herrn, *Der Liebe und dem Leid*, 154.

30. "Gustav, Ritter von Kahr."

31. Heather Leawoods, "Gustav Radbruch: An Extraordinary Legal Philosopher," *Washington University Journal of Law & Policy* 2 (January 2000).

32. Ramsey, "The Rites of Artgenossen," 155.

33. Herrn, *Der Liebe und dem Leid*, 155.

34. Ramsey, "The Rites of Artgenossen," 89.

35. Ramsey, "The Rites of Artgenossen," 97.

36. Thomas A. Knapp, "The German Center Party and the Reichsbanner: A Case Study in Political and Social Consensus in the Weimar Republic," *International Review of Social History* 14, no. 2 (August 1969): 163, 164.

37. Quoted in Herrn, *Der Liebe und dem Leid*, 159.

38. Robert Beachy, *Gay Berlin: Birthplace of a Modern Identity* (Vintage, 2015), 229. It is not verified that Tscheck did in fact join the SA.

39. Sternstein, "The Ruhrkampf of 1923," 108.

40. Herrn, *Der Liebe und dem Leid*, 191–93.

41. Herrn, *Der Liebe und dem Leid*, 193.

42. My account of this period of Dora Richter's life is drawn from her intake interview as recounted in Werner Holz, *Kasuistischer Beitrag zum sogenannten Transvestismus (erotischen Verkleidungstrieb) mit besonderer Berücksichtigung der Ätiologie dieser Erscheinung. Inaugural-Dissertation*, trans. Ulrike Walter-Lipow (Humboldt University, n.d.), 4, 20–21.

43. My account of *Der Steinachfilm* is drawn from Maria Makela, "Rejuvenation and Regen(d)eration: *Der Steinachfilm*, Sex Glands, and Weimar-Era Visual and Literary Culture," *German Studies Review* 38, no. 1 (2015): 39–40.

44. Michael Taylor, Annette Timm, and Rainer Herrn, eds., *Not Straight from Germany: Sexual Publics and Sexual Citizenship since Magnus Hirschfeld* (University of Michigan Press, 2017), 214.

45. Makela, "Rejuvenation and Regen(d)eration," 40.

46. Taylor, Timm, and Herrn, *Not Straight from Germany*, 228.

47. Makela, "Rejuvenation and Regen(d)eration," 40.

48. My account of this period of Dora Richter's life is drawn from her intake interview as recounted in Holz, *Kasuistischer Beitrag*, 4–5, 8, 21.

49. Alex Bakker, Rainer Herrn, Michael Thomas Taylor, and Annette F. Timm, *Others of My Kind: Transatlantic Transgender Histories* (University of Calgary Press, 2020), 59; Rainer Herrn, *Schnittmuster des Geschlechts: Transvestitismus und Transsexualität in Der Frühen Sexualwissenschaft* (Psychosozial-Verlag, 2005).

50. Holz, *Kasuistischer Beitrag*, 21.

51. Herrn, *Schnittmuster des Geschlechts*, 176, 183.

52. Holz, *Kasuistischer Beitrag*, 22, 31.

CHAPTER 10: **LIVES IN TRANSITION**

1. Ludwig Levy-Lenz, *The Memoirs of a Sexologist: Discretion and Indiscretion* (Cadillac, 1954), 463.

2. Levy-Lenz, *Memoirs*, 460–61.

3. Levy-Lenz, *Memoirs*, 8–9.

4. Fredy's story is told in Levy-Lenz, *Memoirs*, 95–97.

5. Levy-Lenz, *Memoirs*, 462.

6. Samuel Dittrich, "Gerd Katter (1910–1995) Trans-Mann, Patient Und Lobbyist," *Communications of the Magnus Hirschfeld Society* no. 64 (February 2020): 18–22.

7. Rainer Herrn, *Schnittmuster des Geschlechts: Transvestitismus und Transsexualität in Der Frühen Sexualwissenschaft* (Psychosozial-Verlag, 2005), 197.

8. Chandak Sengoopta, *The Most Secret Quintessence of Life: Sex, Glands, and Hormones, 1850–1950* (University of Chicago Press, 2006), 118.

9. Sengoopta, *The Most Secret Quintessence of Life*, 121–22, 137–39.

10. Bernhard Zondek, "Mass Excretion of Œstrogenic Hormone in the Urine of the Stallion," *Nature*, no. 133 (1934): 209–10.

11. Rex A. Hess, "Estrogen in the Adult Male Reproductive Tract: A Review," *Reproductive Biology and Endocrinology* 1, no. 1 (2003): 52.

12. Nelly Oudshoorn, *Beyond the Natural Body: An Archaeology of Sex Hormones* (Taylor and Francis, 1994), 26.

13. Jessie K. Cable and Michael H. Grider, "Physiology, Progesterone" (StatPearls, 2023).

14. Sengoopta, *The Most Secret Quintessence of Life*, 144–45.

15. Sengoopta, *The Most Secret Quintessence of Life*, 155, 174.

16. Sengoopta, *The Most Secret Quintessence of Life*, 177.

17. Sengoopta, *The Most Secret Quintessence of Life*, 186.

18. Holger Steinberg, Kenneth Kirkby, and Hubertus Himmerich, "The Historical Development of Immunoendocrine Concepts of Psychiatric Disorders and Their Therapy," *International Journal of Molecular Sciences* 16, no. 12 (December 4, 2015): 28841–69.

19. Rainer Herrn, *Der Liebe und dem Leid: Das Institut für Sexualwissenschaft 1919–1933* (Suhrkamp, 2022), 367.

20. Herrn, *Der Liebe und dem Leid*, 370.

21. Herrn, *Schnittmuster des Geschlechts*, 106.

22. Michael Dillon, *Self: A Study in Ethics and Endocrinology* (William Heinemann, 1946), 53.

23. Herrn, *Schnittmuster des Geschlechts*, 105.

24. Werner Holz, *Kasuistischer Beitrag zum sogenannten Transvestismus (erotischen Verkleidungstrieb) mit besonderer Berücksichtigung der Ätiologie dieser Erscheinung. Inaugural-Dissertation*, trans. Ulrike Walter-Lipow (Humboldt University, n.d.), 8.

25. Herrn, *Schnittmuster des Geschlechts*, 182.

26. Felix Abraham, "Genital Reassignment on Two Male Transvestites," *International Journal of Transgenderism* 2, no. 1 (March 1998): 223–26.

27. Hirschfeld, *Geschlechtskunde* (Berlin: J. Püttmann, 1926), 1:592–93.

28. Abraham, "Genital Reassignment."

29. Herrn, *Der Liebe und dem Leid*, 424.

30. Holz, *Kasuistischer Beitrag*, 21.

31. Levy-Lenz, *Memoirs*, 464.

32. Dr. Kankeleit, "Selbstbeschädigungen und Selbstverstümmelungen der Geschlechtsorgane," *Zeitschrift für die gesamte Neurologie und Psychiatrie* 107, no. 1 (December 1927): 414, 431–36, 459–60.

33. Levy-Lenz, *Memoirs*, 463.

34. Levy-Lenz, *Memoirs*, 489.

35. Levy-Lenz, *Memoirs*, 489.

36. Herrn, *Der Liebe und dem Leid*, 418.

37. Herrn, *Schnittmuster des Geschlechts*, 204.

38. Abraham, "Genital Reassignment."

39. Abraham, "Genital Reassignment."

40. Cleveland Clinic, "Penectomy," April 6, 2022.

41. Abraham, "Genital Reassignment."

42. Lili Elbe, *Man into Woman*, trans. H. J. Stenning (Jarrolds, 1933), 119.

43. Herrn, *Schnittmuster des Geschlechts*, 207.

44. Herrn, *Schnittmuster des Geschlechts*, 195.

45. Elbe, *Man into Woman*, 285–86.

46. Katie Sutton, " 'We Too Deserve a Place in the Sun': The Politics of Transvestite Identity in Weimar Germany," *German Studies Review* 35, no. 2 (2012): 348.

CHAPTER 11: **ALL THE DEVILS ARE HERE**

1. My account of Hitler's trial is drawn from David King, *The Trial of Adolf Hitler: The Beer Hall Putsch and the Rise of Nazi Germany* (W. W. Norton, 2017), 128–46.

2. "Adolf Hitler's Time in Landsberg Prison," Warfare History Network, 2010.

3. "Adolf Hitler: Excerpts from *Mein Kampf*," Jewish Virtual Library (Yad Vashem).

4. Robert Proctor, "Nazi Doctors, Racial Medicine, and Human Experimentation," in George J. Annas and Michael A. Grodin, eds., *The Nazi Doctors and the Nuremberg Code* (Oxford: Oxford University Press, 1993), 18–19, 24.

5. Laurie Marhoefer, *Sex and the Weimar Republic: German Homosexual Emancipation and the Rise of the Nazis* (University of Toronto Press, 2015), 151–52.

6. Proctor, "Nazi Doctors," 22–24; Marhoefer, *Sex and the Weimar Republic*, 175.

7. King, *The Trial of Adolf Hitler*, 159.

8. William Shakespeare, *The Tempest*, Act 1, scene 2.

9. Rainer Herrn, *Der Liebe und dem Leid: Das Institut für Sexualwissenschaft 1919–1933* (Suhrkamp, 2022), 463.

10. Christopher Isherwood, *Christopher and His Kind: 1929–1939* (Farrar, Straus and Giroux, 2015), 18–19.

11. Ludwig Levy-Lenz, *The Memoirs of a Sexologist: Discretion and Indiscretion* (Cadillac, 1954), 464.

12. Herrn, *Der Liebe und dem Leid*, 464.

13. Herrn, *Der Liebe und dem Leid*, 255.

14. Glenn Ramsey, "The Rites of Artgenossen: Contesting Homosexual Political Culture in Weimar Germany," *Journal of the History of Sexuality* 17, no. 1 (2007): 96.

15. Herrn, *Der Liebe und dem Leid*, 256.

16. Ralf Dose and Pamela Eve Selwyn, "The World League for Sexual Reform: Some Possible Approaches," *Journal of the History of Sexuality* 12, no. 1 (2003): 9.

17. Ramsey, "The Rites of Artgenossen," 106.

18. Herrn, *Der Liebe und dem Leid*, 257.

19. Ramsey, "The Rites of Artgenossen," 99.

20. Ramsey, "The Rites of Artgenossen," 100.

21. Ramsey, "The Rites of Artgenossen," 107.

22. Herrn, *Der Liebe und dem Leid*, 257–58.

23. Herrn, *Der Liebe und dem Leid*, 340.

24. Herrn, *Der Liebe und dem Leid*, 338.

25. Charlotte Wolff, *Magnus Hirschfeld: A Portrait of a Pioneer in Sexology* (Quartet, 1986), 255.

26. Herrn, *Der Liebe und dem Leid*, 340.

27. Wolff, *Magnus Hirschfeld*, 256–57.

28. Wolff, *Magnus Hirschfeld*, 257.

29. Herrn, *Der Liebe und dem Leid*, 342.

30. Herrn, *Der Liebe und dem Leid*, 345–47; Volkmar Sigusch, "The Sexologist Albert

Moll—Between Sigmund Freud and Magnus Hirschfeld," *Medical History* 56, no. 2 (April 2012), 195–96.

31. Herrn, *Der Liebe und dem Leid*, 341.

32. Florence Tamagne, *A History of Homosexuality in Europe: Berlin, London, Paris 1919–1939* (Algora, 2006), 82.

33. Wolff, *Magnus Hirschfeld*, 259.

34. Quotes from the WSLR conference resolutions and speeches are drawn from Tamagne, *A History of Homosexuality in Europe*, 82–83.

35. *Weltliga für Sexualreform* (World League for Sexual Reform). "Principal Points of the League's Platform." https://web.archive.org/web/20111122131239/http://www2.hu -berlin.de/sexology/GESUND/ARCHIV/GIF/XWLSR_PL.JPG.

36. Dose and Selwyn, "The World League for Sexual Reform," 1–2.

37. Wolff, *Magnus Hirschfeld*, 257.

38. Wolff, *Magnus Hirschfeld*, 262.

39. Herrn, *Der Liebe und dem Leid*, 387.

40. Herrn, *Der Liebe und dem Leid*, 387.

41. Samuel Dittrich, "Gerd Katter (1910–1995) Trans-Mann, Patient Und Lobbyist," *Communications of the Magnus Hirschfeld Society* no. 64 (February 2020): 21–24.

42. Herrn, *Der Liebe und dem Leid*, 388.

43. Herrn, *Der Liebe und dem Leid*, 389.

44. Marhoefer, *Sex and the Weimar Republic*, 120.

45. Wolff, *Magnus Hirschfeld*, 438.

46. Marhoefer, *Sex and the Weimar Republic*, 120–21.

47. Marhoefer, *Sex and the Weimar Republic*, 128.

48. Marhoefer, *Sex and the Weimar Republic*, 130.

49. Marhoefer, *Sex and the Weimar Republic*, 129.

50. Marhoefer, *Sex and the Weimar Republic*, 131–32.

51. Marhoefer, *Sex and the Weimar Republic*, 134–35.

52. Robert Beachy, *Gay Berlin: Birthplace of a Modern Identity* (Vintage, 2015), 235.

53. Beachy, *Gay Berlin*, 238.

54. Herrn, *Der Liebe und dem Leid*, 398.

CHAPTER 12: **THE END OF EVERYTHING**

1. Material about and quotes from Christopher Isherwood are drawn from Christopher Isherwood, *Christopher and His Kind: 1929–1939* (Farrar, Straus and Giroux, 2015), 12–20.

2. My account of the rise of the Nazis is drawn from Eric D. Weitz, *Weimar Germany: Promise and Tragedy* (Princeton University Press, 2007), 332–49.

3. John Kenneth Galbraith, *The Great Crash 1929: With a New Introduction by the Author.* (Houghton Mifflin, 1988), 1–2.

4. Gary Richardson et al., "Stock Market Crash of 1929," *Federal Reserve History*, November 22, 2013.

5. Julie Marks, "What Caused the Stock Market Crash of 1929?," *The Great Depression*, History.com, April 27, 2021.

6. Galbraith, *The Great Crash 1929*, 15.

7. Richard J. Evans, *The Coming of the Third Reich* (Penguin, 2005), 54.

8. Evans, *The Coming of the Third Reich*, 82.

9. Weitz, *Weimar Germany*, 351–52.

10. Evans, *The Coming of the Third Reich*, 251.

11. Isherwood, *Christopher and His Kind*, 49.

12. Rainer Herrn, *Der Liebe und dem Leid: Das Institut für Sexualwissenschaft 1919–1933* (Suhrkamp, 2022), 413.

13. Details of Hirschfeld's sojourn in the U.S. are drawn from Charlotte Wolff, *Magnus Hirschfeld: A Portrait of a Pioneer in Sexology* (Quartet, 1986), 285.

14. Magnus Hirschfeld, *Magnus Hirschfeld Testament* (Hentrich & Hentric, 2013).

15. Hirschfeld, *Magnus Hirschfeld Testament*.

16. Herrn, *Der Liebe und dem Leid*, 447.

17. Herrn, *Der Liebe und dem Leid*, 449.

18. Herrn, *Der Liebe und dem Leid*, 449–50.

19. Robert Beachy, *Gay Berlin: Birthplace of a Modern Identity* (Vintage, 2015), 239; Simon LeVay, *Queer Science: The Use and Abuse of Research into Homosexuality* (MIT Press, 1996), 37.

20. Eleanor Hancock, " 'Only the Real, the True, the Masculine Held Its Value': Ernst Röhm, Masculinity, and Male Homosexuality," *Journal of the History of Sexuality* 8, no. 4 (April 1998): 616.

21. Joric Center, "Ernst Röhm," Jewish Virtual Library, accessed August 7, 2023.

22. Hancock, "Only the Real," 618–25.

23. Hancock, "Only the Real," 625–26.

24. Ludwig Levy-Lenz, *The Memoirs of a Sexologist: Discretion and Indiscretion* (Cadillac, 1954), 429, 430, 440.

25. Levy-Lenz, *Memoirs*, 432–41.

26. My account of the campaign against Röhm is drawn from Hancock, "Only the Real," 628–35.

27. U.S. National Park Service, "Horst and Graben," April 22, 2020.

28. Mark Edward Harris, "The Czech Republic's West Bohemian Spa Triangle," *Paradise*, January 2, 2023.

29. Hirschfeld, *Magnus Hirschfeld Testament*.

30. "Request for Passport (Národní Archiv), Dora Richter," Dept. 4 No. 57475: Ministry of Foreign Affairs of the Czechoslovak Republic, 1925. As cited in Clara Hartmann, "A Puzzle Piece for the Trans* History – Dora Richter's Baptism Record Found," *Lili-Elbe-Bibliothek Trans* Bücher Und Filme* (blog), accessed June 13, 2023.

31. Weitz, *Weimar Germany*, 353, 356.

32. Hirschfeld, *Magnus Hirschfeld Testament*.

33. Herrn, *Der Liebe und dem Leid*, 451–52; Ralf Dose, *Magnus Hirschfeld: And the Origins of the Gay Liberation Movement*, trans. Edward H. Willis (Monthly Review Press, 2014), 95.

34. Weitz, *Weimar Germany*, 357.

35. Isherwood, *Christopher and His Kind*, 118–25.

36. Hendrik Uhlendahl, Dominik Groß, and Nico Biermanns, "The Ideological Roots of Nazi Eugenics in Pathology and Its Pioneers Martin Staemmler, Ludwig Aschoff, Robert Rössle, and Georg B. Gruber," *Pathology: Research and Practice* 245 (May 2023): 245.

37. Peter Weingart, Jürgen Kroll, and Kurt Bayertz, *Rasse, Blut und Gene: Geschichte der Eugenik und Rassenhygiene in Deutschland* (Suhrkamp, 1988), 189.

38. Corvin Rick and Moritz von Stetten, "Public Health in the Field of Tension between Social Movements and Institutions," *Österreichische Zeitschrift für Soziologie* 48, no. 2 (July 6, 2023): 161–72.

39. Quoted in Siddhartha Mukherjee, *The Gene: An Intimate History* (Scribner, 2017), 138.

40. Susan Bachrach, ed., *Deadly Medicine: Creating the Master Race* (United States Holocaust Museum, 2008); Sheila Faith Weiss, "The Race Hygiene Movement in Germany," *Osiris* 3 (January 1987), 222–24.

41. Mukherjee, *The Gene*, 139.

42. Mukherjee, *The Gene*, 141.

43. Weiss, "The Race Hygiene Movement," 233–34.

44. David Jablonsky, "Röhm and Hitler: The Continuity of Political–Military Discord," *Journal of Contemporary History* 23, no. 3 (July 1988): 367.

45. Hancock, "Only the Real," 669.

46. Eleanor Hancock, "The Purge of the SA Reconsidered: An Old Putschist Trick?," *Central European History* 44, no. 4 (2011): 363.

47. Jablonsky, "Röhm and Hitler," 367.

48. Harry Oosterhuis, "Medicine, Male Bonding and Homosexuality in Nazi Germany," *Journal of Contemporary History* 32, no. 2 (April 1997): 188–89.

49. Harry Oosterhuis, ed., *Homosexuality and Male Bonding in Pre-Nazi Germany: The Youth Movement, the Gay Movement, and Male Bonding before Hitler's Rise* (Harrington Park Press, 1991), 190.

50. Oosterhuis, "Medicine, Male Bonding and Homosexuality in Nazi Germany," 192.

51. Laurie Marhoefer, *Sex and the Weimar Republic: German Homosexual Emancipation and the Rise of the Nazis* (University of Toronto Press, 2015), 171.

52. Oosterhuis, "Medicine, Male Bonding and Homosexuality in Nazi Germany," 196, 195.

53. Oosterhuis, *Homosexuality and Male Bonding in Pre-Nazi Germany*, 203.

54. Oosterhuis, "Medicine, Male Bonding and Homosexuality in Nazi Germany," 194.

55. Mukherjee, *The Gene*, 142.

CHAPTER 13: **INCENDIARY MATTERS**

1. Rainer Herrn, *Der Liebe und dem Leid: Das Institut für Sexualwissenschaft 1919–1933* (Suhrkamp, 2022), 459.

2. Christopher Isherwood, *Christopher and His Kind: 1929–1939* (Farrar, Straus and Giroux, 2015), 129.

3. Ludwig Levy-Lenz, *The Memoirs of a Sexologist: Discretion and Indiscretion* (Cadillac, 1954), 430, 442.

4. Charlotte Wolff, *Magnus Hirschfeld: A Portrait of a Pioneer in Sexology* (Quartet, 1986), 433–34; Isherwood, *Christopher and His Kind*, 129.

5. Herrn, *Der Liebe und dem Leid*, 453.

6. Robert Beachy, *Gay Berlin: Birthplace of a Modern Identity* (Vintage, 2015), 242.

7. Herrn, *Der Liebe und dem Leid*, 467.

8. Volkmar Sigusch, "The Sexologist Albert Moll—Between Sigmund Freud and Magnus Hirschfeld," *Medical History* 56, no. 2 (April 2012), 198.

9. Isherwood, *Christopher and His Kind*, 129.

10. Herrn, *Der Liebe und dem Leid*, 481.

11. Levy-Lenz, *Memoirs*, 442.

12. Heike Bauer, *The Hirschfeld Archives: Violence, Death, and Modern Queer Culture* (Temple University Press, 2017), 86.

13. Robert Proctor, "Nazi Doctors, Racial Medicine, and Human Experimentation," in

George J. Annas and Michael A. Grodin, eds., *The Nazi Doctors and the Nuremberg Code* (Oxford University Press, 1993), 36.

14. "Gohrbandt, Erwin," Traces of War, n.d.
15. Moises Mendez II, "Why Are Social Media Companies Taking Ad Money from a Right-Wing Transphobic Doc?" *Rolling Stone*, June 10, 2022.
16. Matthew Rodriguez, "CPAC Speaker Michael Knowles Says 'Transgenderism Must Be Eradicated'," *THEM*, March 6, 2023.
17. Erin Reed, "This Must Stop: TPUSA's Charlie Kirk Calls for Anti-Trans Violence 'Like in the 50s/60s'," *Erin in the Morning* (blog), February 18, 2023.
18. Anti-Defamation League, "U.S. Antisemitic Incidents Hit Highest Level Ever Recorded, ADL Audit Finds," March 23, 2023.
19. Tim Reid and Ted Hesson, "Trump Does Not Rule Out Building Detention Camps for Mass Deportations," Reuters, April 30, 2024.
20. Eric Cortellessa, "How Far Trump Would Go," *Time*, April 30, 2024.
21. Rebecca Beitsch, "Trump Team Argues Assassination of Rivals Is Covered by Presidential Immunity," *The Hill*, January 9, 2024.
22. Simon LeVay, *Queer Science: The Use and Abuse of Research into Homosexuality* (MIT Press, 1996), 39.

EPILOGUE

1. Clara Hartmann, "A Puzzle Piece for the Trans* History — Dora Richter's Baptism Record Found," *Lili-Elbe-Bibliothek Trans* Bücher Und Filme* (blog), accessed June 13, 2023.
2. These details were discovered by Clara Hartmann in "Volkszählung 1939," Prague National Archives.
3. Oliver von. Noffke, "Dora Ging Nach Böhmen," Rbb/24 [German television news channel], June 2, 2024.
4. These details were discovered by Clara Hartmann in "Volkszählung 1939," Prague National Archives.
5. Clara Hartmann, "New Documents Found on Dora Richter — and Her Later Life Clarified," Lili-Elbe-Bibliothek/Trans* Bücher und Filme, September 11, 2024.

BIBLIOGRAPHY

By Magnus Hirschfeld

Berlins drittes Geschlecht. Hermann Seemann Nachfolger, 1904.
> In English as *Berlin's Third Sex.* Translated by James Conway. Rixdorf Editions, 2017.

Die Homosexualität des Mannes und des Weibes. L. Marcus, 1914.
> In Engish as *The Homosexuality of Men and Women.* Translated by Michael Lombardi-Nash. Prometheus, 2000.

Die Transvestiten: eine Untersuchung über den erotischen Verkleidungstrieb: mit umfangreichem casuistischen und historischen Material. Alfred Pulvermacher & Co., 1910.
> In English as *The Transvestites: The Erotic Drive to Cross-Dress.* Translated by Michael Lombardi-Nash. Urania Manuscripts, 2020.

Geschlechtskunde auf Grund dreissigjähriger Forschung und Erfahrung bearbeitet. J. Püttmann, 1919.
> In English as *Sexual Anomalies and Perversions: Physical and Psychological Development and Treatment.* London, 1937.

Geschlechts-Umwandlungen: (Irrtümer in Der Geschlechtsbestimmung); Sechs Fälle Aus Der Forensischen Praxis. Alder-Verlag, 1912.

Sappho und Sokrates, 1896 (under pseudonym "Th. Ramien").
> In English as *Sappho and Socrates: How Does One Explain the Love of Men and Women to Persons of Their Own Sex?* Translated by Michael A. Lombardi-Nash. Urania Manuscripts, 2019.

Sexualpsychologie und Volkspsychologie. Georg H. Wigand Verlag, 1908.
> In English as *Sexual Pathology: A Study of Derangements of the Sexual Instinct.* Translated by Jerome Gibbs. Emerson Books, 1940.

Sittengeschichte des Weltkriegesm. Verlag für Sexualwissenschaft Schneider & Co., 1920.
> In English as *The Sexual History of the World War.* University Press of the Pacific, 2006.

Magnus Hirschfeld Testament. Heft II. Edited by Ralf Dose. Hentrich & Hentric, 2013.

Selected Sources

Abraham, Felix. "Genital Reassignment on Two Male Transvestites." *International Journal of Transgenderism* 2, no. 1 (March 1998): 223–26.

Ainsworth, Claire. "Sex Redefined: The Idea of 2 Sexes Is Overly Simplistic; Biologists Now Think There Is a Larger Spectrum than Just Binary Female and Male." *Scientific American,* October 22, 2018.

Albertini, Luigi, ed. and trans. *The Origins of the War of 1914, vol. 2, The Crisis of July 1914. From the Sarajevo Outrage to the Austro-Hungarian General Mobilization.* Enigma Books, 2005.

Aldrich, Robert. *The Seduction of the Mediterranean: Writing, Art, and Homosexual Fantasy.* Taylor and Francis, 2002.

Alt, Charlotte. " 'Steel Their Bodies and Minds'—How the Wandervögel Reconciled Nature with Modernity." *Doing History in Public,* March 2022.

Bachrach, Susan, ed. *Deadly Medicine: Creating the Master Race.* United States Holocaust Museum, 2008.

Bakker, Alex, Rainer Herrn, Michael Thomas Taylor, and Annette F. Timm. *Others of My Kind: Transatlantic Transgender Histories.* University of Calgary Press, 2020.

Barnes, Elizabeth. "Ernst Haeckel's Biogenetic Law (1866)." In *The Embryo Project Encyclopedia,* Autumn 2014.

Bauer, Heike. *The Hirschfeld Archives: Violence, Death, and Modern Queer Culture.* Temple University Press, 2017.

Beachy, Robert. *Gay Berlin: Birthplace of a Modern Identity.* Vintage, 2015.

———. "The German Invention of Homosexuality." *Journal of Modern History* 82, no. 4 (December 2010): 801–38.

Berrios, German E. "Historical Epistemology of the Body–Mind Interaction in Psychiatry." *Dialogues in Clinical Neuroscience* 20, no. 1 (2018): 9.

Bisno, Adam. "How Hyperinflation Heralded the Fall of German Democracy." *Smithsonian History* online, May 23, 2023.

Blank, Hanne. *Straight.* Beacon Press, 2012.

Body, N. O. *Memoirs of a Man's Maiden Years.* University of Pennsylvania Press, 2009.

Boyarin, Daniel. *Unheroic Conduct: The Rise of Heterosexuality and the Invention of the Jewish Man.* University of California Press, 1997.

Bristow, Joseph. "The Blackmailer and the Sodomite: Oscar Wilde on Trial." *Feminist Theory* 17, no. 1 (April 2016): 41–62.

Brown-Séquard, Charles-Édouard. *Elixir of Life,* ed. Newell Dunbar. J. G. Cupples Company, 1889.

Brunotte, Ulrike. "Queering Judaism and Masculinist Inventions: German Homonationalism Around 1900." In *Public Discourses About Homosexuality and Religion in Europe and Beyond,* ed. Marco Derks and Mariecke van den Berg. Springer, 2020.

Citino, Robert M. "Meet the *Freikorps*: Vanguard of Terror 1918–1923." National World War II Museum, June 7, 2018.

Clemens, Detlev. "The 'Bavarian Mussolini' and His 'Beerhall Putsch': British Images of Adolf Hitler, 1920–24." *English Historical Review* 114, no. 455 (February 1999): 64–84.

Conradt, David. "Social Democratic Party of Germany." *Encyclopedia Britannica,* May 24, 2023.

Coran, Arnold G., and N. Scott Adzick. *Pediatric Surgery.* 7th ed. Elsevier Mosby, 2012.

Cornwall, Mark. "Conflating Treason and Homosexuality: The Queer History of Colonel Redl." *Proceedings of the European Social Science History Conference,* April 23, 2014.

"Croonian Lectures on the Chemical Correlation of the Functions of the Body, The." *Lancet* 166, no. 4275 (August 1905): 339–41.

Darwin, Charles. *Descent of Man and Selection in Relation to Sex.* Barnes & Noble Books, 2004.

Davies, Peter. "Transforming Utopia: The 'League for the Protection of Mothers and Sexual Reform' in the First World War." In *The Women's Movement in Wartime,* ed. Alison S. Fell and Ingrid Sharp, 211–26. Palgrave Macmillan, 2007.

Dillon, Michael. *Self: A Study in Ethics and Endocrinology.* William Heinemann, 1946.

Dittrich, Samuel. "Gerd Katter (1910–1995) Trans-Mann, Patient Und Lobbyist." *Communications of the Magnus Hirschfeld Society* no. 64, February 2020.

Domeier, Norman. "The Homosexual Scare and the Masculinization of German Politics before World War I." *Central European History* 47, no. 4 (December 2014): 737–59.

Dose, Ralf. *Magnus Hirschfeld: The Origins of the Gay Liberation Movement*, trans. Edward H. Willis. Monthly Review Press, 2014.

———, and Pamela Eve Selwyn. "The World League for Sexual Reform: Some Possible Approaches." *Journal of the History of Sexuality* 12, no. 1 (2003): 1–15.

Edwards, Charles. "The Vienna Institution for Experimental Biology." *Popular Science Monthly*, June 1911.

Elbe, Lili. *Man into Woman*, ed. Niels Hoyer, trans. H. J. Stenning. Jarrolds, 1933.

Elsaesser, Thomas. *Weimar Cinema and After: Germany's Historical Imaginary*. Routledge, 2000.

Epstein, Randi Hutter. *Aroused: The History of Hormones and How They Control Just About Everything*. W. W. Norton, 2018.

Evans, Richard J. *The Coming of the Third Reich*. Penguin, 2005.

Fitzharris, Lindsey. *The Facemaker: One Surgeon's Battle to Mend the Disfigured Soldiers of World War I*. Allen Lane, 2022.

Freud, Sigmund. *Three Essays on the Theory of Sexuality*. Trans. A. A. Brill. 2nd ed. Nervous and Mental Health Diseases Publishing, 1920.

Friedländer, Benedict. "Male and Female Culture: A Causal-Historical View." In *Homosexuality and Male Bonding in Pre-Nazi Germany*, ed. Harry Oosterhuis. Harrington Park Press, 1991.

Fuechtner, Veronika, Douglas E. Haynes, and Ryan M. Jones, eds. *A Global History of Sexual Science, 1880–1960*. University of California Press, 2018.

Funke, Jana. "The Case of Karl M.[artha] Baer: Narrating 'Uncertain' Sex." In *Sex, Gender and Time in Fiction and Culture*, ed. Ben Davies and Jana Funke, 132–53. Palgrave Macmillan, 2011.

Furman, Benjamin L. S., David C. H. Metzger, Iulia Darolti, Alison E. Wright, Benjamin A. Sandkam, Pedro Almeida, Jacelyn J. Shu, and Judith E. Mank. "Sex Chromosome Evolution: So Many Exceptions to the Rules." *Genome Biology and Evolution* 12, no. 6 (June 1, 2020): 750–63.

Galbraith, John Kenneth. *The Great Crash 1929: With a New Introduction by the Author*. Houghton Mifflin, 1988.

Gay, Peter. *Weimar Culture: The Outsider as Insider*. W. W. Norton, 2001.

Gordon, Harold. *Hitler and the Beer Hall Putsch*. Princeton University Press, 1972.

Gordon, Mel. *Voluptuous Panic: The Erotic World of Weimar Berlin*. Expanded edition. Feral House, 2006.

Hancock, Elizabeth. " 'Only the Real, the True, the Masculine Held Its Value': Ernst Röhm, Masculinity, and Male Homosexuality." *Journal of the History of Sexuality* 8, no. 4 (April 1998): 616–41.

Harris, Victoria. "Histories of 'Sex,' Histories of 'Sexuality.' " *Contemporary European History* 22, no. 2 (2013): 295–301.

Hartmann, Clara. "A Puzzle Piece for the Trans* History – Dora Richter's Baptism Record Found." *Lili-Elbe-Bibliothek Trans* Bücher Und Filme* (blog). Accessed June 13, 2023.

Herrn, Rainer. "Arthur Kronfeld." In *Institute of the History of Medicine of the Charité*, n.d.

———. *Der Liebe und dem Leid: Das Institut für Sexualwissenschaft 1919–1933*. Suhrkamp, 2022.

———. *Schnittmuster des Geschlechts: Transvestitismus und Transsexualität in Der Frühen Sexualwissenschaft*. Psychosozial-Verlag, 2005.

Hess, Rex A. "Estrogen in the Adult Male Reproductive Tract: A Review." *Reproductive Biology and Endocrinology* 1, no. 1 (2003): 52.

Heyam, Kit. *Before We Were Trans: A New History of Gender*. Basic Books, 2023.

Hirschauer, Stefan. *Die Soziale Konstruktion Der Transsexualität: Über Die Medizin und Den Geschlechtswechsel.* Suhrkamp, 1993.

Hitler, Adolf. *Mein Kampf.* Trans. Ralf Manheim. Houghton Mifflin, 1999.

Holz, Werner. *Kasuistischer Beitrag zum sogenannten Transvestismus (erotischen Verkleidungstrieb) mit besonderer Berücksichtigung der Ätiologie dieser Erscheinung. Inaugural-Dissertation.* Trans. by Ulrike Walter-Lipow. Humboldt University, n.d.

Isherwood, Christopher. *Christopher and His Kind: 1929–1939.* Farrar, Straus and Giroux, 2015.

Ivory, Yvonne. "The Trouble with Oskar: Wilde's Legacy for the Early Homosexual Rights Movement in Germany." In *Oscar Wilde and Modern Culture: The Making of a Legend,* ed. Joseph Bristow. Ohio University Press, 2009.

———. "The Urning and His Own: Individualism and the Fin-de-Siècle Invert." *German Studies Review* 26, no. 2 (May 2003): 333.

Jablonsky, David. "Röhm and Hitler: The Continuity of Political–Military Discord." *Journal of Contemporary History* 23, no. 3 (July 1988): 367–86.

Joric Center. "Ernst Röhm." *Jewish Virtual Library.* Accessed August 7, 2023.

Kankeleit, Dr. "Selbstbeschädigungen und Selbstverstümmelungen der Geschlechtsorgane." *Zeitschrift für die gesamte Neurologie und Psychiatrie* 107, no. 1 (December 1927): 414–81.

Katz, Jonathan Ned. *The Invention of Heterosexuality.* University of Chicago Press, 2007.

King, David. *The Trial of Adolf Hitler: The Beer Hall Putsch and the Rise of Nazi Germany.* W. W. Norton, 2017.

Knapp, Thomas A. "The German Center Party and the Reichsbanner: A Case Study in Political and Social Consensus in the Weimar Republic." *International Review of Social History* 14, no. 2 (August 1969): 159–79.

Koerber, Amy. *From Hysteria to Hormones: A Rhetorical History.* Pennsylvania State University Press, 2018.

Kosuch, Carolin. *Anarchism and the Avant-Garde: Radical Arts and Politics in Perspective.,* 2020.

Leawoods, Heather. "Gustav Radbruch: An Extraordinary Legal Philosopher." *Washington University Journal of Law & Policy* 2 (January 2000).

Leck, Ralph Matthew. *Vita Sexualis: Karl Ulrichs and the Origins of Sexual Science.* University of Illinois Press, 2016.

Lenman, R. J. V. "Art, Society, and the Law in Wilhelmine Germany: The Lex Heinze." *Oxford German Studies* 8, no. 1 (January 1973): 86–113.

LeVay, Simon. *Queer Science: The Use and Abuse of Research into Homosexuality.* MIT Press, 1996.

Levy-Lenz, Ludwig [as Ludwig L. Lenz]. *The Memoirs of a Sexologist: Discretion and Indiscretion.* Cadillac, 1954.

Linge, Ina. "Sexology, Popular Science and Queer History in *Anders Als Die Andern (Different from the Others)*." *Gender and History* 30, no. 3 (October 2018): 595–610.

Liu, Yongsheng, and Qi Chen. "150 Years of Darwin's Theory of Intercellular Flow of Hereditary Information." *Nature Reviews Molecular Cell Biology* 19 (2018): 749–50.

Makela, Maria. "Rejuvenation and Regen(d)eration: *Der Steinachfilm,* Sex Glands, and Weimar-Era Visual and Literary Culture." *German Studies Review* 38, no. 1 (2015): 35–62.

Mancini, Elena. *Magnus Hirschfeld and the Quest for Sexual Freedom: A History of the First International Sexual Freedom Movement.* Palgrave Macmillan, 2010.

Marhoefer, Laurie. *Sex and the Weimar Republic: German Homosexual Emancipation and the Rise of the Nazis.* University of Toronto Press, 2015.

Mottier, Véronique. "The Invention of Sexuality." In *Chic, chèque, choc,* ed. Françoise Grange Omokaro and Fenneke Reysoo. Graduate Institute Publications, 2012.

Mukherjee, Siddhartha. *The Gene: An Intimate History.* Scribner, 2017.

Murray, Douglas. *Bosie: A Biography of Lord Alfred Douglas.* Hyperion, 2000.

Nelson, Randy Joe, and Lance J. Kriegsfeld. *An Introduction to Behavioral Endocrinology.* 5th edition. Sinauer Associates, 2017.

Nobbs, Patrick. *The Story of the British and Their Weather.* Amberley, 2015.

Nunn, Zavier. "Trans Liminality and the Nazi State." *Past and Present* 260, no. 1 (August 2023): 123–57.

Oosterhuis, Harry, ed. *Homosexuality and Male Bonding in Pre-Nazi Germany: The Youth Movement, the Gay Movement, and Male Bonding before Hitler's Rise.* Harrington Park Press, 1991.

———. "Medicine, Male Bonding and Homosexuality in Nazi Germany." *Journal of Contemporary History* 32, no. 2 (April 1997): 187–205.

———. "Sexual Modernity in the Works of Richard von Krafft-Ebing and Albert Moll." *Medical History* 56, no. 2 (April 2012): 133–55.

Oudshoorn, Nelly. *Beyond the Natural Body: An Archaeology of Sex Hormones.* Taylor and Francis, 1994.

Prichard, James Cowles. "A Treatise on Insanity and Other Disorders Affecting the Mind." In *Embodied Selves*, ed. Jenny Bourne Taylor and Sally Shuttleworth. Oxford University Press, 1998.

Proctor, Robert. "Nazi Doctors, Racial Medicine, and Human Experimentation." In *The Nazi Doctors and the Nuremberg Code*, ed. George J. Annas and Michael A. Grodin. Oxford University Press, 1993.

Ramsey, Glenn. "The Rites of Artgenossen: Contesting Homosexual Political Culture in Weimar Germany." *Journal of the History of Sexuality* 17, no. 1 (2007): 85–109.

Rey, Rudolfo, Nathalie Josso, and Chrystele Racine. "Sexual Differentiation." Endotext, 2020.

Richardson, Gary, Alejandro Komai, Michael Gou, and Daniel Park. "Stock Market Crash of 1929." *Federal Reserve History*, November 22, 2013.

Rick, Corvin, and Moritz von Stetten. "Public Health in the Field of Tension between Social Movements and Institutions." *Österreichische Zeitschrift für Soziologie* 48, no. 2 (July 6, 2023): 161–72.

Rothman, Lily. "How a Speech Helped Hitler Take Power." *Time*, February 24, 2020.

Rush, Homer P. "A Biographic Sketch of Arnold Adolf Berthold: An Early Experimenter with Ductless Glands." *Annals of Medical History* 1, no. 2 (1929): 208–14.

Sengoopta, Chandak. *The Most Secret Quintessence of Life: Sex, Glands, and Hormones, 1850–1950.* University of Chicago Press, 2006.

Sharp, Lesley Alexandra. *Animal Ethos: The Morality of Human–Animal Encounters in Experimental Lab Science.* University of California Press, 2019.

Sigusch, Volkmar. "The Sexologist Albert Moll—Between Sigmund Freud and Magnus Hirschfeld." *Medical History* 56, no. 2 (April 2012): 184–200.

Smith, Adam [pseud. George J. W. Goodman]. "The German Hyperinflation, 1923," in *Paper Money.* Summit, 1981.

Soma, K. K. "Testosterone and Aggression: Berthold, Birds and Beyond." *Journal of Neuroendocrinology* 18, no. 7 (July 2006): 543–51.

Sontag, Raymond J. "German Foreign Policy, 1904–1906." *American Historical Review* 33, no. 2 (January 1928): 278.

Spector Person, Ethel. "As the Wheel Turns: A Centennial Reflection on Freud's Three Essays on the Theory of Sexuality." *Journal of the American Psychoanalytic Association* 53, no. 4 (December 2005): 1257–82.

Stark, Gary D. "Pornography, Society, and the Law in Imperial Germany." *Central European History* 14, no. 3 (1981): 200–29.

Steakley, James D. "Cinema and Censorship in the Weimar Republic: The Case of Anders Als Die Andern." *Film History* 11, no. 2 (1999).

Steinberg, Holger, Kenneth Kirkby, and Hubertus Himmerich. "The Historical Development of Immunoendocrine Concepts of Psychiatric Disorders and Their Therapy." *International Journal of Molecular Sciences* 16, no. 12 (December 4, 2015): 28841–69.

Sternstein, Wolfgang. "The Ruhrkampf of 1923: Economic Problems of Civilian Defence." In *The Strategy of Civilian Defence: Non-Violent Resistance to Aggression*, ed. Adam Roberts. Faber and Faber, 1967.

Štrkalj, Goran, and Nalini Pather. "Beyond the Sex Binary: Toward the Inclusive Anatomical Sciences Education." *Anatomical Sciences Education* 14, no. 4 (July 2021): 513–18.

Stryker, Susan. *Transgender History: The Roots of Today's Revolution.* 2nd ed. Seal Press, 2017.

Sutton, Katie. *Sex between Body and Mind: Psychoanalysis and Sexology in the German-Speaking World, 1890s–1930s.* University of Michigan Press, 2019.

———. "'We Too Deserve a Place in the Sun': The Politics of Transvestite Identity in Weimar Germany." *German Studies Review* 35, no. 2 (2012): 335–54.

Tamagne, Florence. *A History of Homosexuality in Europe: Berlin, London, Paris 1919–1939.* Algora, 2006.

Tata, Jamshed R. "One Hundred Years of Hormones." *EMBO Reports* 6, no. 6 (2005): 490–96.

Taylor, Michael, Annette Timm, and Rainer Herrn, eds. *Not Straight from Germany: Sexual Publics and Sexual Citizenship since Magnus Hirschfeld.* University of Michigan Press, 2017.

Tobin, Robert D. "Queer German Roots of the Alt-Right: Ulrichs, Weininger, Blüher—and Evola." *Monatshefte* 114, no. 3 (2022): 470–88.

Uhlendahl, Hendrik, Dominik Groß, and Nico Biermanns. "The Ideological Roots of Nazi Eugenics in Pathology and Its Pioneers Martin Staemmler, Ludwig Aschoff, Robert Rössle, and Georg B. Gruber." *Pathology: Research and Practice* 245 (May 2023).

Ulrichs, Karl Heinrich. *The Correspondence of Karl Heinrich Ulrichs, 1846–1894*, ed. Douglas Ogilvy Pretsell, trans. Michael A. Lombardi-Nash. Palgrave Macmillan, 2020.

Wald, Chelsea. "Austria's Ahead-of-Its-Time Institute That Was Lost to Nazis." *Nautilus*, April 22, 2014.

Weikart, Richard. "Progress through Racial Extermination: Social Darwinism, Eugenics, and Pacifism in Germany, 1860–1918." *German Studies Review* 26, no. 2 (May 2003): 273.

———. "The Role of Darwinism in Nazi Racial Thought." *German Studies Review* 36, no. 3 (2013): 537–56.

Weingart, Peter, Jürgen Kroll, and Kurt Bayertz. *Rasse, Blut und Gene: Geschichte der Eugenik und Rassenhygiene in Deutschland.* Suhrkamp, 1988.

Weiss, Sheila Faith. "The Race Hygiene Movement in Germany." *Osiris* 3 (January 1987): 193–236.

Weitz, Eric D. *Weimar Germany: Promise and Tragedy.* Princeton University Press, 2007.

Weltliga für Sexualreform (World League for Sexual Reform). "Principal Points of the League's Platform." https://web.archive.org/web/20111122131239/http://www2.hu-berlin.de/sexology/GESUND/ARCHIV/GIF/XWLSR_PL.JPG.

Whisnant, Clayton John. *Queer Identities and Politics in Germany: A History, 1880–1945.* Harrington Park Press, 2016.

Wolff, Charlotte. *Magnus Hirschfeld: A Portrait of a Pioneer in Sexology.* Quartet, 1986.

Young, Harry F. *Maximilian Harden, Censor Germaniae: The Critic in Opposition from Bismarck to the Rise of Nazism.* M. Nijhoff, 1959.

INDEX